HAEMATOLOGY
2nd Edition

HAEMATOLOGY

2nd Edition

Chris Pallister

Managing Director, SciMed Consulting Ltd
formerly, Reader in Haematology,
University of the West of England

and

Malcolm Watson

formerly, Senior Lecturer in Haematology,
University of the West of England

Scion

Second edition © Scion Publishing Ltd, 2011

ISBN 978 1904842 39 2

First edition published in 1999 by Arnold (ISBN 0 750 62457 4)

A CIP catalogue record for this book is available from the British Library.

Scion Publishing Limited
The Old Hayloft, Vantage Business Park, Bloxham Road, Banbury, OX16 9UX
www.scionpublishing.com

Important Note from the Publisher

The information contained within this book was obtained by Scion Publishing Limited from sources believed by us to be reliable. However, while every effort has been made to ensure its accuracy, no responsibility for loss or injury whatsoever occasioned to any person acting or refraining from action as a result of information contained herein can be accepted by the authors or publishers.

Typeset by Phoenix Photosetting, Chatham, Kent, UK
Printed by Thomson Litho, East Kilbride, UK

Contents

Preface

Each generation flirts with the idea that it is nearing the limits of knowledge, that so much has been discovered and defined that there can be little new to learn. However, one of the most powerful lessons of history is that this is nothing more than an arrogant delusion. The 11 years since the first edition of this book have seen such an explosion of knowledge and increased understanding of blood and blood-forming tissues in health and disease that a complete revision of the text was required. In particular, the influence of molecular genetics has informed and expanded our understanding of the mechanisms underlying blood diseases enormously. One important impact of this knowledge has been the development of 'targeted' therapies such as imatinib, bortezomib and rituximab, which have transformed treatment outcomes in hitherto intractable diseases.

However, despite this bewildering and accelerating pace of change, the primary aim of this book remains the same: to explain the science that underpins haematology and the scientific background that informs haematological thinking and understanding. Many excellent texts exist that focus on the practical or clinical aspects of haematological diagnosis and treatment. This book is not intended to replace these essential texts. Instead, its focus is on scientific principles and understanding the 'how?' and the 'why?' rather than the 'what?' of haematology.

As always, although two people are credited with the writing of this book, many people have been closely involved in its genesis, and we want to use this opportunity to thank them. Jonathan Ray and Clare Boomer of Scion Publishing deserve special mention for their patience, encouragement and expertise because, without them, this book would not have been completed. We also thank Donna Pallister for her expertise in creating and adapting the graphics seen in this book. Finally, we offer our sincere thanks to our partners for their forbearance, support and understanding during the long, long months this book took to write.

Chris Pallister and Malcolm Watson
September 2010

Abbreviations

2,3-DPG	2,3-diphosphoglyceric acid	B-ALL	B-lymphoblastic leukaemia / lymphoma
2-PG	2-phosphoglycerate		
ABVD	Adriamycin, bleomycin, vinblastine, dacarbazine	BEACOPP	bleomycin, etoposide, doxorubicin, cyclophosphamide, vincristine, procarbazine, prednisone
ACD	anaemia of chronic disorders		
aCML	atypical CML		
ADCC	antibody-dependent cell-mediated cytotoxicity	BEAM	BCNU, etoposide, cytarabine, melphalan
AEL	acute erythroleukaemia	bFGF	basic fibroblast growth factor
AHD	antecedent haematological disorder	BFU-E	erythroid burst-forming units
		BL	Burkitt lymphoma
AHSP	α haemoglobin stabilizing protein	BMP	bone morphogenetic protein
		B-PLL	B-cell prolymphocytic leukaemia
AIDS	acquired immunodeficiency syndrome		
		BSD	Bernard–Soulier disease
AIF	apoptosis-inducing factor	CALLA	common ALL antigen
AIHA	autoimmune haemolytic anaemias	CAMT	congenital amegakaryocytic thrombocytopenia
AIN	autoimmune neutropenia	CBF	core binding factor
ALK	anaplastic lymphoma kinase	CCV	conductiometric cell volume
ALL	acute lymphoblastic leukaemia	CD	cluster of differentiation
AMegL	acute megakaryoblastic leukaemia	CDA	congenital dyserythropoietic anaemia
AML	acute myeloid leukaemia	CDK	cyclin-dependent kinases
AMMoL	acute myelomonocytic leukaemia	CEL	chronic eosinophilic leukaemia
		CFU-E	erythroid colony-forming units
AMoL	acute monoblastic leukaemia	CGD	chronic granulomatous disease
ANC	absolute neutrophil count	CGP	circulating granulocyte pool
APC	anaphase-promoting complex	CHD	coronary heart disease
APCR	activated protein C resistance	CHR	complete haematological response
APL	acute promyelocytic leukaemia		
APS	anti-phospholipid syndrome	CHS	Chédiak–Higashi syndrome
APTT	activated partial thromboplastin time	CLL	chronic lymphocytic leukaemia
		CML	chronic myeloid leukaemia
AT	antithrombin	CMML	chronic myelomonocytic leukaemia
ATLL	adult T cell leukaemia / lymphoma		
		CMV	cytomegalovirus
ATLS	acute tumour lysis syndrome	CNL	chronic neutrophilic leukaemia
ATRA	all-trans retinoic acid	CNS	central nervous system
AUL	acute undifferentiated leukaemia	CNSHA	congenital non-spherocytic haemolytic anaemia
AvWs	acquired von Willebrand's syndrome		
		CPG III	co-proporphyrinogen III

CPSF	cleavage and polyadenylation specificity factor	G-3-P	glyceraldehyde-3-phosphate
CR	complete response	G-6-PD	glucose-6-phosphate dehydrogenase
CSF	cerebrospinal fluid	G-CSF	granulocyte colony-stimulating factor
CSS	Churg–Strauss syndrome		
CT	computed tomography	GM-CSF	granulocyte–macrophage colony-stimulating factor
CVS	chorion villus sampling		
δ-ALA	δ-aminolaevulinic acid	GPI	glycosylphosphatidylinositol
DAF	decay accelerating factor	GSH	reduced glutathione
DDAVP	1–desamino–8–D–argininylvasopressin	GT	Glanzmann's thrombasthenia
		GvHD	graft versus host disease
DHAP	cisplatin, cytarabine, prednisone	HAART	highly active antiretroviral therapy
DIC	disseminated intravascular coagulation		
		HAT	histone acetyltransferase
DI-IHA	drug-induced immune haemolytic anaemia	[Hb]	haemoglobin concentration
		HBV	hepatitis B virus
DLBCL	diffuse large B cell lymphoma	HC	haptocorrin
dTMP	deoxythymidine-5′-monophosphate	HCD	heavy chain disease
		HCL	hairy cell leukaemia
DTS	dense tubular system	Hct	haematocrit
dUMP	deoxyuridine-5′-mono-phosphate	HD	Hodgkin disease
		HDAC	histone deacetylase
DVT	deep venous thrombosis	HDNB	haemolytic disease of the newborn
EACA	ε-aminocaproic acid		
EBV	Epstein–Barr virus	HE	hereditary elliptocytosis
ECM	extracellular matrix	HEMPAS	hereditary erythroblast multinuclearity with positive acidified serum test
ECP	eosinophil cationic protein		
ECP	eosinophilic cationic protein		
EDN	eosinophil-derived neurotoxin	HGPRT	hypoxanthine guanine phosphoribosyltransferase
EDS	Ehlers–Danlos syndrome		
EFS	event-free survival	HHT	hereditary haemorrhagic telangiectasia
EGF	epidermal growth factor		
EP	eosinophil peroxide	HLA	human leucocyte antigen
EPO	erythropoietin	HNPCC	hereditary non-polyposis colorectal cancer
ESHAP	etoposide, methylprednisolone, cytarabine, cisplatin		
		HPFH	hereditary persistence of fetal haemoglobin
ESR	erythrocyte sedimentation rate		
		HPLC	high performance liquid chromatography
ET	essential thrombocythaemia		
F-1,6-DP	fructose-1,6-diphosphate	HPP	hereditary pyropoikilocytosis
F-6-P	fructose-6-phosphate	HPV	human papillomavirus
FALS	forward angle light scatter	HRT	hormone replacement therapy
FBC	full blood count	HS	hereditary spherocytosis
FDG	fluorine-18 deoxyglucose	HSCT	haemopoietic stem cell transplantation
FIGLU	*N*-formiminoglutamic acid		
FISH	fluorescent *in situ* hybridization	HSP	Henoch–Schönlein purpura
FL	follicular lymphoma	HSt	hereditary stomatocytosis
FM	fibrin monomer	HTLV	human T lymphotropic virus
FPD	familial platelet disorder	HUS	haemolytic uraemic syndrome
FSP	fibrin(ogen) split products	HX	hereditary xerocytosis

ICAM	intercellular adhesion molecule	MIRL	membrane inhibitor of reactive lysis
ICE	ifosfamide, carboplatin, etoposide	MM	multiple myeloma
IF	intrinsic factor	MP	mercaptopurine
IL-1	interleukin-1	MPAL	mixed phenotype acute leukaemia
IM	idiopathic myelofibrosis		
IMiD	immunomodulating agent	MPF	mitosis promoting factor
INR	international normalized ratio	MPN	myeloproliferative neoplasms
IPFP	International Prognostic Factors Project	MPS	mucopolysaccharidosis
		MRI	magnetic resonance imaging
IPSS	International Prognostic Scoring System	MTHFR	methylenetetrahydrofolate reductase
ISI	international sensitivity index	NAD	nicotinamide adenine dinucleotide
ISS	International Staging System		
ITD	internal tandem repeat	NADH	nicotinamide adenine dinucleotide dehydrogenase
ITP	immune thrombocytopenic purpura		
		NAIN	neonatal alloimmune-mediated neutropenia
IWF	International Working Formulation		
		NHL	non-Hodgkin lymphoma
JMML	juvenile myelomonocytic leukaemia	NK	natural killer
		NO	nitric oxide
LAD	leucocyte adhesion deficiency	OPG	osteoprotegerin
LCD	light chain disease	OS	overall survival
LCH	Langerhans cell histiocytosis	PA	pernicious anaemia
LCR	locus control region	PAF	platelet-activating factor
LDH	lactate dehydrogenase	PAGE	polyacrylamide gel electrophoresis
LDT	lymphocyte doubling time		
LFA	leucocyte function-associated antigen	PAI	plasminogen activator inhibitor
		PAP	plasmin–antiplasmin
LP	lymphocyte-predominant	PBG	porphobilinogen
MAHA	microangiopathic haemolytic anaemia	PCD	programmed cell death
		PCH	paroxysmal cold haemoglobinuria
MALT	mucosa-associated lymphoid tissue		
		PCL	plasma cell leukaemia
MBP	major basic protein	PCR	polymerase chain reaction
MCH	mean cell haemoglobin	PCV	packed cell volume
MCHC	mean cell (or corpuscular) haemoglobin concentration	PDGF	platelet-derived growth factor
		PEP	phosphoenol pyruvate
MCL	mantle cell lymphoma	PET	positron emission tomography
MCV	mean cell volume	PFS	progression-free survival
MDR	multi-drug resistance	PIVKA	proteins induced by vitamin K absence or antagonism
MDS	myelodysplastic syndrome		
MDS/MPD	myelodysplastic/ myeloproliferative neoplasms	PK	pyruvate kinase
		PLL	prolymphocytic leukaemia
MDS-U	myelodysplastic syndrome, unclassified	PLZF	promyelocytic zinc finger
		PNH	paroxysmal nocturnal haemoglobinuria
MGP	marginated granulocyte pool		
MGUS	monoclonal gammopathy of undetermined significance	PPG IX	protoporphyrinogen IX
		PRCA	pure red cell aplasia
MHA	May–Hegglin anomaly		

PRPP	5' phosphoribosyl-1-pyrophosphate	SLE	systemic lupus erythematosus
PS	phosphatidylserine	SLL	small lymphocytic lymphoma
PSGL	P-selectin glycoprotein ligand	SPF	S-phase promoting factor
PT	prothrombin time	T-ALL	T-lymphoblastic leukaemia / lymphoma
PTLD	post-transplantation lymphoproliferative disorders	t-AML	therapy-related AML
PUS-1	pseudo-uridine synthase-1	TAR	thrombocytopenia with absent radii
PV	polycythaemia vera	TAT	thrombin–antithrombin
R-5-P	ribose-5-phosphate	TBI	total body irradiation
RA	refractory anaemia	TC	transcobalamin
RAEB	refractory anaemia with excess blasts	TdT	terminal deoxynucleotidyltransferase
RAEB-t	refractory anaemia with excess blasts in transformation	TEC	transient erythroblastopenia of childhood
RALS	right angle light scatter	TF	tissue factor
RARS	refractory anaemia with ring sideroblasts	TFPI	tissue factor pathway inhibitor
		TfR	transferring receptor
RBC	red blood cell	TIA	transient ischaemic attack
RCMD	refractory cytopenia with multilineage dysplasia	TIBC	total iron binding capacity
		TNF	tumour necrosis factor
RCMD–RS	refractory cytopenia with multilineage dysplasia and ring sideroblasts	tPA	tissue plasminogen activator
		T-PLL	T-cell prolymphocytic leukaemia
RCUD	refractory cytopenia with unilineage dysplasia	TPMT	thiopurine methyl transferase
		TPO	thrombopoietin
RE	reticulo-endothelial	TTP	thrombotic thrombocytopenic purpura
REAL	Revised European–American Classification of Lymphoid Neoplasms	u-PA	urokinase-type plasminogen activator
RN	refractory neutropenia	UPG III	uroporphyrinogen III
ROTI	related organ or tissue impairment	VEGF	vascular endothelial growth factor
RT	refractory thrombocytopenia	VSD	ventricular septal defect
Ru-5-P	ribulose-5-phosphate	vWD	von Willebrand's disease
SAHA	suberoylanilide hydroxamic acid	vWF	von Willebrand Factor
SCCS	surface-connected canalicular system	WAS	Wiskott–Aldrich syndrome
		WHO	World Health Organization
SDS	sodium dodecyl sulphate	WM	Waldenström macroglobulinaemia
sIg	surface immunoglobulin		
SK	streptokinase	WPSS	WHO prognostic scoring system

Content of the blood

Learning objectives
After studying this chapter you should confidently be able to:

■ **Describe the cellular and fluid components of normal blood**
The blood is one of the largest organs of the body, with a volume of about five litres. Normal peripheral blood is composed of three types of cell; red cells (erythrocytes), white cells (leucocytes) and platelets (thrombocytes), suspended in a pale yellow fluid called plasma. There are five different types of white cell normally present. Red cells are responsible for gaseous transport, thrombocytes for the arrest of bleeding and white cells for specific and non-specific immune defence against foreign material or organisms.

The blood is one of the largest organs of the body, with a volume of about five litres and a weight of 5.5 kg in an average 70 kg man. Blood circulates throughout the body, supporting the function of all other body tissues. Because blood and bone marrow are sampled easily, the haemopoietic system is probably the most intensively studied organ of the body. This has led to an explosion of knowledge about blood and blood-forming tissue in both health and disease (see also *Box 1.1*).

Box 1.1 Beliefs about the blood

From the time of Hippocrates (460–370 BC), curiosity about the blood and its functions combined with ignorance and mysticism to produce a plethora of mistaken beliefs, myths and legends. The aura of mystery that surrounds the blood has still not completely been dispelled. Examples of the vestiges of primitive belief abound in the work of poets, playwrights and authors. Obvious examples include tales of vampires who must regularly imbibe the blood of virgins to sustain life, and the constant reference to blood to symbolize murder and the pangs of conscience of the anguished Lord and Lady Macbeth following the murder of Duncan.

Our everyday language is enriched by expressions such as 'hot-blooded', which denotes passion or 'cool as a cucumber'. Both are rooted in medieval beliefs about the power and properties of the blood.

Histologically, blood is classed as a connective tissue. However, blood differs from most other connective tissues in having a fluid rather than a gelatinous matrix or 'ground substance'. The fluid component of blood is called plasma. The cells of the blood are suspended in the plasma.

Visualization of the cellular components of blood is most commonly performed by smearing a drop of blood on a glass slide to form a thin film a single cell thick. The smear is then air dried, fixed in alcohol and stained with a type of dye mixture known as a Romanowsky-type stain. It is the stained appearance of blood cells that is the basis of their identification and characterization under a light microscope. This simple technique still forms an important component of haematological diagnosis (see *Box 1.2*).

Box 1.2 Staining characteristics

Specific dye mixtures have been named after their originators, for example Wright, Giemsa, or May–Grünwald (which is not, strictly, a true Romanowsky stain, but is very similar). Romanowsky stains include a basic dye (positively charged) such as methylene blue (or a derivative – see below) and an anionic dye (negatively charged) such as eosin. Methylene blue binds to negatively charged sites in the cells, such as nucleic acid in nuclei and ribosomes, giving them a blue to purple colour. Eosin binds to positively charged sites, for example most cytoplasmic proteins, giving them a pink to red colour. In a strict Romanowsky stain (as against a Romanowsky-*type* stain) methylene blue is oxidized to produce a range of oxidation products, a process called '**polychroming**'. The proportion of the various oxidation products depends on the method of oxidation. The polychromed methylene blue is then mixed with eosin, and the resulting dyes are known as azures. May–Grünwald is not a 'true' Romanowsky stain since it is made from the azures rather than polychromed methylene blue.

1.1 CONTENT OF THE BLOOD

Normal peripheral blood is composed of three types of cell; red cells (erythrocytes), white cells (leucocytes) and platelets (thrombocytes), suspended in a pale yellow fluid called plasma. The cells occupy about 40–50% of the total volume.

Plasma

Plasma occupies about 50–60% of the total blood volume. It is a pale yellow aqueous solution of electrolytes, proteins and small organic molecules such as glucose. The major extracellular cation is Na^+, which has a plasma concentration of about 140 mmol l^{-1}. Other important plasma cations include K^+, Ca^{2+}, Fe^{3+} and Mg^{2+} but these are all found at much lower concentration. The relative concentrations of Na^+ and K^+ in the plasma contrast with their intracellular concentrations where K^+ is present at a higher concentration.

The major plasma anions are Cl^- and HCO_3^-, although SO_4^{2-} and HPO_4^{2-} are also present at lower concentration. Plasma is always electrically neutral, i.e. the concentrations of anions and cations are always such that the total numbers of negative and positive charges exactly balance.

A large number of different plasma proteins exist. The major protein component is albumen, normally comprising around 60% of the total. It is albumen that is primarily responsible for maintaining the osmotic balance between the fluid components of blood and tissue. Like most plasma proteins, albumen is synthesized in the liver. The remainder fall broadly into four distinct families:

- **haemostatic proteins**, such as the coagulation factors, fibrinolytic factors and their inhibitors.
- **immunoglobulins**, which are antibody molecules synthesized by plasma cells. There are five different classes of immunoglobulin (IgA, IgD, IgE, IgG and IgM) which are structurally related but perform distinct biological functions.
- **innate immune system proteins**, which consist of a variety of plasma proteins that are important in the induction of inflammation and immunity against microbial infection, acute phase proteins, complement, interferons and others, all of which are involved with non-specific immunity.
- **transport proteins**, which ferry nutrients, waste products and other substances around the body. These are α and β globulins, and include transferrin (iron), transcobalamin (vitamin B_{12}), and caeruloplasmin (copper), low density lipoproteins that solubilize and transport dietary or stored lipids (which all transport 'nutrients'), hormone-binding proteins that transport steroid hormones and, for example, haptoglobin which transports any haemoglobin that is released into the circulation, thus becoming a 'waste product'.

Myriad other proteins can be found in the plasma, including cytokines, hormones and growth factors, but these are not usually thought of as plasma proteins, as they are simply using the blood as a transport medium.

Red cells

Mature red cells, or erythrocytes, are the most numerous of the blood cells: about 5×10^{12} are normally present in each litre of blood. They constitute about 45% of blood by volume, a measure known as the haematocrit (see *Box 1.3*). Red cells survive in the circulation for about 120 days before being sequestered in the spleen and consumed by the phagocytic cells of the reticuloendothelial system. The normal mature circulating red cell has no nucleus.

The normal red cell is a biconcave discoid shape with a diameter of about 8.4 μm and a volume of about 88 fl (*Figure 1.1*; see also *Box 1.4*). This characteristic shape imparts flexibility to the cell, allowing it to traverse the smallest blood capillaries which have a diameter of only 3 μm, and also facilitates gaseous exchange across the cell membrane by maximizing the surface area:volume ratio of the cell, thereby bringing more haemoglobin molecules closer to the cell surface. The primary function of red cells is to transport oxygen from the lungs to the tissues, but they also play an important role in the reverse transportation of carbon dioxide.

The oxygen-carrying pigment, haemoglobin, is present in high concentration in mature red cells and is responsible for the characteristic red colour of the blood. Haemoglobin consists of two parts, an iron-containing porphyrin, haem, and a protein, globin. As globin is slightly acidic at physiological pH, haemoglobin stains pink with Romanowsky dyes (see *Chapter 6*). There are around 5–6×10^6 molecules of haemoglobin in each red cell, constituting an approximately 33% solution.

Normal circulating red cells contain little other than haemoglobin. They have no nucleus or ribosomes, which means they are incapable of protein synthesis. They also lack mitochondria, which means that they are limited to the anaerobic glycolytic pathway to provide the entire requirement of the red cell for energy and reducing potential (see *Chapter 8*).

Box 1.3 Factitious blood count results

Before the days of automation, three red cell parameters were measured, namely red blood cell count (RBC), haemoglobin concentration (Hb) and packed cell volume (PCV) or haematocrit. PCV was measured by centrifugation under strictly controlled conditions. From these three measured parameters three further parameters were derived, namely mean cell haemoglobin (MCH), which was derived by dividing Hb by RBC, mean cell (or corpuscular) haemoglobin concentration (MCHC), which was derived by dividing Hb by PCV, and mean cell volume (MCV), which was derived by dividing PCV by RBC. MCV, MCH and MCHC are thus, strictly, all derived values and as such cannot be measured directly.

The advent of automation brought huge problems regarding the measurement of PCV. Attempted solutions included conductiometric cell volume (CCV), and continuously spinning flow through centrifugation methods. Neither system proved reliable and accurate.

Paralleling these developments was the development of the Coulter principle, whereby cells were counted as they interrupted the passage of an electric current. Not only did this system allow for the number of cells to be counted, but the size of each interference peak was related to the volume of the cell causing the peak. It rapidly became the standard to measure the size of these peaks and to report this as a measured MCV. However, this method does not measure cell size in plasma, but in an isotonic diluent, so this value is not a true MCV. In some cases, for example in hyperglycaemia, dilution in isotonic saline can cause artefactual swelling of the cells and lead to misreporting of MCV. It is important to be aware of the causes of factitious results like these, many of which are specific to each cell counting system, to be able to spot them and so avoid misreporting and potential misdiagnosis.

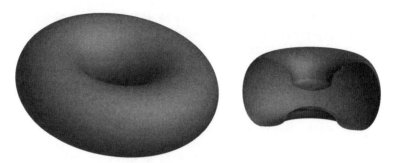

Figure 1.1
The biconcave disc shape of a normal red blood cell.

Box 1.4 Reference values

Reference values for adults:

	Men	Women*
Red blood cells	4.4–5.9 x 10^{12}/l	3.8–5.2 x 10^{12}/l
Haemoglobin	13.3–17.7 g/dl	11.7–15.7 g/dl
Platelets	150–440 x 10^{9}/l	150–440 x 10^{9}/l

*Reference values are for women of child-bearing age

The effective performance of red cell function requires that the cell is capable of traversing the microvascular system without mechanical damage and that it should normally retain a shape that facilitates gaseous exchange. These demands require the red cell membrane to be extremely tough yet highly flexible. During its 120 day lifespan, a red cell travels about 300 miles along blood vessels with a diameter of as little as 3 μm and is subject to the extreme stresses of passage through the heart at least 5×10^5 times. The biconcave shape is readily deformable, assuming an 'arrowhead' conformation to allow passage through narrow capillaries.

The secret of the success of the red cell membrane in meeting the conflicting demands of strength and flexibility lies in the design of its protein cytoskeleton and the way in which the cytoskeleton interacts with the membrane lipid bilayer (see *Chapter 7*).

The main functions of the red cell membrane can be summarized as follows:

- to separate the contents of the cell from the plasma
- to maintain the characteristic shape of the red cell
- to regulate intracellular cation concentrations
- to act as the interface between the cell and its environment via membrane surface receptors

The role of the membrane in separating the contents of the cell from the plasma allows the red cell to control its own internal environment. For example, a constant supply of glucose from the plasma is required by the red cell to supply its energy needs and requirement for reducing potential. The transport of glucose into the red cell is facilitated by a specific transport protein in the membrane. Conversely, it is important that, once inside the cell, the phosphorylated intermediates of glycolysis are retained or the glycolytic pathway would fail in its purpose. Retention is assured because the red cell membrane is impermeable to phosphorylated sugars.

This property of controlling which substances can cross the membrane is called selective permeability and is vital to the economy of the cell.

The red cell membrane contains channels that facilitate the rapid passage of water across the membrane. These channels are formed by a transmembrane protein known as aquaporin-1. This molecule also carries the ABH and Colton blood group antigens (see *Box 1.5*).

Similarly, monovalent anion exchange (e.g. Cl^- and HCO_3^-) is facilitated by a transmembrane anion exchanger protein known as AE1. In contrast, the passage of monovalent cations such as Na^+ and K^+ across the membrane is relatively slow. Large plasma cell concentration gradients exist for these cations. The intracellular Na^+ concentration is relatively low (about 8 mM) while the plasma Na^+ concentration is relatively high (about 140 mM). This results in a slow leakage of Na^+ from the plasma to the cell. On the other hand, the intracellular K^+ concentration is relatively high (about 100 mM) while the plasma concentration is relatively low (about 5 mM). Thus, there is a slow leakage of K^+ from the cell into the plasma. In the absence of some mechanism to counter the leakage of monovalent cations, their concentrations would gradually equalize. However, the red cell membrane contains a protein that acts as a 'cation pump', i.e. it actively pumps Na^+ from the cell into the plasma and pumps K^+ in the opposite direction. The energy required to drive the pump is derived from the conversion of ATP to ADP by a membrane ATPase. The ADP thus formed is utilized by the Embden Meyerhof glycolytic pathway and so is reconverted to ATP (see *Chapter 8*). The activity of the pump is stimulated by a rise in the intracellular Na^+ concentration. The activity rate of the cation pump is controlled in such a way that it precisely balances the rate of leakage of cations across the membrane. Thus, the intracellular Na^+ and K^+ concentrations are maintained within very narrow limits.

Composition of the red cell membrane

The composition of the red blood cell membrane is complex, and is explored further in *Chapter 7*. A brief summary of essential points will suffice here.

Lipids. All of the lipid associated with red cells is present in the cell membrane. The mature red cell has no capacity to synthesize lipid; alterations in membrane lipid content can only occur by exchange with plasma lipids. About 60% of the red cell membrane lipid is composed of one of four different phospholipids: phosphatidyl choline, phosphatidyl ethanolamine, sphingomyelin and phosphatidyl serine. Phospholipid molecules are characterized by a polar head group attached to a non-polar fatty acid tail. The polar head group is hydrophilic (water-loving) while the fatty acid tail is hydrophobic (water-fearing) or lipophilic (fat-loving). Thus, the phospholipid molecules in the cell membrane tend to arrange themselves in a bilayer with their hydrophilic heads pointing towards the inner and outer aqueous phases (the cytoplasm and plasma respectively), while the hydrophobic tails point towards each other as shown in *Figure 1.2*.

Box 1.5 Blood cell antigens

The presence of antigenic material as a component of the RBC membrane was first recognized by Landsteiner in 1901 with the discovery of the ABH blood group system. That these protein components might have some physiological function was not immediately realized, and it was over half a century before their physiological significance began to be appreciated. Up to that point it just seemed that they were there to complicate blood transfusion!

We now realize that the myriad subsequently recognized blood group systems all relate to groups of proteins that have specific physiological function. The specificity within any one system is a demonstration of the detailed structural genetic polymorphism that can exist within substances that often perform the same function, despite these minor differences.

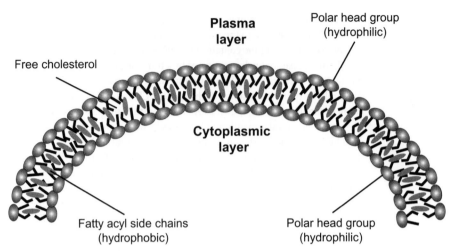

Figure 1.2
Structure of the red cell membrane lipids.

Proteins. Red cell membrane proteins can be grouped into two types:

- **integral proteins**, which penetrate the lipid bilayer and are firmly anchored within it via interactions with the hydrophobic core. Only a relatively small portion of an integral protein molecule is exposed to the inner and outer aqueous phases. About 60–80% of red cell membrane proteins are of this type. Examples of important integral proteins include AE1 (band 3) and the glycophorins. AE1 acts as the anion transport channel while the glycophorins are associated with the MNSs blood group system. Both of the named examples of integral proteins are bound tightly to the protein cytoskeleton.
- **peripheral proteins**, which are in contact with the lipid bilayer but are not strongly attached to it. About 20–40% of red cell membrane proteins are peripheral proteins. Examples of important peripheral proteins include the enzyme glyceraldehyde-3-phosphate dehydrogenase and the cytoskeletal proteins spectrin and actin.

Rh proteins. The Rh proteins are integral membrane proteins and are important blood group antigens from the point of view of blood transfusion and pregnancy. The proteins are associated in the membrane in a multimeric complex that is suspected to interact with the cytoskeleton, influencing cell shape and deformability. A complete absence of Rh proteins (Rh$_{null}$) is associated with red cell shape changes and a shortened red cell lifespan. The Rh proteins are encoded by two genes that are located close to each other on chromosome 1. One gene encodes RhD and the other encodes RhCE. This gives rise to the D, C, c, E and e antigens. However, the *RH* genes are polymorphic and are susceptible to recombination events, resulting in the generation of abnormal or hybrid proteins, giving rise to more than 50 Rh antigens.

Individuals that have a complete deletion of the *RHD* gene or a mutation that renders it completely inactive are said to be 'rhesus negative'. About 15–17% of Caucasians are rhesus negative, mostly due to gene deletion. About 5% of black Africans and 3% of Asians are rhesus negative, but in these cases the genetic basis is more variable and can lead to problems in blood typing for transfusion. Accurate determination of RhD is critical for blood transfusion and the avoidance of haemolytic disease of the newborn.

Surface receptors. Physiologically, the most important surface receptors of red cells are the transferrin receptors TfR1 and TfR2 (see *Chapter 4*). A large variety of other surface receptors have been demonstrated on the red cell membrane, including those for insulin, parathyroid hormone, vitamin E, the complement components C3b and C4b, opiates and oestradiol. In most cases, any function of these receptors in the context of red cell function remains obscure.

Red cell membrane peripheral proteins. The red cell membrane peripheral proteins interact to form a cytoskeleton, which acts as a tough supporting framework for the lipid bilayer. Four proteins play a key role in the structure of the red cell cytoskeleton: spectrin, ankyrin, band 4.1 and actin, although many others play ancillary roles in this complex structure.

Platelets

The second most numerous type of cell in the blood is the platelet or thrombocyte: about 150–440 x 10^9 platelets are present in each litre of blood (see *Chapter 18*). Normal peripheral blood platelets are discoid, anucleate cells, or, more correctly, cell fragments, with a granular cytoplasm. They are derived from cells in the marrow called megakaryocytes, and are produced by a process of budding off from megakaryocyte cytoplasm. They have a volume of about 7 fl, a diameter of about 3 μm and are about 1 μm thick. Platelets survive in the circulation for 10–12 days.

The structure of the platelet plasma membrane is broadly similar to that of the red cell, but is significantly more complex in its detailed structure and function. The external leaflet of the membrane is exceptionally rich in receptors that help to drive the multiple functional processes of platelets. Important platelet receptors include GPIb, a primary receptor for von Willebrand factor (vWF), which serves to mediate the initial adhesion of platelets to sub-endothelium; GPIIb/IIIa which acts as a receptor for fibrinogen, fibronectin, and vWF, thereby mediating platelet aggregation. The platelet membrane also includes receptors for ADP, thrombin, adrenaline (epinephrine) and serotonin, which play a role in platelet aggregation.

Another important feature of the platelet membrane is that the distribution of membrane lipids is asymmetric. The membrane is rich in phospholipids, but phosphatidylserine (PS) is present mainly in the inner cytoplasmic leaflet. This is important because PS is required for formation of the prothrombinase complex during clot formation (see *Chapter 18*). Platelet activation is accompanied by exposure of PS at the platelet surface, which forms a substrate for prothrombinase formation. Because PS normally is 'hidden' from the exterior, resting platelets do not activate coagulation.

The outer surface of the platelet membrane is coated in a layer of glycolipids, mucopolysaccharides and adsorbed proteins called the glycocalyx. This layer confers a negative charge to the platelet surface, which helps to prevent platelet–platelet and platelet–endothelium adhesion in the resting state. The glycocalyx is rich in adhesion molecules and protein receptors, and plays an important role in platelet function. The membrane and glycocalyx make up the peripheral zone of the platelet.

The platelet membrane has multiple contortions that penetrate deeply into the cytoplasm but retain their connection with the cell surface. These structures are collectively known as the surface-connected canalicular system (SCCS) and act as a route for trafficking of molecules between the plasma and platelet interior, including granule release during activation. The SCCS also provides extra intact membrane that allows the platelet to spread and change shape during cell adhesion.

Platelets also contain a dense tubular system (DTS) that, unlike the SCCS, is a closed-channel system. The DTS consists of smooth endoplasmic reticulum and regulates intracellular calcium transport and acts as a site of prostaglandin synthesis. It is the release of calcium from the DTS that triggers platelet contraction and activation of platelets.

The platelet cytoskeleton largely consists of actin, whose assembly and disassembly between globular and filamentous forms provides the motor for platelet filopod formation, spreading and shape change during the early steps of activation and, later, for clot retraction. Beneath the cytoskeleton lies a rim of microtubules that help to maintain platelet shape. The cytoskeleton and microtubule layer constitute the sol-gel zone of the platelet.

Beneath the sol-gel zone lies the organelle zone, which is responsible for the metabolic activities of the platelet. Platelets contain three morphologically distinct types of storage granules; α granules, dense granules and lysosomes. α granules are more common, with each platelet containing up to 200. Dense bodies are less common (2–10 per platelet). These granules act as storage sites for substances required during platelet activation. The contents of both α and dense granules are released during the energy-dependent platelet release reaction. Platelets are rich in mitochondria that provide the energy needed by the platelets.

Adequate numbers of functionally normal platelets are essential for optimal haemostasis. Platelets do not normally adhere to endothelial cells, but they do specifically adhere to underlying tissue matrix should this become exposed by any gaps in the endothelial lining of injured blood vessels. Such binding triggers platelets to release their granule contents, leading to the induction of vasoconstriction, the promotion of aggregation with other platelets to form a plug, and the promotion of fibrin clot formation, all of which contribute to the arrest of haemorrhage. Platelet-derived substances also induce the localized promotion of cell proliferation which facilitates wound healing, and increase vascular permeability which promotes the egress of antibodies and leucocytes to deal with any potentially damaging micro-organisms that may have penetrated the wound. There is also, however, a 'down side', because platelets are also involved in the early stages of the development of atherosclerosis, which can lead to arterial disease and thrombosis.

White cells

The least numerous of the blood cells is the white cell or leucocyte: about 5×10^9 white cells are present in each litre of blood. They consist of a variety of cells specialized for specific and non-specific immune defence against foreign material or organisms. There are five different types of white cell normally present in the peripheral blood: neutrophils, eosinophils, basophils, monocytes and lymphocytes (see also *Box 1.6*).

The neutrophils, eosinophils and basophils are characterized by the presence of cytoplasmic granules and so are known collectively as **granulocytes**. Their names are based on their Romanowsky staining characteristics, which in turn are based on the nature of their specific granule contents. These cells comprise a rapid response force; when triggered by the presence of foreign material, they mount a generalized defensive reaction, involving degradative enzymes, toxins and signalling substances contained within their storage granules. The different granulocytes store different types of secretory substances that contribute to their differing functions. Collectively, the granulocytes make up 50–75% of the total circulating leucocytes.

Box 1.6 Reference values

Reference values (x 10^9/l):

WBC	4.0–11.0	
Neutrophils	2.1–7.2	(55–65%)
Lymphocytes	1.5–4.0	(20–40%)
Monocytes	0.2–0.8	(4–10%)
Eosinophils	0–0.45	(1–3%)
Basophils	0–0.2	(0–1%)

The lymphocytes and monocytes are known as mononuclear leucocytes because they have a non-segmented, round or indented nucleus. These cells are sometimes, incorrectly, known as agranulocytes. This term implies that these cells have no granules but, although they lack the prominent secondary granules that characterize the granulocytes, they can contain fine azurophilic granules.

The monocytes and lymphocytes mount a slower, but more powerful, defensive reaction than the granulocytes. Lymphocytes are responsible for antigen-specific immune responses. Monocytes are non-specific phagocytic cells that are the circulating equivalent of tissue macrophages. The mononuclear cells collectively represent 20–50% of circulating leucocytes.

Neutrophils

The neutrophil is the most numerous white cell in adults: about 60% of circulating white cells are neutrophils (6×10^9 per litre of whole blood). The neutrophil is typically around 12–15 µm in diameter. Its nucleus is divided into a varying number of lobes, joined by thin chromatin strands. Because of this, the neutrophil is sometimes called a polymorphonuclear leucocyte, or 'poly' for short; however, this term is potentially misleading since the other two granulocytes also have polymorphic nuclei, albeit usually with fewer lobes.

Neutrophil cytoplasm contains numerous fine granules, which stain pale pink with Romanowsky dyes. The appearance of these cytoplasmic granules distinguishes the neutrophil from its granulocytic cousins. The granules are of two types, the more abundant, pink-staining, specific or secondary granules, and the larger, reddish-purple staining, azurophilic or primary granules. The neutrophil-specific granules contain a battery of enzymes and other inflammatory substances, including lysozyme which degrades bacterial cell walls, and collagenase which degrades collagen fibres and opens up the tissue matrix. The azurophilic granules also contain digestive enzymes, including lysozyme, glycosidases, proteases, nucleases, and myeloperoxidase. Neutrophils have also been shown to contain tertiary granules and secretory vesicles that contain various membrane proteins that can be expressed during activation and contribute to the anti-microbial role of the cell.

Neutrophils spend about 8–10 hours in the circulation before they exit to the tissues, passing between endothelial cells by a process known as diapedesis. Once in the tissues, neutrophils are responsible for non-specific defence against bacterial and fungal infection. Having left the vessels, neutrophils can survive in the tissues for several days; indeed there are several hundred times more neutrophils in the tissues than there are in the blood at any one time. Neutrophils that do not encounter microbes are thought to undergo apoptosis within 24–48 hours. This mechanism of cell death is important because apoptotic neutrophils are phagocytosed intact by tissue macrophages. This avoids cell lysis, which would release the inflammatory substances within the cell into the surrounding tissues, triggering an inappropriate inflammatory response.

During their time in the peripheral circulation, a proportion of neutrophils, around half under resting conditions, are 'marginated' along the walls of the vascular endothelium or are sequestered in the spleen or lungs (see *Box 1.7*). Marginated neutrophils are perfectly placed both to receive, as early as possible, chemotactic signals radiating from a site of tissue infection, and to respond to such signals by entering the tissues to deal with their source.

Marginated neutrophils are not static; they roll along the vascular endothelial surface. Margination occurs partly due to the hydrodynamic forces of the blood flow and partly to loose interactions between adhesion molecules known as selectins on the neutrophil and endothelial cell surface. Selectins are glycoprotein molecules bearing a free NH_2 terminal lectin domain, and are present on both neutrophils (L-selectins) and endothelial cells (P and E selectins). L-selectins are also present on the surface of monocytes and lymphocytes.

Box 1.7 Neutrophil margination

The margination of neutrophils is a dynamic process, involving continuous interchange between the circulating granulocyte pool (CGP) and the marginated granulocyte pool (MGP). The balance between the CGP and the MGP is dependent on non-turbulent axial flow through the vessels; if these conditions are not met then the CGP expands at the expense of the MGP. Such conditions may arise, for example, when blood vessels passing through muscles are externally squeezed when the muscle becomes active, in so doing dislodging MGP neutrophils into the CGP, temporarily increasing the CGP. It should be noted that when a sample of blood is taken it is taken from circulating cells, so if an accurate WBC count is to be obtained it is essential that the sample is taken under standard conditions, i.e. from an equilibrated, resting patient, otherwise a spuriously high WBC count can result, for example after exercise or even just after a meal.

Localized release of inflammatory mediators such as bacterial lipopolysaccharide or complement components triggers important changes in both the marginated neutrophils and the vascular endothelial cells, including the up-regulation of another family of adhesion molecules called the integrins. Activated neutrophils express the integrins CD11a/CD18 (also known as leucocyte function-associated molecule: LFA-1), CD11b/CD18 (Mac-1 or CR3) and CD11c/CD18 (p150,95 or CR4) on their surface membrane. In parallel with this is an increased expression of CD54, CD102 (intercellular adhesion molecules 1 and 2: ICAM-1 and 2) and CD31 (platelet endothelial cell adhesion molecule: PECAM-1) on the surface of the endothelial cell. These integrin molecules bind tightly to each other (neutrophil CD11a/CD18 and CD11b/CD18 bind to endothelial CD54, and neutrophil CD11b/CD18 binds to endothelial CD102). The result is that the marginated neutrophils stop rolling and begin to respond to the stimulus by crawling along the endothelial surface until they reach a junction, at which point they are able to pass through into the sub-endothelial space by diapedesis. Integrin expression is augmented by interleukin-1 (IL-1), tumour necrosis factor (TNF) and interferon released by responding macrophages and neutrophils (see *Figure 1.3*).

Having passed into the tissues, the neutrophils encounter a concentration gradient of chemoattractants created by radial diffusion from the inflammatory focus. This causes the neutrophil to crawl towards the inflammatory focus, a process known as chemotaxis. The motive force for the neutrophils is provided by assembly and disassembly of actin and myosin fibres within the cytoplasm.

On arrival at their target the neutrophils must first bind to the target, a process involving neutrophil membrane receptors for immunoglobulin (Fc receptors) and the complement protein C3b. Having adhered to the target, the neutrophil then engulfs it by phagocytosis, resulting in the organism being contained within a vacuole in the cytoplasm called the primary phagocytic vacuole. This binding and engulfment is greatly facilitated if the target has been coated in antibodies and the complement system has been activated in a process known as opsonization.

On ingestion of a microbe, the metabolism of the neutrophil undergoes a dramatic and very rapid change, known as the respiratory burst. The previously largely anaerobic metabolism rapidly switches to aerobic systems, the oxygen consumption increasing around 100-fold. This metabolic transformation is mediated via the NADPH–cytochrome oxidase system located in the neutrophil membrane, which is activated by immune complexes, by the *N*-formyl oligopeptides released from micro-organisms and by the complement protein C5a. Also involved in the activation are a series of other cytoplasmic proteins. The outcome of the activation is that potent microbicidal oxidants are produced, including superoxide anion (O_2^-), hydrogen peroxide (H_2O_2) and hypochlorous acid (HOCl), which are released into the phagocytic vacuole.

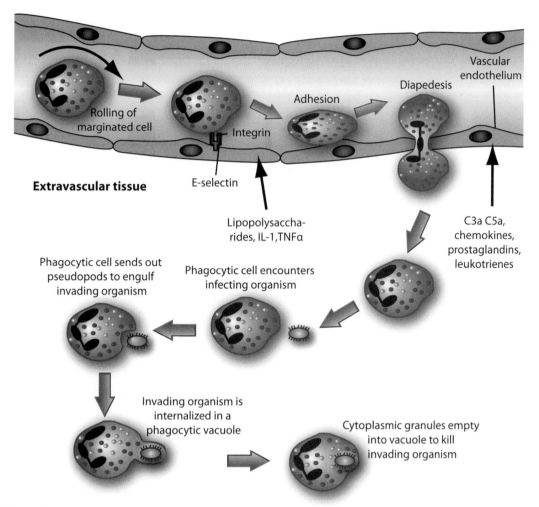

Figure 1.3
Neutrophil function.

In addition to these oxidizing actions, the granules of the neutrophil are also called into play. They migrate through the cytoplasm by a process that is poorly understood. On reaching the phagocytic vacuole, the granule membranes fuse with the vacuole membrane and release their contents. When the specific granules fuse, lysozyme begins to digest polysaccharide in the bacterial cell walls. When the phagocytic vacuoles subsequently fuse with the azurophilic granules, myeloperoxidase catalyses the production of hypochlorite using chloride ions and H_2O_2. This powerful halogenating agent can inactivate most ingested bacteria and some proteins, toxins and viruses. The combination of various digestive enzymes then reduces engulfed foreign material to small molecules, which are used metabolically or diffuse away.

The neutrophil itself is protected from these strong agents by both chemical and physical mechanisms. First, the vacuole is membrane-lined thus containing the digestive process, and secondly the neutrophil possesses powerful anti-oxidants in the form of catalase, which enzymatically reduces H_2O_2, and reduced glutathione (GSH). If the inflammation is sufficiently strong, a considerable localized build-up of neutrophils and monocytes, live, dead and decaying, can build up in a protein-rich liquid, which we call 'pus', sometimes creating the painful swollen area known as an abscess. This powerful toxic mess can be a threat to surrounding tissue, and considerable necrosis can occur before the final clearance is mediated by monocytes and macrophages (see also *Box 1.8*).

Box 1.8 Colour of pus

Pus is characteristically a whitish-yellow colour, but may acquire a distinctly green tinge. This is caused by the presence of neutrophil myeloperoxidase, a digestive enzyme found in neutrophil secondary granules. Other colour changes to pus include a reddish tint if blood is present or a bluish tint in the presence of pyocyanin, a pigment present in the pathogen *Pseudomonas aeruginosa*.

Eosinophils

About 1% of the circulating white cells are eosinophils. This name is derived from the staining characteristics of the large cytoplasmic granules, which stain strongly with the acidic dye eosin. Typically, the eosinophil nucleus is bi-lobed. Eosinophils are responsible for limiting inflammatory responses, particularly helping to dampen any allergic response, and have an important role in defence against parasitic infestation. Tissue eosinophils are also capable of responding, albeit inefficiently, to bacterial and fungal infection in a similar manner to neutrophils. Eosinophils circulate in the bloodstream for about 4–5 hours before they exit to the tissues where they can remain for up to 14 days. Relatively large numbers may be found under epithelial surfaces, such as skin, gut, and the respiratory and urinary tracts, ready to take action against parasites that might enter via these routes.

Attraction of eosinophils to reactive sites is under the influence of various chemokines, including CCL11 (eotaxin-1), CCL24 (eotaxin-2), CCL5 (RANTES), and certain leukotrienes including leukotriene B4 (LTB4). Type 2 cytokines, including IL-5, GM–CSF, and IL-3, released from a specific subset of helper T cells (T_H2) at the reactive site, are responsible for eosinophil activation. Eosinophils are only weakly phagocytic, but they are capable of ingesting and killing micro-organisms in a similar way to neutrophils. They deal with macroparasites that are far too large to ingest by spilling their toxic granule contents directly onto their targets. Eosinophils also ingest antigen–antibody complexes, which are then destroyed by degradative enzymes, and this is an important aspect of their anti-inflammatory, anti-allergic capability.

The strong eosinophilia (acidophilia) of the granules is due to the presence of crystals of MBP (major basic protein), which is rich in the positively charged amino acid arginine. MBP is particularly toxic to many parasites, especially macroparasites such as helminths (worms) and amoebae. The granules also contain a variety of other substances, including enzymes (lysozyme, peroxidase, proteases, lysophospholipase) and chemotactic factors which attract more eosinophils to a reactive site. Eosinophil cationic protein (ECP), another granular protein released into the environment on activation, has the ability to punch holes in the membrane of target organisms, thus permitting the entry of destructive enzymes. Eosinophils also secrete enzymes that inactivate various inflammatory mediators, for instance arylsulfatase and histaminase, which destroy leukotriene and histamine respectively. This is the second important aspect of their anti-inflammatory, anti-allergic capability.

Finally, on activation eosinophils release cell signalling compounds of various kinds, including eicosanoids (leukotrienes including LTC_4, LTD_4 and LTE_4, and prostaglandins including PGE_2), growth factors including TGFβ, VEGF and PDGF, and cytokines including IL-1, IL-2, IL-4, IL-5, IL-6, IL-8, IL-13 and TNFα.

Basophils

Basophils are the least numerous circulating white cell; less than 1% of circulating white cells are basophils. The large cytoplasmic granules are characterized by their avidity for the basic dye methylene blue due to their content of the anionic polysaccharide, heparin. The granules also contain histamine and other inflammatory mediators (e.g. chemotactic factors, proteases, and cytokines). Basophils are involved in anaphylactic, hypersensitivity and inflammatory reactions. They release their granule contents when surface receptors bind IgG or IgE antibodies, the complement components C3a and C5a, basic polypeptides such as bradykinin and neurotensin, or histamine-releasing factors such as RANTES or IL-8.

Chemotactic factors that are released attract eosinophils and more basophils to the site. In this way a very quick defensive reaction (immediate hypersensitivity reaction) is mounted against foreign antigens. In some cases this is experienced as an allergic response, such as hay fever or asthma. Some of the substances released serve to limit the extent of tissue damage and to begin repair processes. For example, heparin acts as an anticoagulant, while other factors regulate vascular permeability, blood flow, tissue oedema and fibroblast differentiation. Mast cells are probably more closely involved in the post-injury phase than basophils.

Basophils can be thought of as the circulating equivalent of fixed tissue mast cells, although mast cells arise from a distinct precursor and are not derived from emigrant basophils. Mast cells have the disadvantage of being fixed in tissue sites, whereas basophils can move responsively and rapidly to inflammatory sites, and can reach high concentration at such sites, where they mount immediate hypersensitivity responses.

Lymphocytes

Lymphocytes are the second most common white cell in the peripheral blood: in adults about 33% of circulating white cells are lymphocytes. They are responsible for specific immunity to recognized molecules, known as antigens, through the responsive production of antibodies specific to the antigens. Morphologically, there are two populations of lymphocytes. Small lymphocytes are consistently sized at 10–12 μm in diameter, and thus form a useful size scale when examining peripheral blood films. They have much less cytoplasm than monocytes. Small lymphocyte cytoplasm often appears as a thin perinuclear rim, rich in ribosomes. In contrast to the monocyte, the lymphocyte nucleus is round, intensely basophilic and almost fills the cell. A few lymphocytes; the so-called 'large lymphocytes', have more abundant cytoplasm, and can mimic monocytes; however, they may be differentiated both by their cytoplasmic colour and by their nuclear shape. Lymphocytes have a variable lifespan of between a few days and many years. The biology of lymphocytes is hugely complex and beyond the scope of this text – readers should consult a specific immunology text for more detail.

There are three different main functional types of lymphocytes, each with several subtypes, which play distinct roles in specific immunity; the functional subtypes do not correlate with morphological types.

B lymphocytes normally account for 10–30% of the circulating blood lymphocytes and play a central role in humoral (i.e. antibody-mediated) immunity (see also *Box 1.9*). B lymphocytes carry antigen receptors on their cell surface and when they encounter and recognize foreign

---

Box 1.9 Why B lymphocytes?

B lymphocytes are so called because, in chickens, they are 'educated' in a specialized organ known as the Bursa of Fabricius. Glick and associates defined the importance of this organ in 1961, when 'bursectomized' chickens were shown to fail to synthesize antibody and to succumb rapidly in response to *Salmonella* infection. In humans, B lymphocyte education occurs predominantly in the bone marrow.

antigen, they migrate to lymph nodes where they undergo a proliferative burst that results in the generation of a clone of identical B cells, which subsequently mature into clonal plasma cells that synthesize and secrete antibody specific to the inducing antigen. A minority of the stimulated B lymphocytes mature to form long-lived memory cells that are capable of mounting a rapid antibody response on a second encounter with antigen. B lymphocytes also play a role in processing and presenting antigen to T cells.

T lymphocytes account for 40–80% of the circulating blood lymphocytes and are responsible for cell-mediated immunity. The thymus gland is responsible for T cell education (see *Box 1.10*). Several T lymphocyte subsets have been identified, each with a distinct immune function. T lymphocytes carry surface antigen receptors that are analogous to those on B cells. Encounter with a specific antigen triggers an immune response. Important T lymphocyte subsets include:

- T helper (T_H) lymphocytes, which secrete cytokines that regulate the immune response.
- T cytotoxic (T_C) lymphocytes, which directly kill tumour cells and virus-infected cells and play a central role in transplant rejection.
- memory T lymphocytes, which are long-lived and can trigger a rapid immune response on a second encounter with specific antigen.
- regulatory or suppressor T (T_S) lymphocytes, which are responsible for maintenance of immune tolerance.

Natural killer cells (NK cells) are a type of large granular cytotoxic lymphocyte that play an important role in fighting cancer and viral infections. NK cells have cytoplasmic granules that contain cytotoxins such as perforin and granzyme. They kill target cells by engagement and direct release of these proteins, triggering target cell apoptosis.

Box 1.10 Why T lymphocytes?

The pivotal role of the thymus gland in cellular immunity was first demonstrated in 1961 when it was shown that thymectomized mice had a greatly impaired capacity to fight infection. T lymphocytes are named to show that they are educated in the thymus gland.

Monocytes

About 5% of circulating white cells are monocytes; the vast majority are the precursors of fixed tissue macrophages, the remainder being immature dendritic cells, the two types of cells being morphologically indistinguishable. Blood monocytes circulate for about 10 hours before they exit to the tissues where they mature into and join the pre-existing population of actively phagocytic tissue macrophages, which are responsible for the removal and processing of aged red cells and other debris. They may undergo limited proliferation in the tissues, and can exist there for periods of months or even years. There is a degree of specialization of tissue macrophages that is determined largely by the influence of the various interleukins and other cell signalling compounds that individually and collectively effect the maturation in response to specific need. Dependent on location, tissue macrophages and dendritic cells are known by different names in different locations (e.g. Küpffer cells in liver, Langerhans cells in skin, microglial cells in brain, osteoclasts in bone, etc.). Together, the monocytes, the fixed tissue macrophages and their precursors constitute the reticulo-endothelial (RE) system.

The blood monocyte is a large cell (16–22 μm in diameter) with a kidney-shaped or distinctly cleft nucleus and a scattering of delicate azurophilic granules in the cytoplasm, giving it an overall grey-blue appearance. They can resemble large lymphocytes; however, their cytoplasm is typically more grey-blue in colour, their nucleus is less intensely stained, shows a more uniform granularity and often appears 'folded over' to give a kidney or more complex shape. They are a heterogeneous population.

Tissue macrophages play several important roles, primarily in the non-specific immune system. Although less numerous than the neutrophils, they are actively phagocytic and have a much wider spectrum of digestive enzymes within their lysosomes, enabling them to be active against a much wider range of targets, including soluble target materials, which they remove in a process known as pinocytosis. On their surface they carry a range of receptors, which trigger the ingestion of bound ligands, an example being the Fc receptor, which promotes the ingestion of opsonized targets. They respond to a variety of chemotactic signals, which attract them to areas of inflammation, and they release a variety of growth factors and cytokines, which regulate responses of other cell types. On activation they, like neutrophils, undergo a respiratory burst, and thus produce both reactive oxygen and reactive nitrogen species, which, together with the large array of enzymes, enable them to be effective against a wide variety of targets.

Tissue macrophages also play an important role in specific immunity, since they are involved in the processing and presentation of antigen to T lymphocytes. However, it is in this role that dendritic cells predominate. They display fragments of digested material on their surface, in combination with specific receptors for lymphocytes, in a process called 'antigen presentation'.

SUGGESTED FURTHER READING

Bain, B.J. (2006) *Blood Cells: a Practical Guide.* Blackwell Publishing, Oxford.
ASH Image Bank – http://ashimagebank.hematologylibrary.org/
Bloodline Image Atlas – www.bloodline.net/external/image-atlas.html

SELF-ASSESSMENT QUESTIONS

1. Which of the following statements are true?
   a. The plasma Na^+ concentration is lower than the K^+ concentration.
   b. The red cell Na^+ concentration is lower than the K^+ concentration.
   c. Plasma is always electrically neutral.
   d. The major plasma protein component is immunoglobulin.
2. Approximately how many red cells are present in each litre of blood in an adult male?
   a. $4.4–5.9 \times 10^9$.
   b. $4.4–5.9 \times 10^{12}$.
   c. $3.8–5.2 \times 10^{12}$.
   d. $3.8–5.2 \times 10^9$.
3. Aged red cells are sequestered by which organ?
4. Is red cell spectrin an integral or a peripheral protein?
5. Name the second most numerous blood cell in a healthy person.
6. Fill in the blanks in the text below:
   The outer surface of the platelet membrane is coated in a layer of glycolipids, mucopolysaccharides and adsorbed proteins called the _____. This layer confers a _____ charge to the platelet surface, which helps to prevent platelet–platelet and platelet–endothelium adhesion in the resting state. The membrane and glycocalyx make up the _____ zone of the platelet.
7. Platelets contain two channel systems, the SCCS and the DTS. Which of these is a closed-channel system?
8. Name the three morphologically distinct types of storage granules found in platelets.
9. Name the most numerous white cell in a healthy person.

10. Which white cell is most closely associated with defence against parasitic infestation?
11. Which granulocyte is most closely associated with anaphylaxis?
12. Fill in the blanks in the text below:

    B lymphocytes normally account for 10–30% of the circulating blood lymphocytes and play a central role in _____ (i.e. _____-mediated) immunity. B lymphocytes also play a role in processing and presenting antigen to _ cells. T lymphocytes account for 40–80% of the circulating blood lymphocytes and are responsible for _____-mediated immunity. The _____ gland is responsible for T cell education. NK cells play an important role in fighting _____ and _____ infections.

Haemopoiesis

Learning objectives
After studying this chapter you should confidently be able to:

■ **Describe the various sites of haemopoiesis throughout life**
Haemopoiesis is conducted at a number of different anatomical sites during the process of development from embryo to adult. The earliest recognizable red cell precursors are demonstrable in 2 week old embryos. Haemopoiesis occurs in the fetal liver at 6 weeks gestation, and this organ is the primary source of fetal blood cells until about 30 weeks gestation. The fetal spleen is a secondary source of haemopoietic cells. Bone marrow rapidly becomes the sole source of blood cells by 40 weeks gestation and remains so throughout life.

■ **Discuss the physiological significance of the haemopoietic stem cell compartment**
Blood cells are produced continuously throughout life. This requires a population of precursor cells that are capable of both self-renewal and differentiation – the stem cell compartment. The common ancestral cell of all mature blood cells in humans is the totipotent stem cell. This cell can differentiate to form lymphoid or myeloid pluripotent stem cells. These stem cells retain the dual capacity for self-renewal and differentiation. Pluripotent stem cells are capable of differentiating into a number of different unipotent stem cells that are committed to a single cell line, e.g. BFU-E can only differentiate into mature red cells.

■ **Outline the mechanisms of regulation of haemopoiesis**
Haemopoiesis is a closely regulated process. The bone marrow micro-environment is important for supporting cell growth and differentiation, but the main regulatory role lies with a large family of glycoproteins known as cytokines or, more precisely, haemopoietic growth factors. The impact of growth factors on the regulation of haemopoiesis *in vivo* is highly complex and incompletely understood.

■ **Outline the importance of the haemopoietic micro-environment**
The bone marrow contains a mixture of haemopoietic and non-haemopoietic cells anchored within a structural network known as the extracellular matrix (ECM). The complete structure comprising the ECM and all of the cells of the bone marrow is known as the haemopoietic micro-environment, because all of these cells and structures interact to provide an optimal micro-environment for haemopoiesis. The non-haemopoietic cells of the haemopoietic micro-environment constitute the marrow stroma.

Under normal physiological conditions, the number of circulating blood cells is maintained within remarkably narrow limits. Because all blood cells have a limited lifespan, a dynamic equilibrium must exist between cell loss due to senescence or normal function and the synthesis and release of their replacements. The process of blood cell production is known as haemopoiesis (see *Box 2.1*). The maintenance of circulating blood cell numbers is an example of physiological homeostasis (see *Box 2.2*).

Box 2.1 Definition of haemopoiesis

Haemopoiesis is the blanket term that covers the production of all blood cells. The production of the different blood cell lineages is known as erythropoiesis (red cells), myelopoiesis (granulocytes and monocytes), granulopoiesis (granulocytes), monopoiesis (monocytes), and thrombopoiesis (platelets). The production of lymphocytes (lymphopoiesis) is also strictly part of haemopoiesis, but there are features of lymphocyte production that are markedly different from the production of the other lineages. The most significant difference is that circulating lymphocytes are not end-stage cells. When they encounter antigen they undergo a second proliferative burst that generates a clonal response.

Box 2.2 Homeostasis

The concept of homeostasis is arguably the single most profound and powerful idea that has emerged within physiology over the last 150 years. It was the French physiologist Claude Bernard, the founder of modern experimental physiology, who in 1865 first expounded the importance of the consistency of the internal environment for the continued normal functioning of the human body, with the words '*La fixité du milieu intérieur est la condition d'une vie libre et indépendante*' ('The constancy of the internal environment is the condition for a free and independent life'). This seminal observation remains the cornerstone of modern biological thought.

It was the American physiologist Walter Cannon who coined the word *homeostasis* in his book *The Wisdom of the Body* (1932). The concept of the negative feedback homeostatic loop as a mechanism for maintaining the consistency of any variable that is subject to perturbation from factors outside the feedback system itself (so-called external variables), is now recognized as being, in various forms, the mechanism whereby the vast majority of all physiological 'constants' are maintained.

Haemopoiesis is regulated by an array of protein growth factors that have been shown to stimulate the proliferation and/or differentiation of haemopoietic progenitor cells to produce the different blood cell types in precisely the proportions required to maintain normal circulating cell counts. For example, a significant haemorrhage leads to a reduction in circulating red blood cells. This triggers secretion of a red cell growth factor called erythropoietin that influences haemopoietic progenitor cells to preferentially produce red cells until the reduced red blood cell count is corrected (see also *Box 2.3*).

Box 2.3 Astonishing facts about haemopoiesis

The maintenance of a stable population requires an astonishing capacity for haemopoiesis. An average 70 kg man has a total blood volume of about 5 litres which contains a total of 25×10^{12} red cells. Since normal red cells survive for an average of 120 days, maintenance of a constant cell number requires the replacement of more than 2×10^{11} red cells every day! If the destruction and replacement of the other blood cells is taken into account, the total daily requirement for new blood cells is about 5×10^{11}. This rate of production must be maintained without pause for an average of 70 years, during which time the bone marrow will have released more than 1×10^{16} mature blood cells which, for an average 70 kg man, would weigh about 7 tonnes!

2.1 ONTOGENY OF HAEMOPOIESIS

Haemopoiesis is conducted at a number of different anatomical sites during the process of development from embryo to adult (*Figure 2.1*). Changes in the primary site of haemopoiesis

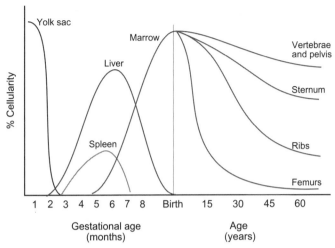

Figure 2.1
Sites of haemopoiesis throughout life.

are accompanied by simultaneous changes in the morphology of the cells produced and in the types of haemoglobin molecule synthesized within the red cell precursors.

Embryonic haemopoiesis

The earliest recognizable red cell precursors are large, nucleated cells and are demonstrable in 2 week old embryos (see *Box 2.4*). The major haemoglobin present in these cells is haemoglobin Gower I ($\zeta_2\varepsilon_2$; see *Chapter 6*). Leucopoiesis and thrombopoiesis do not commence until about 6 weeks gestation, when megakaryocytes and granulocytes can be seen in the yolk sac. In contrast to other blood cells, lymphocytes are not formed in the yolk sac, but in the lymph sacs, which begin to develop at about 7 weeks gestation. Activation of the α and γ genes occurs at about 5 weeks gestation when haemoglobin Portland ($\zeta_2\gamma_2$) and haemoglobin Gower II ($\alpha_2\varepsilon_2$) are synthesized. These three embryonic haemoglobins are undetectable by routine methods after about 10 weeks gestation. This is coincident with the end of the yolk sac phase of erythropoiesis. Haemopoietic cells share a common precursor, the haemangioblast, with endothelial cells. It is believed that it is these cells that seed the spleen, liver and bone marrow.

Box 2.4 Embryonic anatomy

The earliest recognizable blood cell precursors are demonstrable in 2 week old embryos. At this stage of development, the embryo consists of little more than two sacs – the **amniotic sac** and the **yolk sac** – separated by a wedge of tissue called the **embryonic plate**. At this stage the yolk sac is the main site of haemopoiesis. As the embryo develops, the amniotic sac expands greatly to fill the entire uterus, and the placenta is formed. The yolk sac is compressed by the expanding amniotic sac into a narrow stalk that forms the core of the umbilical cord. The embryo develops from the embryonic plate.

Fetal haemopoiesis

Haemopoietic activity is first demonstrable in the fetal liver at 6 weeks gestation. This organ is the primary source of fetal blood cells until about 30 weeks gestation. Hepatic haemopoietic activity ceases at about 40 weeks gestation. The major haemoglobin synthesized during the hepatic phase of fetal haemopoiesis is haemoglobin F ($\alpha_2\gamma_2$).

The fetal spleen begins production of blood cells at about 10 weeks gestation and continues throughout the second trimester of pregnancy. However, even at the height of its activity, the fetal spleen is of secondary importance as a haemopoietic organ.

Bone cavities begin to form at about 20 weeks gestation and provide such an ideal environment for haemopoietic activity that the bone marrow rapidly becomes the sole source of blood cells in humans, a process complete by 40 weeks gestation. This process is associated with a gradual replacement of haemoglobin F by haemoglobin A ($\alpha_2\beta_2$).

Haemopoiesis in the developing child and adult

In the developing child, there are two demands placed on haemopoiesis: the ongoing need for replacement of senescent cells, and the pressure to increase the bone marrow volume and total blood cell pool to meet growth demands.

At birth, haemopoietically active, or red, marrow completely fills the available marrow space. This means that infants have no reserve haemopoietic capacity that can be called upon in times of increased demand. The only response open to a neonate in such circumstances is to expand the marrow volume. This is the cause of the skeletal deformities that develop in severe haemolytic states such as thalassaemia.

During early childhood, marrow volume increases in parallel with the increased marrow space made available by increased stature. The bone marrow volume in an average 3-year-old child has expanded to about 1500 ml. This is still entirely composed of active red marrow and is sufficient to meet the normal demands for blood cells of an adult. Thus, as the child grows into an adult, and the available bone marrow space expands, there is no requirement for a concurrent increase in volume of active red marrow. The expanding marrow space becomes progressively filled with inactive, or yellow, marrow. This process begins in the peripheral diaphyses of the long bones and continues until, in an adult, three-quarters of the red marrow is found in the pelvis, vertebrae, sternum and scapulae. The remainder is distributed between the skull, ribs and the epiphyseal ends of the long bones. Yellow marrow is mainly located in the middle portion of long bones. The changes in the extent of active marrow as the body matures are shown in *Figure 2.2.*

Yellow bone marrow consists mainly of fat cells (adipocytes) and serves as a fat store for the body. In times of excess haemopoietic demand that cannot be met by the existing red bone

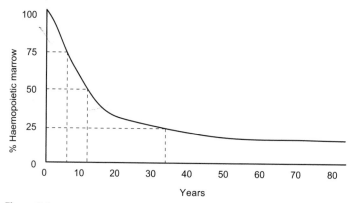

Figure 2.2
Changes in the extent of active marrow over time.

marrow, yellow bone marrow can be converted to red bone marrow to increase haemopoietic capacity. This means that adults have a reserve haemopoietic capacity of about six times normal.

In conditions where the bone marrow is unable to meet the demands of the body for blood cells, e.g. when the bone marrow space is occupied by metastatic tumours, haemopoiesis may revert to fetal sites, namely the spleen and liver. This phenomenon is known as extramedullary haemopoiesis. The most likely mechanism triggering extramedullary haemopoiesis is seeding of circulating haemopoietic stem cells in the spleen, liver or other site.

2.2   SEQUENCE OF DIFFERENTIATION OF BLOOD CELLS

Blood cells are produced in vast numbers throughout life, with no apparent sign of exhaustion of their source. This requires the existence of a population of precursor cells that are capable of both self-renewal and differentiation – the stem cell compartment. The common ancestral cell of all mature blood cells in humans is the totipotent stem cell (*Figure 2.3*). This cell can differentiate to form either a lymphoid stem cell (CFU-L) or a myeloid stem cell (CFU-GEMM). These cells are said to be pluripotent, i.e. they have the capacity to differentiate along several different cell lines but their choice is limited, as shown in *Figure 2.3* (see also *Box 2.5*). These stem cells retain the dual capacity for self-renewal and differentiation. Pluripotent stem cells are capable of differentiating into a number of different unipotent stem cells; these are committed to differentiation along a single cell line, e.g. BFU-E can only differentiate into mature red cells.

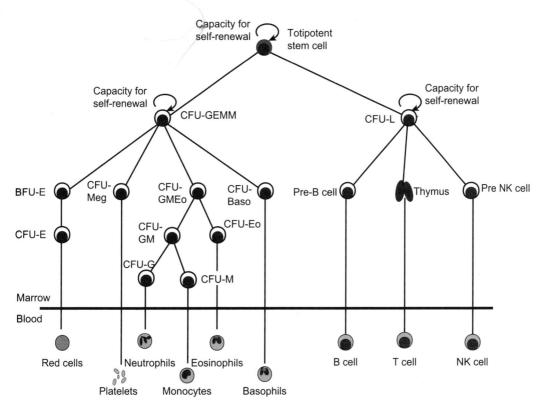

Figure 2.3
Differentiation of mature blood cells from stem cells.

Box 2.5 Pluripotent stem cells

The first unequivocal demonstration of the existence of pluripotent stem cells came in 1961 when Till and McCulloch performed experiments to determine the sensitivity of mouse bone marrow to damage by irradiation. Briefly, mice were subjected to a dose of ionizing radiation sufficient to destroy their haemopoietic capacity, and bone marrow cells from genetically identical mice were immediately transfused. After about 7 days the spleens of these mice had developed numerous macroscopic nodules which consisted of haemopoietic tissue. Subsequent experiments showed that these nodules were clonal in nature, i.e. each was derived from a single stem cell, which was given the name colony forming unit spleen or CFU-S. Under different experimental conditions, CFU-S could be influenced to produce granulocyte–macrophage colony forming units (CFU-GM), erythroid colony forming units (CFU-E) or megakaryocyte colony forming units (CFU-Meg) or a mixture of more than one cell line.

2.3   CONTROL OF HAEMOPOIESIS

Much of our current knowledge of the activities of haemopoietic growth factors has been derived from a mixture of animal experiments, tissue culture experiments and molecular biology. However, there is still much to learn and it is uncertain how much of the experimental data are applicable to the human *in vivo* setting.

Haemopoiesis is a closely regulated process. The bone marrow micro-environment is important for supporting cell growth and differentiation, but the main regulatory role lies with a large family of glycoproteins known as cytokines or, more precisely, haemopoietic growth factors.

Cytokines comprise a diverse family of soluble proteins and peptides that function as humoral regulators of the functions of individual cells, of the interactions between cells, and of various processes in the extracellular environment. They can act via autocrine, paracrine, juxtacrine and retrocrine mechanisms (see *Box 2.6*). In many respects, cytokines bear comparison with classical hormones, although cytokines generally impact on a wider range of cells and their secretion is not restricted to specialized glands. Haemopoietic growth factors are a subset of cytokines that exert important regulatory functions in blood cell proliferation and differentiation. Some of the most important haemopoietic growth factors are shown in *Table 2.1*.

The impact of growth factors on the regulation of haemopoiesis *in vivo* is highly complex and incompletely understood. It is clear that the naïve view: one cellular source – one cytokine – one target cell – one effect, is over simplistic. A single cell type can secrete many different cytokines in response to various stimuli. Each of the cytokines can impact on many different cell types. Each cytokine can exert many different effects on different target cells. Each of these effects can be exerted by more than one cytokine. Finally, the impact of a given cytokine can

---

Box 2.6 Cell signalling definitions

Autocrine – a form of cell signalling in which a cell secretes a hormone or cytokine that exerts its activity on the same type of cell.

Paracrine – a form of cell signalling in which a cell secretes a hormone or cytokine that exerts its activity on cells that are close to, but not in contact with the secreting cell.

Juxtacrine – a form of cell signalling in which a cell secretes a hormone or cytokine that exerts its activity on cells that are in contact with the secreting cell.

Retrocrine – a type of cell signalling in which soluble forms of cytokine receptors are shed by cells that interact with distant target cells expressing the relevant cytokine on their surface membranes.

differ, depending on whether it is acting alone or in concert with other cytokines and also on the sequence of cytokine activity. In short, the reality of cytokine regulation of haemopoiesis is extraordinarily complex. A simplified indication of which cytokines exert important positive effects on haemopoiesis is shown in *Figure 2.4*.

Table 2.1 Selected important haemopoietic growth factors

Growth factor family	Growth factor	Primary target	Gene locus	Source
Interleukins				
	IL-1	Stem cells, T-helper cells, B cells, NK cells, endothelial cells	IL-1α 2q13 IL-1β 2q13–21	Monocytes, activated macrophages
	IL-3	Haemopoietic progenitor cells	5q23–31	Activated T cells
	IL-4	Activated B cells, basophils	5q23–31	Activated T-helper 2 cells
	IL-5	Eosinophils, thymocytes	5q23–31	T cells
	IL-6	B cells, plasma cells, multiple non-haemopoietic cells	7p21–p1	Monocytes, fibroblasts, endothelial cells
	IL-7	B cell progenitors, NK cells, T cell progenitors	8q12–q13	Stromal cells, thymic cells
	IL-8	Neutrophils, basophils, B cells	4q12–q21	Monocytes, multiple non-haemopoietic cells
	IL-9	T-helper cells, mast cells, fetal thymocytes	5q31–32	T-helper cells
Colony stimulating factors				
	G-CSF	CFU-G, CFU-GM	17q21–q22	Monocytes, macrophages, activated neutrophils
	GM-CSF	CFU-GM, CFU-GEMM, endothelial cells	5q22–31	T cells, macrophages
	M-CSF	CFU-M, CFU-GM	5q33	Monocytes, granulocytes, fibroblasts, endothelial cells
Hormones				
	Erythro-poietin	Erythroid progenitor cells, megakaryocyte progenitor cells	7q21–22	Renal tubular, juxtatubular and interstitial cells
	Thrombo-poietin	Megakaryocyte progenitor cells	3q26–27	Liver, kidney

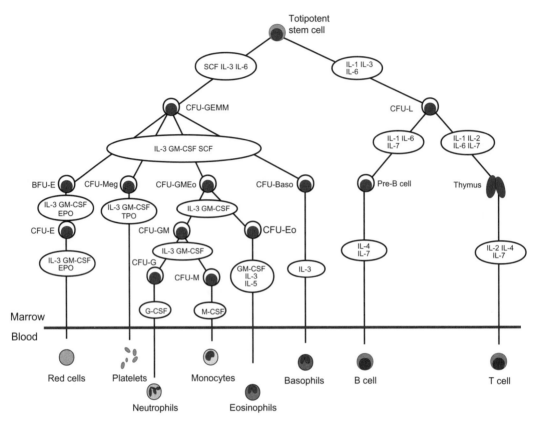

Figure 2.4
Simplified view of cytokine-mediated regulation of haemopoiesis.

One of the key features of the currently accepted model of the stem cell compartment is that a small population of self-renewing stem cells can give rise to the large number of different blood cells produced every day as shown schematically in *Figure 2.5*.

Until relatively recently the haemopoietic stem cell was regarded purely as a progenitor of blood cells but this is now known to be only part of the story. Adult haemopoietic stem cells have been shown experimentally to be capable of differentiating into a wide range of non-haemopoietic cell types, a phenomenon known as stem cell plasticity (see *Figure 2.6* and *Box 2.7*). The therapeutic potential of this observation is the focus of much scientific and clinical research. It is hoped that harvesting of haemopoietic or mesenchymal stem cells may provide a means to effect repair of damaged tissue throughout the body. If this can be achieved by differentiation of patient-derived haemopoietic stem cells, it should also avoid problems associated with immune rejection.

2.4 THE HAEMOPOIETIC MICRO-ENVIRONMENT

The bone marrow contains a mixture of haemopoietic and non-haemopoietic cells anchored within a structural network known as the ECM. Among the non-haemopoietic cells present are myofibroblasts, adipocytes, osteoblasts, osteoclasts, mesenchymal stem cells and endothelial stem cells (see *Figure 2.7*). In addition, the bone is penetrated by a

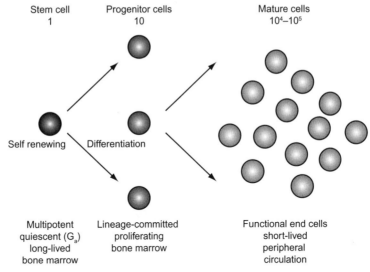

Figure 2.5
Schematic representation of stem cell expansion.

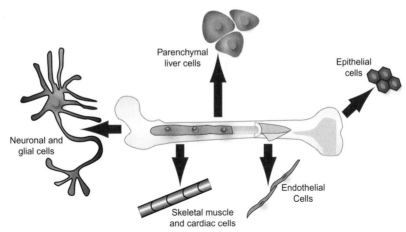

Figure 2.6
Illustration of haemopoietic stem cell plasticity.

Box 2.7 Stem cell plasticity

The first reported transplant of a human organ grown from adult haemopoietic stem cells was performed in 2008 in a cooperative effort involving researchers from Barcelona, Padua, Bristol and Milan. The patient, Claudia Castillo, had suffered a collapsed trachea due to tuberculosis, just at the point where it entered her lungs. To engineer a replacement, a section of trachea was harvested from a cadaveric donor and stripped of cells to create a skeleton of cartilage.

Haemopoietic stem cells harvested from Ms Castillo were then seeded onto the cartilage and grown on to form a new organ. The new section of trachea was successfully transplanted, without the need for immunosuppressive anti-rejection medication. This technique offers the prospect of transforming transplantation surgery.

network of blood vessels that both supply blood to the bone and form a route of egress for mature blood cells. The ECM comprises a network of fibrous proteins, glycoproteins and proteoglycans including various forms of collagen, fibronectin, laminin, haemonectin, tenascin and thrombospondin. The complete structure comprising the ECM and all of the cells of the bone marrow is known as the haemopoietic micro-environment, because all of these cells and structures interact to provide an optimal micro-environment for haemopoiesis. The non-haemopoietic cells of the haemopoietic micro-environment constitute the marrow stroma.

Several important facets of haemopoiesis are regulated by the marrow stroma, as follows.

■ Many of the stromal cells (e.g. endothelial cells, fibroblasts, macrophages) are important sources of haemopoietic growth factors. The close proximity of the stromal cells to the haemopoietic progenitors facilitates paracrine growth factor activity.

■ The ECM plays an important role in supporting haemopoiesis by providing a structural framework within the marrow that cells can adhere to and grow on. It may also be involved in compartmentalization of haemopoietic tissue within the marrow space.

■ The marrow micro-environment plays a central role in the regulation of the release of mature blood cells to the circulation. The endothelium that lines the bone marrow sinuses is tightly packed and so normally permits only the most mature cells (e.g. red blood cells, neutrophils, platelets) to exit the marrow space. To enter the bloodstream, cells must

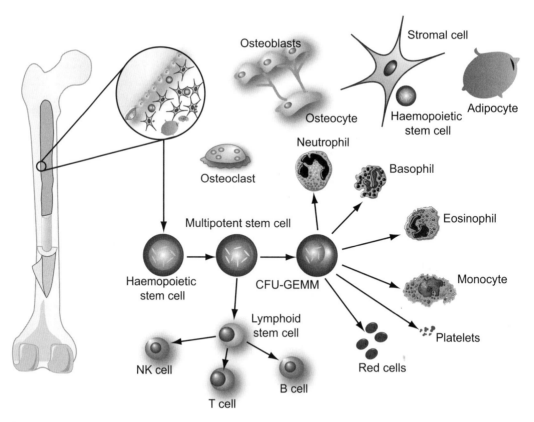

Figure 2.7
Cells of the haemopoietic micro-environment. The term stromal cell encompasses fibroblasts, endothelial cells and marrow macrophages. In some settings, the term stromal cell is used to encompass all non-haemopoietic cells found in the bone marrow.

traverse pores in the marrow vascular endothelium that are much smaller in diameter than a red blood cell. Only anucleate cells (red blood cells, platelets) or cells with a highly distensible nucleus (granulocytes) can ordinarily leave the marrow. All of the maturing blood elements have large, rigid nuclei that restrict them to the marrow.

■ The adhesion molecules present on cells and the ECM also play a critical role in retaining immature cells within the marrow.

■ Elements of the marrow haemopoietic micro-environment are important for the phenomenon known as stem cell 'homing'. Circulating haemopoietic stem cells are selectively attracted to and retained by the bone marrow, where they can proliferate optimally. This mechanism is important because it ensures that haemopoiesis occurs in the most hospitable environment. It is this process that is thought to govern the transfer of the sites of haemopoiesis from embryonic yolk sac to fetal liver, and from spleen to fetal bone marrow during early development. Homing is also important clinically (see *Box 2.8*).

■ The ECM can be induced to selectively release haemopoietic stem cells into the circulation in response to injury or inflammation. These stress events trigger activation of neutrophils, resulting in the release of proteolytic enzymes including elastase and matrix metalloproteinases. These substances degrade and inactivate adhesion molecules, including SDF-1, VLA-4 and P/E selectins, responsible for selectively binding haemopoietic stem cells to the ECM. As a result, haemopoietic stem cells are released into the circulation. This process, known as stem cell mobilization, is exploited clinically to harvest haemopoietic stem cells for transplantation. Treatment of a donor with recombinant granulocyte colony-stimulating factor (G–CSF) markedly increases the number of haemopoietic stem cells in the peripheral blood. These can be collected by apheresis, avoiding the need for bone marrow sampling.

■ The bone marrow serves as an important reservoir for mature neutrophils. In a healthy individual, over 95% of the mature neutrophils in the body are in the bone marrow, ready to be released rapidly when required, e.g. in response to bacterial infection. These neutrophils are said to be in the bone marrow's neutrophil storage pool. Bacterial endotoxin, immune complexes, and cytokines like GM–CSF and G–CSF are all capable of stimulating rapid release of the marrow storage pool of neutrophils into the peripheral blood.

Box 2.8 Homing and haemopoietic stem cell transplantation

The phenomenon of stem cell homing is exploited clinically in haemopoietic stem cell transplantation. In essence, patients with haematological malignancies are treated with high-dose chemotherapy to partially or completely ablate their bone marrow and they are then 'rescued' by venous infusion of allogeneic or autologous haemopoietic stem cells. The stem cells circulate in the blood only for a short time before they home to the bone marrow spaces and repopulate haemopoiesis.

2.5 ERYTHROPOIESIS

Maintenance of the circulating red cell mass within the narrow limits seen in health is achieved by a feedback mechanism, which senses body oxygen demands (tissue hypoxia) and delivery, and adjusts the rate of erythropoiesis accordingly. This feedback mechanism, mediated by the glycoprotein hormone erythropoietin is, for reasons explored in the next chapter, imperfect in pathological conditions but, when working physiologically, does so as follows.

- A fall in the circulating red cell mass leads to decreased haemoglobin, which in turn leads to reduced delivery of oxygen to the tissues, and hypoxia develops.
- Tissue hypoxia is sensed by an enzyme-linked mechanism in the kidney (see *Box 2.9*) and increased synthesis of erythropoietin (EPO) by the peritubular endothelial cells of the kidney is stimulated. There are other minor sites that can be called into play, but this is the main one by far.
- EPO binds to specific receptors on BFU-E and CFU-E in the bone marrow, resulting in a shortening of cell-cycle time, an increased rate of maturation and an increased rate of release of red cells from the bone marrow.
- The resulting increased red cell mass, and hence [Hb], improves oxygen delivery to the tissues, the hypoxia is corrected and EPO synthesis is decreased.

The EPO gene is located at 7q21–q22. The feedback regulation of erythropoiesis is considered in more detail in *Chapter 3*. *Figure 2.8* shows a lineage tree for normal erythropoiesis and the progenitor cells that are influenced by EPO.

Box 2.9 Erythropoietin and hypoxia

The question of how the kidney senses tissue hypoxia and triggers transcription of erythropoietin has recently been elucidated. The first step came in 1992 when Semenza and Wang identified a novel transcription factor that bound to the EPO gene and induced transcription. They called this new protein hypoxia inducible factor-1 (HIF-1). It was subsequently shown that, in the presence of oxygen, hydroxylation of specific proline residues in the α chain of HIF-1 triggers binding of von Hippel–Lindau tumour suppressor protein (VHL). The resulting complex is rapidly degraded by the proteasome. In the absence of oxygen, prolyl hydroxylation and proteasomal degradation are slowed, resulting in stabilization and accumulation of HIF-α. The HIF-α subunit translocates to the nucleus where it dimerizes with HIF-β, binds to the hypoxia response elements of HIF-target genes (such as EPO), and activates their transcription. We now know that HIF proteins are closely involved in many different physiological responses to hypoxia, including glycolysis, inflammation and neutrophil apoptosis.

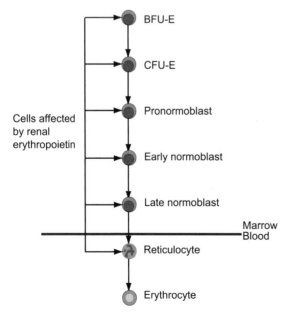

Figure 2.8
The impact of erythropoietin on erythropoiesis.

2.6   GRANULOPOIESIS AND MONOPOIESIS

Granulocyte and monocyte production is regulated by the combined actions of haemopoietic growth factors. IL-3 and GM–CSF act together on CFU-GEMM to stimulate production of CFU-GMEo. The action of G–CSF on these cells stimulates neutrophil production, M–CSF stimulates monocyte production and IL-5 stimulates eosinophil production. Basophil production is stimulated by the action of IL-3 on CFU-GEMM. A lineage tree for normal granulopoiesis and monopoiesis is shown in *Figure 2.9*.

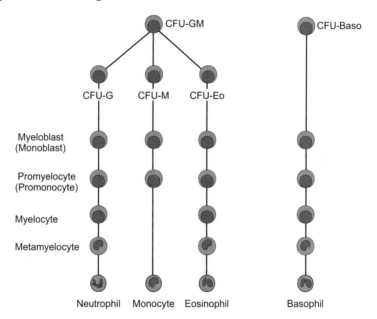

Figure 2.9
Lineage tree for granulopoiesis and monopoiesis.

2.7   THROMBOPOIESIS

Megakaryoblasts are formed from CFU-Meg by a unique process called **endomitotic replication**. In this process, DNA replication and expansion of cytoplasmic volume occur, but not cellular division. Thus, with each complete cycle of endomitosis, the cell becomes progressively larger and increasingly polyploid. Morphologically recognizable megakaryocytes may have up to $64n$ DNA content (i.e. 32 times the normal diploid ($2n$) content).

Once endomitotic replication has ceased, the megakaryocyte nucleus becomes lobulated and the cytoplasm matures, with the formation of ribbon-like structures that project through the endothelium into the venous sinus. It is from the ends of these projections that the platelets are shed into the circulation. This process is estimated to take from 2 to 3 days. Each megakaryocyte is capable of producing between 2000 and 7000 platelets.

Megakaryocyte proliferation and differentiation is stimulated by a glycoprotein hormone called thrombopoietin (TPO). This hormone is synthesized in the liver by parenchymal cells and sinusoidal epithelial cells, and in the kidney by proximal convoluted tubule cells. TPO is also synthesized by striated muscle and bone marrow stromal cells. The TPO gene is located at 3q26.3–27. Abnormalities of 3q are frequently found in a range of haematological malignancies.

A lineage tree for normal thrombopoiesis is shown in *Figure 2.10*.

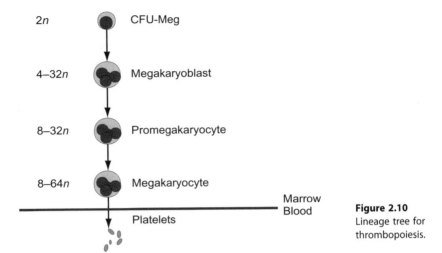

Figure 2.10
Lineage tree for thrombopoiesis.

2.8 LYMPHOPOIESIS

In contrast to the other forms of haemopoiesis, lymphopoiesis is not a one-way process of differentiation and maturation into end-stage cells. Two distinct phases of lymphopoiesis are distinguishable:

- antigen-independent differentiation, in which the lymphoid stem cell differentiates to form mature antigen-committed lymphocytes. This process occurs in the primary lymphoid organs: T lymphocyte differentiation occurs in the thymus gland, while B lymphocyte differentiation takes place in the fetal liver and adult bone marrow. As the name suggests, antigen-independent differentiation is the process that populates the body with B and T cells that are capable of responding to antigen, but is not driven by antigen exposure. The T and B cells produced by this process are known as naïve or virgin cells because they have not yet encountered antigen.
- antigen-dependent differentiation occurs when a naïve T or B cell encounters and recognizes a foreign antigen. Binding of an antigen triggers the T or B cell to undergo a process called 'blast transformation' that includes a burst of proliferation to form a clone of cells specifically able to target the offending antigen. This process is an important component of the immune response to a foreign antigen. Antigen-dependent differentiation occurs in secondary lymphoid tissue such as the spleen, lymph nodes and mucosa-associated lymphoid tissue (MALT).

B lymphopoiesis

Antigen-independent B cell differentiation

During antigen-independent B cell differentiation, there are a series of important changes in the developing cells that prepare them for their role in immune surveillance. A central feature of the human immune system is that, for every conceivable foreign antigen, a B cell already exists that carries a specific surface receptor that can recognize it. This requires that there are hundreds of millions of different B cell receptor molecules available and, because each B cell only carries one type of receptor, that there are millions of distinct B cells circulating around the body.

As shown in *Figure 2.11*, the different stages of B cell differentiation include:

- precursor B cells that have undergone immunoglobulin gene rearrangement, but are not yet expressing immunoglobulin in their cytoplasm and carry no surface immunoglobulin receptor;
- immature B cells in which immunoglobulin heavy chains are expressed in the cytoplasm of the cell but not on the cell surface;
- naïve B cells, which represent the final stage of antigen-independent B cell differentiation. These cells carry two forms of immunoglobulin surface receptor: IgM and IgD, and are capable of recognizing and responding to, but have not yet been exposed to, foreign antigen.

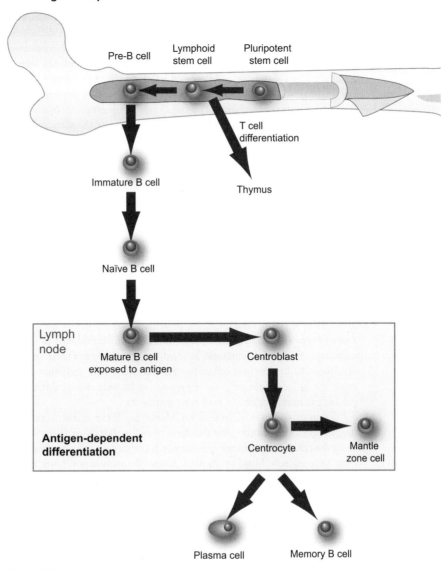

Figure 2.11
The stages of B cell differentiation.

Naïve B cells circulate in the bloodstream and are also found in relatively small numbers in primary lymphoid follicles and follicle mantle zones.

Antigen-dependent B cell differentiation

As the name suggests, antigen-dependent B cell differentiation represents a second wave of differentiation following encounter of a naïve B cell with foreign antigen, and is an important component of the immune response.

Following engagement of a B cell receptor with antigen, the cell proliferates to form a clone of lymphocytes that mature into plasma cells and which mount a specific antibody response to the inducing antigen. This stage of antigen-dependent B cell differentiation, sometimes known as the immunoblastic reaction, occurs in the paracortical region of lymph nodes, and leads to IgM-producing plasma cells accumulating in the medullary cords.

Within a few days of the immunoblastic reaction a second reaction, known as the germinal centre reaction, occurs. During this reaction, proliferating B cells differentiate into centroblasts and undergo a process called somatic hypermutation of the immunoglobulin genes, that increases the antigen affinity of the antibody that they will eventually secrete.

Centroblasts mature into centrocytes, which no longer proliferate. These cells interact with T cells in the germinal centres of lymph nodes and differentiate into high-affinity immunoglobulin-secreting plasma cells and memory B cells. Some B cells generated by the germinal centre reaction migrate outwards from the lymphoid follicle to populate the marginal and mantle zones of the lymphoid follicle. These post-germinal centre B cells are capable of rapid immune responses if re-challenged with their inducing antigen.

Some of the pre-plasma cells formed by the germinal centre reaction migrate from the lymph node to the bone marrow, where they mature into antibody-secreting plasma cells. A proportion of the pre-plasma cell population become resident in the lymph node and mature to form nodal plasma cells.

All of the B cell differentiation processes described for lymph nodes also occur in mucosa-associated lymphoid tissue (MALT), such as Waldeyer's ring, Peyer's patches, and mesenteric nodes. B cells and plasma cells formed in MALT circulate but return preferentially to their site of origin rather than to lymph nodes.

B cell markers

Throughout B cell development, the proteins expressed within the cell cytoplasm and on its surface membrane evolve and change. This fact can be exploited in the laboratory to identify each stage of B cell differentiation, by identifying the pattern of these 'cell markers' carried by the cell. These markers include cell surface receptors, enzymes, and other proteins in the cytoplasm or on the surface of the cell, whose presence or location change during differentiation and the presence of immunoglobulin gene rearrangements.

The most common technique for identifying these markers, immunophenotyping, uses 'tagged' monoclonal antibodies that bind to and enable visualization of the markers present in or on the cell. Immunophenotyping can be performed on cell suspensions or on biopsy material from bone marrow, blood or lymphoid tissue. The ways in which some of the most useful B cell markers change during differentiation is shown in *Figure 2.12*.

The earliest change that marks a precursor cell as belonging to the B cell lineage is the rearrangement of the μ immunoglobulin heavy chain genes located on chromosome 14q32. This is followed by rearrangements of the κ immunoglobulin light chain genes on chromosome 2p12, and the λ immunoglobulin light chain genes on chromosome 22q11. The defining feature of the pre-B cell is the appearance of μ immunoglobulin heavy chains in the cytoplasm of the cell. As the pre-B cell continues to differentiate, intact IgM and IgD immunoglobulin are expressed on the cell surface, which act as the B cell antigen receptor.

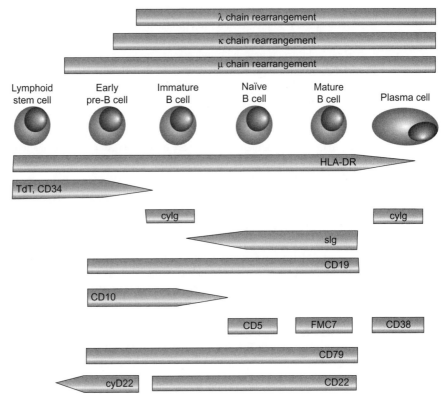

Figure 2.12
Changes in B cell markers during B cell differentiation (adapted from Rezuke *et al.* 1997).

A variety of cellular antigens are expressed in a predictable way as B cells differentiate. These are designated by CD (cluster of differentiation) numbers, e.g. CD10 as shown in *Figure 2.12*. The earliest antigens expressed in B cells are the nuclear enzyme terminal deoxynucleotidyltransferase (TdT), and the cell surface antigen HLA-Dr. Neither of these antigens is specific to B cells; they can also be found in other cell types. However, their presence is a useful indicator of the stage of differentiation. As the cell matures, antigens that are specific to B cells such as CD19, CD20, and CD10 are expressed. The terminally differentiated plasma cell can be recognized by the absence of the majority of B cell-associated antigens and the presence of the CD38 antigen.

T cell differentiation

Antigen-independent T cell differentiation
All T cells are derived from haemopoietic stem cells in the bone marrow. During fetal development, T lymphoid stem cells (CFU-L) populate the subcapsular region of the thymus gland where, under the influence of epithelial nurse cells they proliferate and differentiate. The progeny of these lymphoid stem cells progress through the cortical and medullary regions of the thymus and, from there, enter the circulation as mature T cells. During their journey, the T cells acquire surface receptors that are responsible for the specificity of their function.

In the process of differentiation into fully mature T cells, cortical T lymphoblasts progress through four distinct phases. The most primitive cortical T lymphoblasts express the intranuclear enzyme TdT and the surface marker CD7. The earliest events in the process of differentiation are the rearrangement of the T cell receptor genes in a manner analogous to immunoglobulin gene rearrangement in B cells, and the expression of the adhesive molecule CD2. These markers of differentiation are associated with large cortical thymocytes. The next stage of differentiation involves the acquisition and simultaneous expression of the accessory molecules CD4 and CD8. CD4 is responsible for recognition of MHC class II molecules while CD8 recognizes MHC class I molecules. These accessory molecules play an important role in the 'selection' of T cells within the thymus gland.

T cell selection is an important protective mechanism that helps to ensure that circulating T cells do not react against self-antigens. The vast majority of T cells produced in the thymus die in the process of maturation and are never released into the circulation. It is thought that all immature T cells are predestined to undergo apoptosis in the thymus unless they are specifically selected for 'rescue'. There are two stages in this selection process.

1. Positive selection occurs in the thymic cortex where the CD3+ CD4+ CD8+ thymocytes are exposed to MHC class I and II molecules on the surfaces of cortical epithelial cells. Any T cell that fails to recognize self-MHC molecules will undergo apoptosis. This step ensures that circulating T cells can only recognize foreign antigens expressed in association with self-MHC class I or II molecules on the surface of antigen-presenting cells.
2.. Negative selection occurs in the thymic medulla and involves T cells at the next stage of differentiation when they express either CD4 or CD8, never both. Here, they come into contact with antigen-presenting cells that carry processed host antigens in association with self-MHC molecules. Any T cell that recognizes and binds strongly to self-antigen undergoes apoptosis. This step ensures that circulating T cells do not recognize self-antigens expressed in association with self-MHC class I or II molecules on the surface of antigen-presenting cells.

Thymocytes that survive both positive and negative selection exit the thymus as naïve T cells and are characterized by expression of CD62L and absence of the activation markers CD25, CD44 and CD69. These cells circulate in the blood but are preferentially attracted to lymph nodes and other secondary lymphoid tissues, a process known as 'homing'.

Antigen-dependent T cell differentiation

Foreign antigen is recognized and processed by antigen-presenting cells such as dendritic cells, which then migrate to lymph nodes and other secondary lymphoid tissues where they present processed antigen to naïve T cells. If a naïve T cell binds strongly to a presented antigen, it undergoes a burst of proliferation to produce an expanded clone of cells capable of binding to the inducing antigen. These activated T cells undergo further differentiation and migrate to sites of inflammation where they help to direct various facets of the immune response.

NK cell differentiation

NK cells are derived from haemopoietic stem cells, but the stages involved in their differentiation are not well understood. They function to directly kill tumour cells and virus-infected cells. Precisely how NK cells recognize target cells is unclear, but recognition of an 'altered-self' state has been proposed.

NK cells do not respond to antigen in the same way as T and B cells. Instead, they carry a more primitive surface receptor that recognizes a component of all antibodies, which enables them to recognize and kill cells that have bound antibody. They also express receptors that recognize cells with low concentrations of MHC class I molecules. NK cells are activated by, and undergo proliferation in response to cytokines released during the immune response such as interferon.

SUGGESTED FURTHER READING

Bain, B.J. (2006) *Blood Cells: a Practical Guide.* Blackwell Publishing, Oxford.

Byrne, J.L. & Russel, N.H. (2005) Haemopoietic growth factors. In: *Postgraduate Haematology* (Hoffbrand, A.V., Catovsky, D. & Tuddenham, E.G.D., eds), pp. 303–317. Blackwell Publishing, Oxford.

Craig, F. & Foon, K. (2008) Flow cytometric immunophenotyping for hematologic neoplasms. *Blood,* **111**: 3941–3967.

Gordon, M. (2005) Stem cells and haemopoiesis. In: *Postgraduate Haematology* (Hoffbrand, A.V., Catovsky, D. & Tuddenham, E.G.D., eds), pp. 1–12. Blackwell Publishing, Oxford.

Higgs, D.R. & Wood, W.G. (2005) Erythropoiesis. In: *Postgraduate Haematology* (Hoffbrand, A.V., Catovsky, D. & Tuddenham, E.G.D., eds), pp. 13–25. Blackwell Publishing, Oxford.

Rezuke, W.N., *et al.* (1997) Molecular diagnosis of B- and T-cell lymphomas: fundamental principles and clinical applications. *Clin. Chem.* **43**: 1814–1823.

Wickrema, A. & Kee, B. (eds.) (2009) *Molecular Basis of Hematopoiesis.* Springer, New York.

Zon, L.I. (ed.) (2001) *Hematopoiesis – a Developmental Approach.* Oxford University Press, New York.

SELF-ASSESSMENT QUESTIONS

1. Where are the earliest recognizable blood cell precursors formed?
2. Name the three different embryonic haemoglobins and show their globin structure.
3. What is the functional difference between red and yellow marrow in adults? Where are these found?
4. Place the following in order of increasing maturity: promyelocyte; myelocyte; myeloblast; CFU-GEMM.
5. Why is chronic renal failure associated with anaemia?
6. Complete the following: post-natal antigen-independent differentiation in B cells occurs in the _____ _____, while for T cells it occurs primarily in the _____ _____.

Anaemia

Learning objectives
After studying this chapter you should confidently be able to:

■ **Define anaemia**
Anaemia is functionally defined as an insufficient red cell mass to adequately deliver sufficient oxygen to peripheral tissues to meet physiological needs. However, this is impractical to measure so, in practice, anaemia is frequently defined as a haemoglobin concentration ([Hb]), red blood cell count (RBC) or haematocrit (Hct) outside of the reference range.

■ **Explain the relationship between anaemia and the reference range for haemoglobin**
Defining anaemia simply as a blood parameter value outside of the reference range can be misleading in several ways (e.g. following acute blood loss, in pregnancy, following severe burns, in dehydration, with chronic hypoxia, in inherited haemoglobin disorders or due to postural changes). The astute haematologist needs to be aware of these situations to avoid misdiagnosis.

■ **Describe in outline the broad morphological classes of anaemia**
In morphological terms, anaemia can be described in terms of red cell size (as microcytic, normocytic or macrocytic) and in terms of colour intensity (as hypochromic or normochromic; the term hyperchromic is not used). Variation in red cell size, colour and shape are known as anisocytosis, polychromasia and poikilocytosis respectively. Many abnormal cell shapes have specific descriptive names, e.g. spherocyte, ovalocyte, sickle cell and target cell.

■ **Outline the pathophysiology of anaemia**
The basic problem in all anaemias is the inability to deliver sufficient oxygen to permit normal function. The most common presenting features are reduced exercise tolerance, shortness of breath after minimal exertion and palpitations. The severity of these symptoms is related to the severity of the anaemia, the speed with which anaemia developed and the presence of co-morbidity. Acute anaemia may be associated with obvious, acute symptoms such as shortness of breath, tachycardia, vertigo, orthostatic hypotension and a sensation of extreme fatigue. Conversely, very gradual onset of anaemia can permit gradual physiological compensation to offset the development of symptoms.

■ **Outline the mechanisms leading to microcytic, hypochromic anaemia and macrocytic, normochromic anaemia**
Red cell size is determined by the number of mitotic divisions during development. Broadly, cell size decreases with each mitotic division and maturation phase. Intracellular haemoglobin concentration increases with red cell maturity but synthesis stops when a critical intranuclear concentration is reached. Macrocytic anaemias result when nuclear maturation is retarded, leading to fewer cell divisions before maturity. Conversely, microcytic, hypochromic anaemias arise when haemoglobin synthesis is retarded, allowing more cell divisions before maturity.

3.1 DEFINING ANAEMIA

The definition of anaemia is not as simple as it might at first appear. Anaemia is functionally defined as an insufficient red cell mass to adequately deliver sufficient oxygen to peripheral tissues to meet physiological needs. However, this is impractical to measure so, in practice, anaemia is frequently defined as a haemoglobin concentration ([Hb]), red cell count (RBC) or haematocrit (Hct) outside of the reference range (see *Box 3.1*). For the most part, this definition serves as a useful screening tool to identify people with anaemia, but there are many circumstances in which a single measurement of Hb, RBC or Hct can be misleading. The astute haematologist must be aware of these circumstances to avoid misinterpretation and hence missed diagnosis.

Box 3.1 Reference values

Subject	Hb (g/dl)	RBC (x 10^{12}/l)	Hct (l/l)
Neonate	13.5–19.5	3.9–5.3	0.42–0.60
Infant	9.5–13.5	3.1–4.5	0.29–0.41
Adolescent	11.5–14.5	4.0–5.2	0.35–0.45
Adult male	13.3–17.7	4.4–5.9	0.37–0.49
Adult female*	11.7–15.7	3.8–5.2	0.36–0.46

*Values are for females of child-bearing age

[Hb] and acute blood loss

Acute blood loss is a common reason for requesting a full blood count, and this provides an excellent example of the need for careful interpretation of isolated haemoglobin measurements. The immediate response to significant acute blood loss is vasoconstriction, so an early haemoglobin measurement may be normal. After about six hours, there is a shift of tissue fluid into the bloodstream to restore the total blood volume, so a haemoglobin measurement will be reduced due to the dilution effect. A reticulocyte response will be seen in healthy individuals after 24–48 hours and the red cell count and haemoglobin level will be restored gradually. So which of these haemoglobin values is 'correct' and can be used to determine the presence and severity of anaemia?

In reality, determination of anaemia in the presence of acute blood loss should be based on symptoms and signs of decreased tissue oxygen supply, because none of the haemoglobin values on their own will truly reflect the clinical state of the patient. In an otherwise healthy individual, acute blood loss of up to 20% of their total blood volume can be compensated for without significant reduction in tissue oxygen delivery. The body possesses several compensatory mechanisms, including shifting the haemoglobin oxygen dissociation curve (see *Chapter 6*) to increase oxygen delivery, increased synthesis of intracellular 2,3-DPG (see *Chapter 8*), decreasing vascular resistance and increasing cardiac rate and stroke volume. In practice, the maintenance of circulatory pressure through rapid restoration of blood volume with colloid solutions is more important than the correction of haemoglobin concentration. In patients with co-morbidity such as cardiopulmonary disease, hypertension or a history of heavy smoking, physiological compensation may be impaired and blood transfusion may be appropriate.

In summary, diagnosis of anaemia must be made only after considering the blood count, other haematological signs of anaemia (see later in this chapter) and the clinical picture. An isolated haemoglobin measurement can be seriously misleading.

[Hb] and pregnancy

Anaemia is common in pregnancy and can be caused by the excess nutritional demands (mainly iron and folate) placed on the mother by the growing fetus. However, there are significant changes in plasma volume and red cell mass in pregnancy; typically, the red cell mass of a pregnant woman increases, primarily to serve the increased need for oxygen of the fetus. Plasma volume also increases, particularly in the third trimester. The increase in plasma volume is usually greater than the increase in red cell mass. The dilution effect that results causes an apparent reduction in [Hb], RBC and Hct, but does not reflect a true anaemia.

This haemodilution may also be physiologically desirable because it reduces the amount of iron lost by haemorrhage at delivery and also enhances the ease of perfusion of the placenta, thus improving oxygen delivery to the fetus.

[Hb] and severe burns

Severe and extensive burns are associated with loss of plasma through the injured skin, which can spuriously increase the measured [Hb], RBC and Hct, even in the presence of a normal red cell mass. If anaemia is present, it can be masked by this effect. In addition, red cells are highly susceptible to thermal injury and a degree of haemolysis is usually present in severe, extensive burns cases.

[Hb] and dehydration

Dehydration due, for example, to protracted and severe diarrhoea and vomiting, or prolonged sweating, can cause spuriously high [Hb], RBC and Hct and may mask the presence of anaemia. This effect is more likely in infants.

[Hb] and hypoxia

The physiological response to chronic hypoxia caused by living at altitude or by cardiopulmonary disease is to increase the red cell count to meet oxygen demands. In these circumstances, a normal [Hb] might actually represent anaemia. Consideration of the complete clinical picture is required in such cases.

[Hb] and thalassaemia

Thalassaemia is an inherited condition in which there is impaired synthesis of one globin chain (see *Chapter 6*). Patients with thalassaemia frequently present with a low [Hb] and a high RBC. Because of physiological compensation, thalassaemia patients may have mild–moderate reduction in [Hb] without having true anaemia. Conversely, the presence of anaemia may be missed because of the expectation of a low [Hb].

[Hb] and structural haemoglobinopathy

Some abnormal haemoglobin variants have an altered oxygen affinity, and this can be associated with physiologically appropriate changes in [Hb]. For example, Hb Yakima has an increased oxygen affinity and so presents as a raised [Hb]. In these patients, a normal [Hb] might reflect anaemia. Conversely, Hb Kansas has a decreased oxygen affinity and so a lower than normal [Hb]. In this case, the reduced [Hb] does not represent anaemia because oxygen delivery to the tissues is increased.

[Hb] and posture

When normal individuals lie down, the Hct falls by 5–10% within an hour or so due to shifts in plasma volume from the lower limbs. When the individual stands up, their previous Hct is restored within about 15 minutes. Obviously, neither of these changes reflects anaemia.

[Hb] and the reference range

The interpretation of any clinical laboratory test (e.g. [Hb]) involves comparing the patient results with the appropriate reference range. The reference range is defined as the mean ± 2 standard deviations, assuming a Gaussian distribution of values in the relevant population (see *Figure 3.1*). This definition means that 95% of the defined population in whom the reference range was determined (e.g. adult males) will have a test result that falls within the reference range. Conversely, this means that 5% of the population will have test results that fall outside of the range, but do not represent 'abnormal' results! Accordingly, a haemoglobin value that falls below the reference range does not automatically define anaemia, even if none of the confounding factors described above is present. However, such results should be investigated further to exclude the presence of anaemia. Similarly, a haemoglobin value that falls within the reference range is not a guarantee that anaemia is absent.

This explains why the term 'reference range' is preferred over the term 'normal range'.

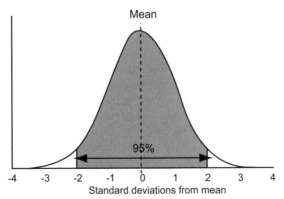

Figure 3.1
Derivation of a reference range.

Anaemia as a clinical disorder

Anaemia is probably the most commonly encountered of all clinical disorders globally. Strictly, anaemia is a sign of a disorder rather than a disorder in its own right, since anaemia is invariably secondary to some underlying cause. Whatever the cause, there are a variety of signs and symptoms that are associated with anaemia, their severity depending both on the specific cause and on the severity of the disorder (see *Box 3.2*).

The basic problem in all anaemias is the inability to deliver sufficient oxygen to permit normal function. The most common presenting features of the anaemic patient are reduced exercise tolerance, shortness of breath after minimal exertion, and palpitations. The severity of these

---

Box 3.2 Symptoms and signs

In a medical sense, signs and symptoms of disease have distinct meanings. A symptom is a manifestation of disease recognized and reported by the patient, e.g. lack of energy or pain. A sign is a manifestation recognized by an examining doctor, e.g. pallor of nail beds is a sign of anaemia.

---

symptoms is related to the severity of the anaemia, the speed with which anaemia developed and the presence of co-morbidity. Acute anaemia may be associated with obvious acute symptoms such as shortness of breath, tachycardia, vertigo, orthostatic hypotension and a sensation of extreme fatigue. Conversely, very gradual onset of anaemia can permit gradual physiological compensation to offset the development of symptoms. Severe anaemia can occasionally be found in patients who are unaware of their condition because of physiological compensation. The presence of co-morbidity can modulate the severity of anaemia symptoms. For example, patients with cardiopulmonary disease typically have a much lower tolerance of anaemia.

Symptoms of anaemia include:

- Cardiopulmonary symptoms such as dyspnoea, palpitations, tachycardia, vertigo, systolic murmur and orthostatic hypotension. These symptoms may be present at rest in severe anaemia, acute onset of anaemia or in the presence of cardiopulmonary co-morbidity. In chronic anaemia of slow onset these symptoms may be minimal.
- Pallor is a sign of anaemia but can be ambiguous. For example, some people naturally have a pale complexion that can obscure anaemia-related pallor. Anaemia can cause faints, but fainting is accompanied by pallor even in the absence of anaemia. Hypothyroidism is associated with pallor and symptoms of lethargy even in the absence of anaemia. On the other hand, pallor can be masked by skin pigmentation, jaundice or cyanosis. The last two of these signs may be indicative of certain types of anaemia. The most reliable way to determine the presence of pallor is to ignore the skin colour and to examine the mucous membranes, conjunctivae, nail beds and palmar creases.
- Jaundice can be indicative of certain types of anaemia, provided the more obvious cause of hepatobiliary disease is excluded. Haemoglobin released from destruction of red cells is metabolized to bilirubin (a yellow pigment), so accelerated red cell destruction may be accompanied by jaundice. Classically, one of the signs of pernicious anaemia is said to be a distinct, lemon-yellow tinge to the complexion, caused by the combination of pallor due to anaemia and an increased level of circulating unconjugated bilirubin.
- Other changes that might indicate anaemia include thinning of the skin, premature greying of the hair (pernicious anaemia), nail changes such as easy breaking and concavity (koilonychia), inflammation of the tongue with depapillation (glossitis), fissures at the edges of the mouth (angular stomatitis), and the development of chronic lower leg ulcers.
- In severe anaemia, neuromuscular changes can include headache, excessive sleepiness, restlessness, peripheral neuropathy and paraesthesia (particularly in vitamin B_{12} deficiency).
- Retinal haemorrhage and visual loss.
- Gastrointestinal symptoms frequently accompany anaemia, some of these contribute to the development of the anaemia and some are caused or exacerbated by the anaemia itself. Chronic bleeding from a hiatus hernia, duodenal or gastric ulcer, or from a gastric or colonic tumour, is a relatively common cause of anaemia. Ulceration, infection and inflammation of the oral cavity may be seen in bone marrow failure states or haematological malignancy. Difficulty in swallowing with choking and aspiration may be associated with iron deficiency (Plummer–Vinson syndrome or Paterson–Brown-Kelly syndrome), although the significance of the association has been questioned.

3.2 MECHANISMS OF ANAEMIA

There are a great many causes of anaemia and, in individual cases, there may be many contributory factors. For example, a patient with chronic haemolysis may develop a deficiency of folic acid and, if they have haemorrhoids, they may also be deficient in iron. Any discussion of the broad causes of anaemia must be simplistic and so should be interpreted intelligently.

Figure 3.2 illustrates the processes involved in the regulation of erythropoiesis and provides a useful way of thinking about the different ways in which anaemia can develop:

- ■ if the bone marrow is appropriately stimulated with erythropoietin, the outcome *should* be more RBC (A)
- ■ if there are more RBCs, the outcome *should* be an increased circulating haemoglobin level (B)
- ■ if there is more haemoglobin, the outcome *should* be enhanced oxygen transport and delivery (C)
- ■ the synthesis of erythropoietin is regulated by tissue oxygen tension; hypoxia *should* stimulate erythropoietin synthesis (D).

Each of these processes can go wrong and lead to the development of anaemia. These mechanisms of anaemia are outlined briefly below and then in detail in the following chapters.

Process A. This is dependent on an adequate supply of the raw materials needed to make red cells. Problems arise when there is a shortage of stem cells, as in bone marrow failure or myelofibrosis, when the number of normal stem cells is reduced by the presence of a malignant clone or where nutrients required for replication, e.g. vitamin B_{12} or folic acid, are deficient.

Process B. This requires an appropriate rate of haemoglobin synthesis and normal survival of the released red cells. A reduced rate of globin synthesis is the hallmark of the thalassaemias. Abnormalities of haem synthesis are present in the porphyrias and in deficiency of iron, vitamin B_6 deficiency or copper. Loss of red cells due to bleeding is a common cause of failure at this stage. Finally, a reduction in the lifespan of red cells due to intrinsic or extrinsic defects can cause failure of the haemoglobin concentration to rise, despite adequate red cell production. Among the intrinsic abnormalities that lead to shortened red cell survival are inherited abnormalities of membrane structure, haemoglobin structure and metabolism. Extrinsic abnormalities include

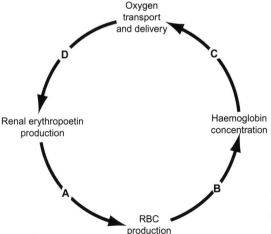

Figure 3.2
The processes involved in regulation of erythropoiesis (see text for explanation).

infection or infestation, e.g. malaria or microbial toxins, immune mechanisms, disseminated intravascular coagulation, physical causes including extremes of heat or cold, mechanical causes such as march haemoglobinuria, or turbulence associated with early prosthetic heart valves and chemical causes such as heavy metal poisoning.

Process C. This can be disrupted by the presence of an abnormal haemoglobin with altered oxygen affinity. Haemoglobin with an increased affinity will be reluctant to part with oxygen on reaching the tissues, leading to reduced oxygen delivery and tissue hypoxia. The response to this is polycythaemia (increased RBC and [Hb] rather than anaemia). A similar response occurs with reduced atmospheric oxygen tension (see *Box 3.3*) and during cardiopulmonary disease (see *Box 3.4*). Conversely, haemoglobin with a reduced oxygen affinity reduces the drive for erythropoietin production and leads to a reduced [Hb] with adequate oxygen delivery.

Process D. This requires an ability to respond to hypoxia with an increase in erythropoietin synthesis. Patients with renal impairment cannot synthesize sufficient erythropoietin, resulting in chronic anaemia. Conversely, increased synthesis of erythropoietin is found in some rare malignant conditions, resulting in polycythaemia. The erythropoietin produced acts on erythroid stem cells in the bone marrow, completing the cycle.

Box 3.3 Erythropoiesis and sport

Elite athletes, particularly cyclists and long distance runners, can exploit the physiological response to low oxygen tension by training at altitude. The erythropoietic response that ensues temporarily enhances the ability to transport oxygen to muscles. If the training is conducted sufficiently close to an event, the enhanced oxygen delivery potential and enhanced performance will be retained until after the event. Injecting synthetic erythropoietin can induce a similar effect, although this practice is banned. The downside is, of course, that blood viscosity is increased, and this leads to a need for increased cardiac work. The short-term consequences of this increased cardiac work in a young, elite athlete are probably negligible, but whether the risks are worthwhile is open to debate.

Box 3.4 Cardiopulmonary function and [Hb]

Haemoglobin oxygenation is critically dependent on adequate cardiopulmonary function. If the heart does not pump blood efficiently, oxygen delivery to the tissues is impaired. Similarly, if blood is not adequately oxygenated in the lungs, oxygen delivery to the tissues is reduced. In both cases, tissue hypoxia will stimulate a compensatory erythropoiesis, leading to a rise in [Hb]. However, erythrocytosis can lead to an increase in blood viscosity, which can further impair the capacity of the heart to pump blood efficiently around the body, thereby creating a vicious cycle. This topic is discussed in *Chapter 14*.

3.3 DESCRIBING RED CELLS

Understanding the terms used to describe the morphology of red cells is fundamental to any study of anaemia, since anaemias are often described in terms of the morphological appearance of the red cells. There are three basic morphological characteristics of red cells: size, colour and shape. Of these, size is the simplest. Red cells may be normal in size (**normocytic**), larger than normal (**macrocytic**) or smaller than normal (**microcytic**). Occasionally there may be variation in cell size, which is known as **anisocytosis**. Finally, it may sometimes, for example during haematinic therapy, appear that there is more than one population of red cells present, based on their size (and often on their colour too). This is known as a **dimorphic blood picture**.

The colour of red cells can similarly be described, in that normal coloured cells (those that contain a normal concentration of haemoglobin) are described as being **normochromic** and cells that lack normal colour, i.e. where the normal area of central pallor is too large due to a lack of haemoglobin, are described as being **hypochromic**. As the normal red cell has an area of central pallor, it might be thought that there would be an equivalent term where there is too much colour, i.e. where there is no area of central pallor. Such a situation does occur, but it is not because the cell has too much haemoglobin, rather it is due to a change of shape from the normal biconcave shape into a more spheroidal shape. Thus the term hyperchromia is not used. The final colour descriptor is **polychromasia**. This term is used when some of the red cells display a bluish colouration. This results from the presence of acidic material (RNA) and indicates the presence of slightly immature red cells known as reticulocytes. Thus polychromasia is an indication of higher than normal red cell production, and may occur, for example, in a haemolytic state or when a patient is responding to haematinic therapy.

The greatest range of descriptors is concerned with red cell shape. A few are self-explanatory, for example:

- **spherocytic** means the cells are spheroidal rather than biconcave discs
- **ovalocytic** or **elliptocytic** means that the cells are oval rather than round
- **sickle cells** (**drepanocytes**) means the cells are the shape of a crescent moon, as found in sickle cell disease
- **target cells** means that the cells have the appearance of targets due to a bulge in the middle of the biconcavity producing a pink centre in the normal area of central pallor

Many terms are, however, less simple. Just as anisocytosis describes variation in cell colour, so **poikilocytosis** is the term used to describe variation in cell shape. The variation of shape that may be exhibited in different red cell disorders is quite wide. Many have specific descriptors, for example:

- **leptocytes** are unusually thin cells, similar to target cells
- **schistocytes** are red cell fragments, often seen in haemolytic anaemias
- **dacrocytes** are tear-drop shaped cells, seen in several different states, including myelofibrosis
- '**bite cells**' look as though they have had a bite taken out of them, and are seen in some haemolytic states
- **stomatocytes** are cells with a central slit of pallor
- **pencil cells/cigar cells** are, unsurprisingly, pencil or cigar shaped
- **acanthocytes** or **spur cells** display a few (2–20) spicules, whereas cells that display rather more spicules are known as **echinocytes** or **burr cells**. The former are associated with, for example, liver disease, whereas the latter are associated with, for example, burns.

Red cells may not always appear as separate entities on film examination. Two possible appearances are rouleaux and agglutination. **Rouleaux** is where the cells associate to give an appearance that has been likened to stacks of coins that have been knocked over. This phenomenon is usually associated with multiple myeloma. **Agglutination** may be seen in an immune disorder, where antibodies are causing the red cells to adhere to one another in irregular clumps.

In various states it is possible for RBCs to display inclusion bodies. **Howell Jolly bodies** are nuclear remnants and are found in, for example, post-splenectomy patients. **Heinz bodies** are precipitated aggregates of denatured, oxidized globin adhering to the cytoskeleton of the red cell and are found in some haemoglobinopathies, or in conditions where the haemoglobin is subjected to oxidative damage such as in abnormalities of red cell metabolism. **Malarial parasites** are very important causes of red cell destruction in tropical parts of the world, and can be seen within red cells in affected patients. **Punctate basophilia** (or **basophilic stippling**) is the term given to the presence of fine blue dots within the cytoplasm of red cells. It is usually caused by mitochondrial poisoning by, for example, heavy metals. **Pappenheimer bodies** and **siderotic granules** are discrete iron-containing particles found within the red cell cytoplasm in various anaemias, especially those where iron utilization is impaired, for example, sideroblastic anaemia. **Cabot rings** are unusual cytoplasmic inclusions, red–violet in colour, and in the shape of a ring or a figure eight. They are sometimes found in megaloblastic anaemias and other cases of dyserythropoiesis, and are thought to be remnants of microtubules.

Finally, it must be remembered that all of the above are dependent on the observed morphology being genuine rather than artefactual. A well-made film from fresh blood is essential for accurate morphological descriptions, since technique, age of sample and anticoagulants can all cause various artefacts that can mimic several of the above abnormalities of morphology.

Anaemia and red cell morphology

There are many examples where the morphology of red cells is associated with specific causes of anaemia. One example of this is that microcytosis and hypochromia are associated with iron deficiency, but this morphology is not diagnostic because there are several other, less common causes. Instead, recognition of microcytic, hypochromic anaemia should trigger secondary investigations of iron status to confirm the correct diagnosis.

Similarly, macrocytic anaemia is most closely associated with deficiency of folic acid and/or vitamin B_{12}, but there are many other causes of macrocytosis. *Figure 3.3* presents a schematic

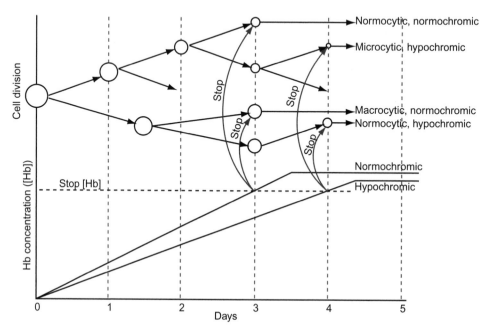

Figure 3.3
A conceptual depiction of the interaction between red cell development and morphology.

explanation of why iron deficiency is associated with microcytosis and vitamin B_{12} deficiency is associated with macrocytosis.

Figure 3.3 shows two interacting effects. The effect of the number of mitotic divisions during development on cell size is illustrated at the top of the figure. Broadly, cell size decreases with each mitotic division and maturation phase. Therefore, if developing red cells undergo fewer divisions, the result will be larger (macrocytic) cells released into the circulation. Conversely, an increase in the number of divisions will result in smaller (microcytic) cells. The lower part of the figure illustrates the effect of the rate of haemoglobin synthesis. In general, intracellular haemoglobin concentration increases with red cell maturity. Haemoglobin is present in the nucleus of the cell as well as the cytoplasm. When it reaches a critical nuclear concentration, haemoglobin reacts with nuclear histones, triggering chromosomal inactivation and signalling the end of cell division. The nucleus is extruded soon thereafter, producing a mature red cell. From this point, no more RNA can be produced and that which already exists has a limited lifespan, thus limiting the period over which more globin, and hence haemoglobin synthesis can occur. This time period is independent of the rate of haemoglobin synthesis. This means that, if the rate of haemoglobin synthesis is reduced, the final concentration within the mature red cell will be lower than normal. The red cell thus produced will be hypochromic. In addition, retardation of haemoglobin synthesis increases the time taken to reach the critical 'stop' haemoglobin concentration, allowing a greater number of mitotic cycles to have taken place. The resultant mature red cells will be both microcytic and hypochromic. This effect occurs irrespective of the cause of the retarded haemoglobin synthesis, so iron deficiency, thalassaemia and vitamin B_6 deficiency all result in microcytic hypochromic cells.

An adequate supply of vitamin B_{12} and folate co-enzymes is essential for optimal DNA and RNA synthesis. The most significant effect of a deficiency of either of these vitamins is to retard DNA synthesis. The result is that fewer cell divisions have occurred by the time that the critical 'stop' haemoglobin concentration is reached. This explains the macrocytic anaemia that is the hallmark of vitamin B_{12} and folate deficiency. Because RNA synthesis is slowed to a lesser extent, the macrocytic red cells are fully 'haemoglobinized', and so are normochromic.

Finally, a co-deficiency of iron and either vitamin B_{12} or folate can sometimes 'fool' automated cell counters to report a normal MCV, when the true picture is of a twin population of microcytes and macrocytes. Modern cell counters typically recognize this situation and will flag marked anisocytosis. Examination of a blood film will reveal the cause of the anomaly in these cases.

3.4 APPROACH TO ANAEMIA DIAGNOSIS

Accurate diagnosis of anaemia requires a consideration of the full clinical picture as well as knowledge of the mechanisms and markers of the different forms of anaemia. *Figure 3.4* illustrates a simplified flow chart showing one approach to the early stage of differentiating the causes of anaemia. *Chapters 4–8* explore the different forms of anaemia in detail and provide the knowledge required to direct more advanced diagnostic investigations.

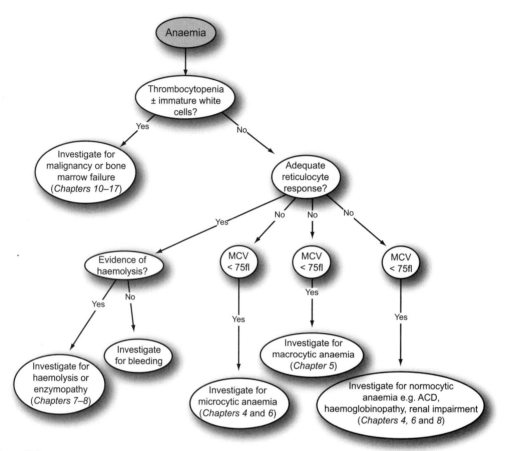

Figure 3.4
A simplified approach to the characterization of the anaemias.

SUGGESTED FURTHER READING

ASH Image Bank at http://ashimagebank.hematologylibrary.org/.
Bain, B.J. (2006) *Blood Cells: a Practical Guide.* Blackwell Publishing, Oxford.
Uthman, E. (1998) *Understanding Anemia.* University Press of Mississippi, Jackson.

SELF-ASSESSMENT QUESTIONS

1. Why can a single haemoglobin measurement in the last trimester of pregnancy be a poor indicator of anaemia?
2. What proportion of a population will have an [Hb] outside of the reference range for that population?
3. Which of the following are common features of acute, severe anaemia?
   - Fatigue
   - Hypertension
   - Tachycardia

- Bradycardia
- Vertigo
4. Name the hormone responsible for stimulation of red cell production.
5. What word can be used to describe variation in red cell size on a blood film?
6. What word can be used to describe variation in red cell shape on a blood film?
7. What word can be used to describe the variation in red cell colour seen in reticulocytosis?
8. Is thalassaemia a microcytic or a macrocytic anaemia?
9. Why is folate deficiency associated with macrocytosis?

Disorders of iron metabolism

Learning objectives
After studying this chapter you should confidently be able to:

■ **Describe the importance of iron for optimal blood cell production and physiological function**
Iron plays a vital role in the normal function and metabolism of virtually every cell of the body. Iron-containing compounds include the haem-containing compounds haemoglobin, myoglobin and the cytochromes, and the non-haem iron compounds nicotinamide adenine dinucleotide dehydrogenase (NADH) and succinic dehydrogenase.

■ **Review the control mechanisms that govern iron absorption**
Inorganic iron uptake is regulated by altering the expression of DMT-1: in iron deficiency, synthesis of DMT-1 is up-regulated and iron uptake from the gut is increased. Conversely, iron overload down-regulates DMT-1 expression. This represents the first level of control over iron absorption. The export of iron from the enterocyte into the portal plasma is regulated by ferroportin, which is in turn regulated by hepcidin. Binding of hepcidin to ferroportin triggers internalization and degradation of ferroportin and so leads to reduced export of intracellular iron. Hepcidin synthesis is down-regulated by hypoxia, iron deficiency and ineffective erythropoiesis, leading to increased iron export from the enterocyte. This represents the second layer of control of iron absorption.

■ **Differentiate between iron deficiency, thalassaemia and anaemia of chronic disorders**
Iron deficiency presents as a microcytic, hypochromic anaemia with the combination of a raised total iron binding capacity (TIBC) and reduced transferrin saturation. Differentiation between iron deficiency and other, superficially similar microcytic anaemias relies on laboratory assessment of iron status, coupled with clinical features.

■ **Outline the classification of the sideroblastic anaemias**
The sideroblastic anaemias are a heterogeneous group of disorders characterized by disordered incorporation of iron into haem within developing erythroblasts. They are classified according to their aetiology as hereditary/congenital, acquired clonal, and acquired secondary (reversible) types.

■ **Differentiate clearly the iron overload states**
Hereditary haemochromatosis results from mutations of genes that regulate iron absorption, release and transport. Type 1 haemochromatosis results from mutation in the *HFE* gene. Type 2 haemochromatosis is caused by mutations in the haemojuvelin gene (type 2a) or the hepcidin gene (type 2b). Type 3 haemochromatosis is caused by mutation in the *TfR-2* gene. Type 4 haemochromatosis is caused by mutation in the ferroportin gene. Haemosiderosis results from chronic transfusion regimes.

Adequate nutrition is an essential requirement for the maintenance of normal bodily function, growth and repair. The nutritional requirements for optimal blood cell production are similar to those of the other cells of the body. Because of this, nutritional deficiencies seldom cause problems that are restricted to the blood. However, because of the rapid turnover of blood components, the blood is frequently a good early indicator of such deficiencies.

4.1 IRON

Iron plays a vital role in the normal function and metabolism of virtually every cell of the body. An adequate daily dietary intake of iron is essential for optimal health.

The role of iron within the body

Iron-containing compounds can be divided into two groups according to their role within the body: those that play a role in cellular metabolism and those that are required for iron transport and storage. Most of the iron-containing compounds that play a role in cellular metabolism contain iron in the form of a haem group. The haem-containing compounds include haemoglobin and myoglobin, the oxygen-carrying pigments of red cells and muscle respectively, and the cytochromes which are a family of electron-transport enzymes that play a variety of roles in oxidative metabolism. Non-haem iron compounds such as the enzymes nicotinamide adenine dinucleotide dehydrogenase (NADH) and succinic dehydrogenase are also important in cellular metabolism. The substances required for iron transport and storage are described in detail in this chapter.

Body iron distribution

A normal 70 kg male has a total body iron content of about 4 g. Almost three-quarters of this is found in the form of haemoglobin and myoglobin, while most of the remainder is held in reserve in the body stores (*Figure 4.1*). The tiny proportion of total body iron that is found in the cytochromes belies their pivotal role in oxidative metabolism within the body.

Daily iron requirements

Iron has been described as a 'one-way element' within the body. This means that iron is absorbed from the diet but that no substantial mechanism for iron excretion exists (see also *Box 4.1*). On the contrary, the body possesses elaborate mechanisms to prevent loss of iron. In the normal steady state, daily iron requirements consist of the amount required to replace the small amount lost in sweat, tears, urine and faeces plus the amount required for growth (*Figure 4.2*).

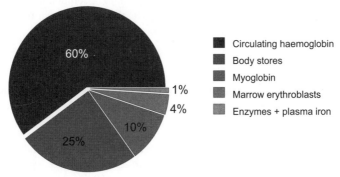

Figure 4.1
Body iron distribution.

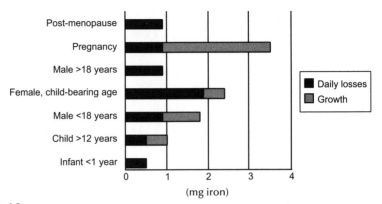

Figure 4.2
Daily iron requirements.

Box 4.1 Vitamins

One of the most important sources of vitamins and minerals in the average, highly-processed Western diet is breakfast cereals which are fortified with these nutrients during manufacture. An average (30 g) serving of a well known brand of cornflakes contains almost one-third of the recommended daily intake for an adult of iron and vitamins B_1, B_2, B_6, B_{12} and C.

The excess requirement in females of child-bearing age is due to the monthly blood loss, which contains up to 30 mg of iron in total. The very high iron requirement in pregnancy consists of three components: the growth requirement of the fetus and placenta, the expansion in maternal blood volume, and haemorrhage at delivery, although this last loss is mitigated to some extent by the physiological haemodilution that occurs towards the end of pregnancy. The figure quoted is a representative average value over the duration of pregnancy; the actual daily requirements vary according to the stage of pregnancy.

Iron absorption

Because iron deficiency and iron overload are both associated with morbidity, the body must strictly regulate body iron (see also *Box 4.2*). There is no mechanism for excretion of excess iron from the body. Indeed, there are several mechanisms designed to prevent significant loss of iron. Instead, the body regulates iron by closely controlling absorption from the diet according to current iron stores: when the body is iron replete, absorption is down-regulated and conversely iron deficiency triggers enhanced absorption.

Box 4.2 Minerals

Copper is widely distributed in food and the daily requirement of 2 mg is readily met by the average Western diet. Deficiency of copper impairs iron metabolism and leads to a lack of usable iron in the blood and so is manifest as a microcytic, hypochromic anaemia.

Cobalt is required by micro-organisms for the synthesis of vitamin B_{12}. Cobalt deficiency does not appear to cause impairment of health in man but is associated with neurological problems in ruminant farm animals.

Small amounts of zinc are present in both red cells and plasma but its role remains obscure. Zinc deficiency is not associated with the development of anaemia but may predispose to microbial infection.

Dietary sources of iron

A normal, mixed daily diet in the UK contains about 18 mg of iron, far in excess of normal body requirements (see also *Box 4.3*). The main dietary sources are liver, red meat, some green vegetables such as spinach, cereals (which are supplemented with iron during processing), and fish. Dietary iron falls into one of two categories: inorganic iron which is mainly present in cereals and vegetables, and haem iron which is found in the haemoglobin and myoglobin of meat products.

Box 4.3 Spinach and iron – part 1

Spinach is commonly regarded as an extremely rich source of iron. In fact, a 100 g serving of boiled spinach contains around 3 mg of iron (around twice as much as most green vegetables). However, spinach is also rich in oxalate, which markedly reduces the bioavailability of the iron. It really is doubtful then, whether spinach deserves its reputation as a rich source of iron.

The myth about spinach and its high iron content may be traceable to a Dr E. von Wolf who published his analysis of the iron content of spinach in 1870. Unfortunately, he misplaced the decimal point, leading to publication of an iron content that was ten times too high. The mistake was not corrected until 1937 and, by then, the belief that spinach was an especially good source of iron was unshakeable.

Site of iron absorption

Inorganic (non-haem) iron in food is released by the combined action of proteolytic enzymes and hydrochloric acid in the stomach. The low pH environment of the stomach encourages the reduction of Fe^{3+} ions to Fe^{2+} ions, which are absorbed more readily. Iron is absorbed maximally from the duodenum and upper jejunum. Absorption of inorganic iron is enhanced by any factor that increases its solubility. For example, Fe^{2+} compounds are generally more soluble than their Fe^{3+} counterparts, so the presence of reducing agents such as ascorbic acid (vitamin C) improves absorption. Conversely, alkaline pancreatic secretions, phosphates and phytates decrease solubility and strongly retard inorganic iron absorption.

The iron in animal products (haem iron) is absorbed, probably via a specific receptor on duodenal enterocytes called HCP-1. The luminal factors described above have little influence on the absorption of haem iron. Haem groups are absorbed intact by the intestinal mucosal cell, and subsequently broken down for release into the portal bloodstream.

Control of iron absorption

The regulation of iron homeostasis is complex and the mechanisms involved have only begun to be unravelled in the last few years. To effectively regulate iron homeostasis, mechanisms are required that:

- sense the changing demand for iron
- finely regulate the amount of iron absorbed from the diet
- regulate the trafficking of iron between the duodenum, the body stores and the tissues.

In essence, there are two major mechanisms that govern iron homeostasis, as follows.

- The concentration of iron regulates the synthesis of several proteins involved in iron storage and transport, including the iron storage protein ferritin, the iron transporter transferrin, and the transferrin receptor. For example, synthesis of transferrin receptor is increased by iron deficiency and reduced in the presence of excess iron.
- Several other proteins, including hepcidin, ferroportin and DMT-1 interact to regulate the transport of iron into and out of cells where it is absorbed and stored.

Inorganic iron (Fe^{2+}) in the gut binds to the divalent metal ion transporter DMT-1, which is expressed on the apical surface of duodenal enterocytes. DMT-1 is a transporter protein that is responsible for internalization of iron into the enterocyte. This transporter can only bind Fe^{2+} ions; the Fe^{3+} in food must be converted to Fe^{2+} by a membrane ferrireductase called DcytB before it can be absorbed. The expression of DMT-1 appears to be altered in response to changing iron stores: in iron deficiency, synthesis of DMT-1 is up-regulated and iron uptake from the gut is increased. Conversely, iron overload down-regulates DMT-1 expression. Regulation of intestinal uptake of iron represents the first level of control over body iron absorption.

The export of iron from the enterocyte into the portal plasma is regulated by another transmembrane protein, ferroportin. The concentration of ferroportin on the enterocyte membrane is regulated by hepcidin, an antimicrobial peptide synthesized in the liver. Binding of hepcidin to ferroportin triggers internalization and degradation of ferroportin and so leads to reduced export of intracellular iron from the enterocyte into the portal circulation. Hepcidin synthesis is, in turn, down-regulated by hypoxia, iron deficiency and ineffective erythropoiesis. Down-regulation of hepcidin in these circumstances leads to a physiologically appropriate response, increased iron export from the enterocyte (see also *Box 4.4*). This represents the second, and more important, layer of control of iron absorption.

Hepcidin expression is regulated by three proteins: HFE, haemojuvelin and transferrin-receptor-2.

- HFE is a regulator of the uptake of transferrin-bound iron from plasma. Classical haemochromatosis, an autosomal recessive iron overload disorder, is most often caused by mutation in the *HFE* gene.
- Haemojuvelin is a transmembrane co-receptor of bone morphogenetic protein (BMP). Mutations of the haemojuvelin gene are the most common cause of juvenile (type 2) haemochromatosis and a minority of cases of classical haemochromatosis.
- Transferrin-receptor-2 acts as a sensor of transferrin saturation: low saturation stimulates hepcidin synthesis. Mutations of the *TfR-2* gene are responsible for type 3 haemochromatosis.

Hepcidin synthesis is also increased in inflammatory states in response to interleukin-6 stimulation. This may serve to reduce iron availability for microbial growth and so might represent a crude mechanism of defence against infection.

The third level of control over iron homeostasis is the regulation of iron release from storage in macrophages, which is under hepcidin–ferroportin control.

The mechanisms that regulate iron absorption are depicted in *Figure 4.3*.

Iron transport

Iron absorbed from the duodenum is released into the bloodstream where it is bound to a specific carrier protein called transferrin. Transferrin is a β globulin with a molecular weight

---

Box 4.4 Hepcidin

Hepcidin was isolated from human urine and blood and identified as having antimicrobial properties. Hepcidin is mainly expressed in the liver but is also present in the heart and brain. The name hepcidin is derived from **hep**atic bacteri**cid**al prote**in**. Recognition of the central role of hepcidin in iron homeostasis hinged on two observations: genetically modified mice engineered to overexpress hepcidin die shortly after birth due to severe iron deficiency, and the discovery that two patients in the USA with liver cancer, and a severe microcytic anaemia that was refractory to iron therapy, had tumours that overexpressed hepcidin. Surgical excision of these tumours effectively cured their anaemia.

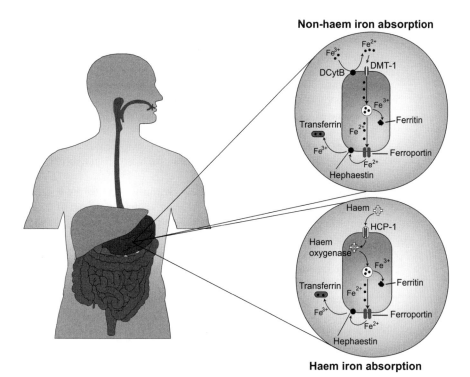

Non-haem iron absorption

Haem iron absorption

Figure 4.3
The mechanisms of iron absorption.

of 74 000 which can carry up to two Fe^{3+} ions per molecule. Transferrin can only bind Fe^{3+}. The Fe^{2+} released from enterocytes is converted to Fe^{2+} by a membrane ferroxidase called hephaestin. Iron is transported, bound to transferrin, to the bone marrow where it is fed to developing erythroblasts for incorporation into haemoglobin via specific transferrin receptors.

There are two forms of transferrin receptor (known as transferrin-receptor-1 and transferrin-receptor-2, TfR1 and TfR2, respectively) embedded in the erythroblast membrane. The better characterized form TfR1 is a homodimer that binds diferric transferrin with high affinity, monoferric transferrin with intermediate affinity, and has a low affinity for apotransferrin. TfR2 is less well characterized but is highly expressed in liver and erythroblasts. Mutation of TfR2 is associated with hereditary haemochromatosis. TfR expression on erythroblasts varies with the stage of maturation (and the requirement for iron incorporation). Low levels of TfR are found on erythroid burst-forming units (BFU-E), with slightly more found on erythroid colony-forming units (CFU-E). The TfR concentration then increases and peaks at the intermediate normoblast stage of maturation. As late normoblasts mature into reticulocytes and mature red cells, the TfR is shed by proteolytic cleavage. Measurement of the plasma TfR concentration provides a sensitive indicator of red cell mass and tissue iron deficiency.

TfR–transferrin complexes are internalized within the erythroblast by invagination of clathrin-coated pits and formation of endocytic vesicles. The pH of these vesicles is reduced to facilitate release of iron from the transferrin and to temporarily strengthen the affinity of the TfR for apotransferrin. The iron is once again converted to the Fe^{2+} state by an endosomal ferrireductase called STEAP2, before transport into the cytoplasm via DMT-1. The TfR–transferrin complexes are then recycled to the cell surface where the physiological pH reduces the affinity of TfR for apotransferrin, facilitating its release into the circulation. Cytosolic iron is transported to mitochondria for incorporation into protoporphyrin IX by the enzyme ferrochelatase as the final step of haem biosynthesis. Iron entry into mitochondria is mediated by a transmembrane iron transport protein called mitoferrin.

Normal plasma contains sufficient transferrin to bind about 300 µg of iron per dl. This figure is called the total iron binding capacity (TIBC) and is one of the useful measures in the assessment of iron status. Typically, plasma transferrin is about 33% saturated with iron.

Newly absorbed iron represents only about 5% of the iron utilized for haem synthesis. About 90% of the iron required each day for this purpose is derived by recycling iron from the haemoglobin of senescent red cells. Any shortfall in iron requirement is met by continuous slow release from the body iron stores.

Synthesis of transferrin receptor and ferritin is regulated by body iron status. Erythroid precursors contain iron-responsive element-binding proteins (IRE-BP) that can bind to sequences called iron-responsive elements on transferrin receptor and ferritin mRNA. When IRE-BP binds to ferritin mRNA, it impedes its translation. Conversely, IRE-BP binding to transferrin receptor mRNA stabilizes the molecule and so promotes its translation. IRE-BP only binds to mRNA when it is not bound to iron. This means that, in the iron-replete cell, IRE-BP binding to transferrin receptor and ferritin mRNA is reduced. This has the effect of up-regulating ferritin synthesis, but down-regulating transferrin receptor synthesis, i.e. cellular iron uptake is reduced and storage is increased. Conversely, in the iron-deficient cell, IRE-BP binding to transferrin receptor and ferritin mRNA is increased, thereby down-regulating ferritin synthesis (storage), but up-regulating transferrin receptor synthesis (cellular uptake).

Iron storage

About one-quarter of the total body iron is in storage, mainly in the liver, tissue macrophages and bone marrow. Two forms of storage iron exist: ferritin and haemosiderin. Ferritin exists as a spherical structure with a diameter of about 5 nm and hydrated Fe^{3+} phosphate at its core. Typically, ferritin contains up to 20% of iron by weight. Each ferritin complex can contain up to 5000 iron ions. About two-thirds of body iron stores are present in this form. Different tissues are associated with slightly different forms of ferritin or isoferritins, which vary somewhat in their chemical and physical properties but share the same basic molecular shape. Plasma ferritin is derived from tissue macrophages and its estimation provides the single most useful indicator of iron status.

Like transferrin receptor, synthesis of ferritin is also regulated by body iron status (see *Box 4.5*). In the presence of iron deficiency, synthesis of apoferritin is reduced, whereas in iron-replete states synthesis is increased. This is physiologically appropriate: when there is not

---

Box 4.5 Measuring iron stores

The most common method of assessing body iron stores involves the measurement of the serum concentration of ferritin. In most cases, this provides a fair reflection of the state of the body iron stores; however, serum ferritin is an acute phase protein, i.e. its concentration is (possibly markedly) increased during the acute phases of inflammatory conditions such as rheumatoid arthritis and cancer. In these circumstances, the serum ferritin concentration bears little relationship to the state of the body iron stores.

A definitive estimation of body iron stores is best obtained by taking a small liver biopsy. The iron content of the biopsy can be assessed by dehydration and acid digestion of the tissue, followed by colorimetric assay using bathophenanthriline sulphonate. Because of its invasive nature, this technique is reserved for suspected cases of iron overload, when it can be combined with microscopic examination to assess the level of tissue damage present.

much iron around, the body down-regulates storage and attempts to enhance cellular uptake. Conversely, when iron is plentiful, storage is favoured over cellular uptake.

The other form of storage iron, haemosiderin, is not a single substance but a variety of different, amorphous iron–protein complexes. Typically, it contains about 37% of iron by weight. Haemosiderin probably represents ferritin in various stages of degradation. Haemosiderin in bone marrow can be visualized under light microscopy using Perls' stain, and this is one method for estimating body iron stores. Iron in haemosiderin can be released to plasma transferrin under the influence of the copper protein caeruloplasmin.

4.2 IRON DEFICIENCY

Iron deficiency is by far the most common cause of anaemia worldwide. Most frequently, iron deficiency is observed as a secondary manifestation of another primary pathological state and may even be the presenting feature. Because iron is essential to the function of every cell of the body, iron deficiency causes a wide range of adverse physiological effects: anaemia is simply the best recognized and most obvious of these.

The state of iron deficiency is defined as a reduction below normal limits of the total body iron content. Iron deficiency anaemia, the most severe manifestation of iron deficiency, develops slowly and insidiously through a series of successive stages, although progression from one stage to the next is not inevitable. When the rate of absorption of iron from the diet is insufficient to meet the daily requirement, iron is mobilized from the body stores to meet the shortfall. If this negative iron balance persists, the body iron stores become depleted, a state known as latent iron deficiency. In this state, the body is deficient in iron but erythropoiesis is still normal and no adverse physiological effects are obvious. Many people exist for prolonged periods in latent iron deficiency and never develop anaemia. If the negative iron balance persists once the body iron stores are exhausted, iron-deficient erythropoiesis ensues and the characteristic changes that accompany severe iron deficiency gradually develop (see also *Box 4.6*). The final stage in this sequence of events is the development of iron deficiency anaemia. Because iron deficiency anaemia develops gradually, the body is able to adapt to the falling haemoglobin level and clinical symptoms often do not appear until the anaemia is moderately severe.

The converse is also true. During iron replacement therapy for iron deficiency anaemia, the blood cell parameters normalize before iron stores are replete.

Box 4.6 Iron deficiency and literature

In the seventeenth century, iron deficiency was known as 'the green sickness' or chlorosis and was believed to be associated with being in love. One common treatment for the condition was to drink wine (sherris) in which iron filings had been steeped. The effects of drinking this potion are described in Shakespeare's *Henry IV Part 2*:

Falstaff: "… for thin drink doth so over-cool their blood, and making many fish meals, that they fall into a kind of male green-sickness … A good sherris-sack hath a two-fold operation in it; it ascends me into the brain, dries me there all the foolish, and dull, and crudy vapours which environ it, makes it apprehensive, quick, forgetive, full of nimble, fiery, and delectable shapes, which delivered o'er to the voice, the tongue, which is the birth, become excellent wit. The second property of your excellent sherris is the warming of the blood, which, before cold and settled, left the liver white and pale, which is the badge of pusillanimity and cowardice. But the sherris warms it, and makes it course from the inwards to the parts extreme. It illumineth the face, which as a beacon gives warning to all the rest of this little kingdom, man, to arm; and then the vital commoners, and inland petty spirits, muster me all to their captain, the heart; who, great and puffed up with this retinue, doth any deed of courage. And this valour comes of sherris."

Causes of iron deficiency

Iron deficiency arises where absorption of iron does not meet daily requirements. This can occur where the supply of iron is decreased or where the daily requirement for iron is increased.

Decreased supply of iron

A sustained decrease in the supply of iron to the body can be caused by two main conditions:

- inadequate diet
- malabsorption of iron from the diet

Inadequate diet. The average adult mixed diet in the UK contains about 18 mg of iron per day: apparently more than enough to meet normal demands. However, much of this is not readily bioavailable. Despite this, inadequacy of the diet is seldom the sole cause of iron deficiency in this age group, although it is commonly a contributing factor to the more rapid onset of iron deficiency due to another primary cause. Breast milk and its artificial substitutes are relatively deficient in iron. Newborn babies have significant body stores of iron that were accumulated *in utero*. Normally, these are sufficient to meet the relatively low demand for iron in the first weeks of life. However, introduction of a mixed diet that has a greater iron content is required to meet the increased demands imposed by growth. Prolonged breast or bottle-feeding may lead to iron deficiency in toddlers. Inadequacy of the diet is often a significant contributory factor in the development of iron deficiency in the Third World, particularly when the iron demand is raised, for example in pregnancy.

Malabsorption of dietary iron. Iron deficiency secondary to malabsorption is a relatively common complication of diseases of the upper alimentary tract such as coeliac disease. Malabsorption of dietary folate commonly exacerbates the anaemia in this disorder. Partial gastrectomy predisposes strongly to the development of iron deficiency because the absence of stomach acid impairs absorption of dietary iron. The malabsorption is aggravated by the rapid gastrojejunal food transit times that result from removal of part of the stomach. It seems doubtful whether reduced gastric acid (achlorhydria) alone results in iron deficiency, because prolonged treatment of heartburn with proton pump inhibitors such as omeprazole does not appear to be associated with the development of this condition.

Increased requirement for iron

There are three main causes of an increase in daily iron requirement:

- loss of blood
- growth and pregnancy
- loss of iron

Blood loss. Chronic blood loss from the gastrointestinal and genito-urinary tracts is the most common cause of iron deficiency (2 ml of blood contains about 1 mg of iron). The effect of menstrual blood loss on iron requirements in adult females has been described earlier in this chapter. The most common cause of bleeding in tropical areas is infestation of the gut with the hookworms *Ancylostoma duodenale* or *Necator americanus*. It is estimated that about 500 million people carry hookworms in their guts. Each worm consumes a tiny quantity of blood from its host but infestations can be very heavy (a female *Ancylostoma* produces 30 000 eggs each day!).

Outside of the tropics, the most common causes of pathological blood loss are carcinoma, duodenal ulcer, hiatus hernia, haemorrhoids and menorrhagia. Other than in menorrhagia, frank blood loss is usually absent: a loss of only 3–5 ml of blood per day, if sustained, will eventually lead to iron deficiency. Even smaller losses can result in iron deficiency if the diet is poor or if malabsorption is present.

Growth and pregnancy. The increased requirement for iron during periods of accelerated growth makes iron deficiency very common in adolescence and in pregnancy. For example, in a normal uncomplicated pregnancy, maternal total red cell mass increases by between 20 and 40%. This imposes an extra requirement for iron of up to 500 mg. The developing fetus, which always has first call on available iron, requires about 300 mg of iron. These dual excess demands for iron are greatest during the second and third trimester of pregnancy, when the daily demand for iron can rise to 6–7 mg! The delicate iron balance that this inevitably causes is compounded by maternal blood loss at delivery. Small amounts of iron are also lost in breast milk. The excess requirement for iron in pregnancy is offset partially by the temporary cessation of menstruation (amenorrhoea), which saves about 200 mg of iron in total.

Loss of iron. Chronic intravascular haemolysis can result in the loss of considerable amounts of iron as haemosiderin in the urine. In severe cases, this can contribute to the development of iron deficiency.

Pathophysiology

A wide range of clinical manifestations accompanies severe iron deficiency anaemia. These can be considered under three broad headings:

- effects caused by the primary precipitating condition (these are beyond the scope of this book)
- effects that are manifest in the blood and blood-forming tissue
- effects that are manifest in other tissues

Effects on the blood and blood-forming tissue

Depletion of the iron stores means that there is insufficient iron available for incorporation into the haemoglobin of developing erythroblasts and iron-deficient erythropoiesis ensues. This is manifest as a reduced MCHC and an increased concentration of free protoporphyrin within the cell (see also *Box 4.7*). The major determinant of the volume of a mature red cell is the number of mitotic divisions it undergoes before the nucleus is poisoned by the increasing concentration of

---

Box 4.7 Red cell indices

Using the measured red cell parameters of haemoglobin concentration ([Hb]), mean red cell volume (MCV) and red cell count (RBC), three red cell indices can be calculated, as follows.
Packed cell volume (PCV, Hct):

$$PCV\ (l/l) = MCV\ (fl) \times RBC\ (\times 10^{12})$$

Mean cell haemoglobin:

$$MCH\ (pg) = [Hb]\ (g/dl)\ /\ RBC\ (\times 10^{12})$$

Mean cell haemoglobin concentration:

$$MCHC\ (g/dl) = [Hb]\ (g/dl)\ /\ PCV\ (l/l)$$

Some analysers measure the PCV and calculate the MCV:

$$MCV\ (fl) = PCV\ (l/l)\ /\ RBC\ (\times 10^{12})$$

Artefactual changes in the MCV measured by electronic counters can be caused by many factors, including delays in processing, changes in plasma osmolality and the presence of cold agglutination. Such artefacts are carried through to the calculated indices. Careful microscopic examination of a stained blood film can reveal many of these artefacts.

haemoglobin. In iron deficiency, haemoglobin synthesis is retarded and an extra mitotic division occurs before the erythroblast nucleus dies. This results in a mature red cell that is smaller than normal. Thus, the anaemia that typically accompanies iron deficiency is hypochromic and microcytic.

The condition most likely to be confused with iron deficiency anaemia on morphological grounds is β-thalassaemia. The differential diagnosis of these two conditions is described in *Chapter 6*. The main laboratory features of iron deficiency anaemia are shown in *Table 4.1*.

One of the biochemical hallmarks of iron deficiency is the combination of a raised TIBC and reduced transferrin saturation. The relationship between TIBC and transferrin saturation in a range of conditions is shown in *Figure 4.4*.

Table 4.1 Laboratory and physiological features of iron deficiency

Blood cell features
  Microcytosis and hypochromia
  Reticulocytopenia (see *Box 4.8*)
  Poikilocytosis (pencil forms)
  Defective neutrophil function
  Reduced percentage of T lymphocytes in children
Bone marrow features
  Erythroid hypoplasia
  Normoblasts have ragged cytoplasm
  Decreased stainable iron deposits
Biochemical features
  Raised TIBC
  Decreased % transferrin saturation
  Raised catecholamine levels
  Reduced serum ferritin levels
Physiological features
  Impaired ability to maintain body temperature
  Depressed muscle function
  Abnormal thyroid hormone metabolism

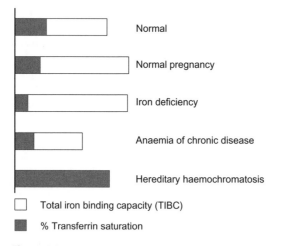

Normal

Normal pregnancy

Iron deficiency

Anaemia of chronic disease

Hereditary haemochromatosis

☐ Total iron binding capacity (TIBC)

■ % Transferrin saturation

Figure 4.4
The relationship between total iron binding capacity and % transferrin saturation in a range of conditions.

General effects of iron deficiency anaemia

There are three main types of generalized effect of iron deficiency:

- changes that are directly attributable to anaemia but not specific to iron deficiency
- changes in epithelial tissue
- changes in behaviour

A reduction in circulating haemoglobin causes a reduction in oxygen-carrying capacity and leads to the most widely recognized changes seen in anaemia, i.e. pallor of skin and mucous membranes and reduced exercise tolerance. The body responds to anaemia by increasing cardiac output and increasing synthesis of red cell 2,3-DPG, thereby maintaining oxygen delivery to the tissues under basal conditions. However, there is an exaggerated response to exercise, which causes shortness of breath on exertion and palpitations, the most common presenting features of iron deficiency anaemia.

Severe iron deficiency causes deficiency of iron-containing enzymes such as cytochromes in a wide range of tissues. The effect of this is manifest most severely in epithelial cells, which ordinarily are turning over relatively rapidly. Characteristic changes include:

- **koilonychia** – flattening or 'spooning' of the finger nails
- **angular stomatitis** – atrophic lesions at the corners of the mouth
- **glossitis** – smooth, inflamed tongue
- **atrophic gastritis** – inflammation of the lining of the stomach
- **achlorhydria** – lack of hydrochloric acid secretion in the stomach
- **dysphagia** – difficulty in swallowing caused by the development of oesophageal webs; this rare condition is known as the Plummer–Vinson syndrome and may progress to oesophageal carcinoma

Iron deficiency in early childhood is associated with impairment of intellectual ability and hyperactivity (see also *Box 4.9*). Most studies have shown that these effects are at least partially reversed by suitable iron therapy.

Box 4.8 Understanding haematology terms

The suffix –*penia* implies a low number of the given cell type, e.g. thrombocytopenia means a low platelet count.

The suffix –*osis* means an increased number of the given cell type, e.g. reticulocytosis means an increase in the reticulocyte count.

The suffix –*plasia* means formation, e.g. erythroid hypoplasia means a reduction in the rate of erythropoiesis, erythroid hyperplasia implies an increased rate of red cell production, and aplasia means a complete arrest of production.

Box 4.9 Spinach and iron – part 2

The association between spinach and strength and vigour was brought to life for most people when Max Fleischer invented the cartoon character Popeye. The pugnacious sailor has been a popular character with children of all ages since the 1930s.

In 1971, Dr R. Hunter published in *The Lancet* his observations that laboratory animals fed on a high folate diet became tense and irritable. Perhaps it was the high folate content of spinach that caused Popeye to become so quarrelsome and to pick fights with Bluto!

Another characteristic, but poorly understood, behavioural abnormality in iron-deficient subjects is manifest as a strong desire to eat unusual substances such as soil (geophagia), ice (pagophagia) or even carpet fluff. In some cases, this obsessive behaviour, known as pica, may exacerbate the iron deficiency (see also *Box 4.10*). For example, ingestion of clay soil can impair intestinal absorption of dietary iron.

Iron deficiency is not a disease but, rather, it is a sign of disease. Effective treatment of iron deficiency requires that the primary precipitating cause be removed. Excluding pregnancy and menorrhagia, the most common underlying cause of iron deficiency is occult blood loss from the gastrointestinal tract.

Replacement of body iron stores is best achieved by supplementation of the diet using ferrous sulphate or, less commonly, by intramuscular injection of iron–dextran. Appropriate oral supplementation should induce a reticulocyte response within 3 or 4 days and a sustained rise in circulating haemoglobin concentration. Failure of response to an adequate dose of oral iron suggests that the underlying cause has not been removed, that patient compliance is poor, or that iron deficiency is not the cause of the anaemia. It should be remembered that iron deficiency is only one of many causes of microcytic, hypochromic anaemia.

If iron replacement therapy is effective, it should be continued beyond the time of normalization of [Hb] to ensure that the body iron stores are replenished.

Box 4.10 Pica and pregnancy

It has been suggested that pica may be at least part of the explanation for the unusual dietary cravings experienced by some pregnant women. A number of studies have shown that the more exaggerated cases of this phenomenon correlate with depletion of the iron stores.

4.3 ANAEMIA OF CHRONIC DISORDERS

Chronic inflammatory or malignant disorders are frequently accompanied by a normocytic, normochromic anaemia that is refractory to all treatment except that which causes regression of the primary condition. This form of anaemia is known as the anaemia of chronic disorders (ACD).

Chronic inflammation causes activation of tissue macrophages with a consequent up-regulation of surface apotransferrin receptors. Binding of significant quantities of apotransferrin to macrophages reduces the TIBC of the plasma as shown in *Figure 4.4*. Inflammation also stimulates neutrophils to synthesize and release large quantities of apolactoferrin, which acts as an iron-binding protein. The apolactoferrin is bound to specific surface receptors on activated tissue macrophages and acts like a magnet for circulating iron. Any iron that is bound to the apolactoferrin–receptor complex is internalized by the macrophage and stored as ferritin. Thus, tissue iron stores are increased. It is this apparent anomaly of reduced TIBC and transferrin saturation, accompanied by normal or increased body iron stores, which is the hallmark of ACD.

Hepcidin expression is increased in inflammatory states and contributes to the anaemia by down-regulating release of iron from macrophages.

There is clear evidence of suppression of erythropoietic activity in ACD. There have been sporadic reports of the presence of specific inhibitors of erythropoiesis in individuals but in most cases the suppression is likely to be caused by the release of growth inhibitors such as interleukin-1, γ-interferon and TNF in response to the primary condition. A slight reduction in red cell lifespan has also been reported in a minority of cases of ACD.

4.4   SIDEROBLASTIC ANAEMIAS

The sideroblastic anaemias are a heterogeneous group of disorders that are characterized by disordered incorporation of iron into haem within developing erythroblasts. The resulting toxic accumulation of iron within the mitochondria of late erythroblasts leads to some degree of ineffective erythropoiesis. Demonstration of iron-laden mitochondria encircling the nuclei of late erythroblasts, the so-called 'ringed sideroblast', is the hallmark of sideroblastic anaemia. However, ringed sideroblasts are not specific indicators of sideroblastic anaemia: they are frequently found in leukaemia, megaloblastic anaemia and alcoholism amongst other conditions. The sideroblastic anaemias are classified according to their aetiology as hereditary/congenital, acquired clonal, and acquired secondary or reversible types, as shown in *Table 4.2*.

Table 4.2 Classification of the sideroblastic anaemias

Hereditary/congenital
X-linked pyridoxine-responsive (e.g. δ-ALA synthase mutations)
X-linked pyridoxine resistant (e.g. ABC-7 mutation)
Rare autosomal types exist (e.g. PUS-1 mutations)
Congenital due to mitochondrial DNA deletion
Acquired clonal
Subtype of myelodysplastic syndrome (RARS ± thrombocytosis)
Associated with clonal haematological disorder (e.g. myeloproliferative disease, acute erythroleukaemia)
Acquired secondary (reversible)
Drug treatment (e.g. isoniazid, chloramphenicol)
Intoxication (e.g. alcoholism, lead poisoning)
Copper deficiency
Hypothermia

Hereditary sideroblastic anaemia

Most cases of hereditary sideroblastic anaemia have shown an X-linked recessive pattern of inheritance. Affected males have hypochromic, dimorphic anaemia with mild ineffective erythropoiesis and erythroid hyperplasia (see *Box 4.11*). Most commonly, these cases are caused by heterogeneous point mutations in the gene that encodes δ-aminolaevulinic acid (δ-ALA) synthase. Many of these respond to the administration of vitamin B_6 (pyridoxine), but such responses are, at best, partial and are usually temporary. A less common X-linked sideroblastic anaemia with non-progressive cerebellar ataxia is caused by mutation of the *ABC-7* gene.

Rare autosomal forms of inherited sideroblastic anaemia also exist, including a neuromuscular syndrome with impaired oxidative phosphorylation (mitochondrial myopathy) that is associated with pseudo-uridine synthase-1 (PUS-1) mutations. Sideroblastic anaemia also occurs as a component of a number of rare congenital syndromes such as Roger syndrome and Pearson syndrome.

Box 4.11 Ineffective erythropoiesis

Ineffective erythropoiesis means the production of red cells that die within the bone marrow, i.e. the production is ineffective because it does not increase the circulating red cell count.

Roger syndrome is an autosomal recessive disorder characterized by megaloblastic anaemia, diabetes mellitus, progressive sensorineural deafness with ring sideroblasts and variable neutropenia and thrombocytopenia. The condition is caused by mutations of the thiamine transporter gene *SLC19A2*. Accordingly, the megaloblastic anaemia often responds to thiamine administration.

Pearson syndrome is a multisystem disorder that presents in the first few months of life with a variable mix of severe anaemia, metabolic acidosis, exocrine pancreatic insufficiency and hepatic/renal failure. The condition is caused by deletion, rearrangement or duplication of mitochondrial DNA with consequent mitochondrial dysfunction.

Acquired clonal sideroblastic anaemia

Acquired clonal sideroblastic anaemia is primarily a disease of the middle-aged and elderly and is the most common of the sideroblastic anaemias. It is associated with a clonal abnormality of haemopoietic progenitor cells that confers a growth advantage and so is most commonly classed as a myelodysplastic syndrome. Most cases are classified as refractory anaemia with ring sideroblasts (RARS). Characteristic dyserythropoietic changes include macrocytosis, poikilocytosis, basophilic stippling and the appearance of ringed sideroblasts affecting all stages of erythroblast development. Cytogenetic abnormalities are demonstrable in about 50% of cases. If dysplastic features are also present in other cell lines, the condition is classified as refractory cytopenia with multilineage dysplasia and ring sideroblasts (RCMD–RS). The presence of leucocytosis, thrombocytosis, or both is suggestive of a mixed myelodysplastic/myeloproliferative disease. Sideroblastic anaemia is also seen in acute leukaemia, particularly erythroleukaemia.

Secondary (reversible) sideroblastic anaemia

Drug-induced sideroblastic anaemia

The most common cause of secondary sideroblastic anaemia is the administration of drugs such as isoniazid or chloramphenicol. Isoniazid inhibits biochemical reactions that involve pyridoxal 5′-phosphate, including synthesis of δ-ALA, the first and rate-limiting step in the haem biosynthetic pathway. Chloramphenicol inhibits the synthesis of δ-ALA synthase and ferrochelatase. The blood picture in drug-induced or alcohol-induced sideroblastic anaemia closely resembles that of the hereditary form. All of the sideroblastic changes are reversible by withdrawal of the offending substance.

Alcohol

Alcohol also inhibits several biochemical reactions involved in the synthesis of haem, and chronic abuse can produce a similar clinical picture to isoniazid-induced sideroblastic anaemia. However, anaemia in alcoholics is usually multifactorial: folate and/or iron deficiency are also frequently found where nutrition is chronically suboptimal, or when chronic bleeding from the gastrointestinal tract is present.

Lead poisoning

Chronic lead poisoning was a relatively common condition when most drinking water was supplied via lead pipes and lead pigments were commonly used in paints (see also *Box 4.12*). Most cases nowadays are associated with occupational exposure. Lead is absorbed by ingestion or inhalation. Most absorbed lead accumulates in bone and bone marrow. In the bone marrow, lead is associated particularly with mitochondrial membranes of developing erythroblasts. The presence of lead in the mitochondria severely disrupts haem synthesis and leads directly to sideroblastic change. Lead also causes damage to red cell membranes and inhibits glycolytic

---

Box 4.12 Lead poisoning

The ancient Romans made heavy use of lead. They used it in their water pipes (the name plumber is derived from the Latin for lead, *plumbum*), their pottery drinking vessels were lead-glazed, and their cooking utensils were commonly lined with lead. Archaeological evidence shows high concentrations of lead in bones found at Roman sites such as York and Cirencester. Some historians believe that the increasing sophistication of the Romans' use of lead contributed to the fall of the Roman Empire because of a presumed high incidence of lead-induced dementia.

---

activity. These two activities result in mild haemolysis, which contributes significantly to the anaemia of chronic lead poisoning.

Typically, the blood picture in chronic lead poisoning is microcytic and hypochromic with prominent basophilic stippling and a reticulocytosis. The basophilic stippling is the result of the accumulation of pyrimidine nucleotides in the cell cytoplasm and is only present in the youngest red cells. The accumulation of pyrimidine nucleotides is caused by the inhibition of the enzyme pyrimidine 5'-nucleotidase by lead.

Copper deficiency

Copper deficiency is relatively rare in humans because requirements are low and copper is plentifully available. Recorded causes have included prolonged parenteral nutrition in the absence of copper supplementation, chelation therapy and prolonged zinc ingestion. Copper deficiency interferes with haem synthesis and mitochondrial function. Most cases demonstrate sideroblastic anaemia with variable neutropenia, but some also have neurological manifestations. Zinc ingestion can cause copper deficiency because it induces metallothionein, which binds copper.

Hypothermia

Hypothermia can induce transient erythroid hypoplasia with ring sideroblasts and thrombocytopenia, probably due to impaired mitochondrial function at low temperatures. As the body temperature returns to normal, these changes remit.

4.5 IRON OVERLOAD

There are three commonly seen forms of chronic iron overload:

- hereditary haemochromatosis
- transfusion-associated haemosiderosis
- dietary causes

Hereditary haemochromatosis

Hereditary haemochromatosis results from an irregularity of intestinal iron absorption in which feedback control over the rate of absorption of dietary iron is impaired. The inexorable accumulation of iron within the body that results damages vital organs and, if untreated, is fatal. There are several genetic forms of haemochromatosis, as follows.

- **Type 1 or classical haemochromatosis** is an autosomal recessive disorder, most commonly caused by a mutation in the *HFE* gene at 6p21.3. *HFE* acts as a negative regulator of transferrin receptor-mediated uptake or handling of transferrin-bound iron. When the *HFE* gene mutates, this 'brake' on iron absorption is lost and cellular iron uptake proceeds unabated. Screening studies have estimated that hereditary haemochromatosis affects approximately 1 in every 125–333 individuals in the normal populations of the United States, Northern Europe, and Australia.

■ **Type 2 or juvenile haemochromatosis** is also autosomal recessive and is caused by mutations in the haemojuvelin gene at 1q21 (type 2a haemochromatosis) or the hepcidin gene (type 2b haemochromatosis) at 19q13. Mutations of either of these genes leads to reduced availability of hepcidin and failure of ferroportin inactivation, which causes unregulated iron release into the plasma.

■ **Type 3 haemochromatosis** is an autosomal recessive disorder and is caused by mutation in the gene encoding TfR-2 at 7q22.

■ **Type 4 haemochromatosis** is an autosomal dominant disorder and is caused by mutation in the gene (*SLC40A1*) that encodes ferroportin at 2q32.

Absorption of dietary iron typically exceeds normal by about 2 mg per day in haemochromatosis homozygotes and is unrelated to iron requirements. Because of this, an affected adult male may have accumulated a total body iron content of over 20 g. However, in contrast to transfusion-associated haemosiderosis, bone marrow macrophages are not grossly overloaded with storage iron. Most of the excess iron is stored in the parenchymal cells of the liver and other organs.

Laboratory investigation

Diagnosis of haemochromatosis requires the demonstration, in tissue and/or blood, of excess stores of iron. The most useful screening test to assess systemic iron overload is measurement of transferrin saturation. In haemochromatosis homozygotes, transferrin saturation is >45% in more than 95% of cases. Because transferrin saturation levels can be affected by diurnal variation, dietary factors, laboratory imprecision, or concomitant disease states such as inflammation or hepatitis, an elevated result should be confirmed in a fasting sample. Second level screening requires exclusion of other likely causes of increased transferrin saturation and estimation of serum ferritin levels. A serum ferritin of >200 μg/l for premenopausal women or >400 μg/l for men, in the presence of a persistently elevated transferrin saturation, implies primary iron overload.

The key to successful treatment of haemochromatosis is early diagnosis. Although the rate of clinical progression varies widely in haemochromatosis patients, most will show elevated serum ferritin levels by early adulthood. If the suspicion of haemochromatosis in an individual is high, a serum ferritin level below these values does not exclude a diagnosis and they should be followed by repeated testing at least every other year.

The definitive diagnostic test for hereditary haemochromatosis is demonstration of a mutation in the *HFE*, haemojuvelin, hepcidin or transferrin receptor genes. Liver biopsy can provide definitive demonstration of parenchymal iron loading but this invasive procedure is no longer considered essential for a diagnosis.

Pathophysiology

One of the early signs of hereditary haemochromatosis is greatly increased saturation of circulating transferrin as shown in *Figure 4.4*. Thus, when iron is absorbed inappropriately and released into the portal circulation, some may be unable to bind to the iron transport protein transferrin because it is already fully saturated. Iron that cannot bind to transferrin circulates as hydrated complexes of ferrous and ferric ions until binding sites become available. About 30% of the circulating plasma iron exists as hydrated ionic complexes in haemochromatosis heterozygotes. These hydrated ionic complexes of iron can act as a catalyst for the formation of toxic oxygen radicals in the presence of NADPH. Oxygen radicals are short-lived and extremely reactive molecular species that are capable of causing extensive localized tissue damage. The principal villain in this regard is hydroxyl radical (OH•).

Accumulated organ damage results in the major clinical features of hereditary haemochromatosis: hepatic cirrhosis, skin pigmentation, diabetes and progressive congestive cardiomyopathy, which is the leading cause of death. In about 30% of cases, hepatic cirrhosis progresses to hepatoma.

Because the iron accumulates very slowly in hereditary haemochromatosis, tissue damage is seldom debilitating before the age of 30 years (except for the juvenile form of the condition). If the diagnosis is made early, severe tissue damage can be avoided by a programme of weekly venesection involving the removal of at least 500 ml of blood on each occasion. The aim of this programme of venesection is to deplete the excess body iron stores over a 12–18 month period. Once depleted, a less energetic programme involving bimonthly venesection can prevent reaccumulation. Recent experience suggests that, provided that treatment is started early and controlled carefully, life expectancy is returned to normal.

Transfusion-associated haemosiderosis

As described in *Chapter 6*, β-thalassaemia homozygotes are completely dependent on a programme of regular blood transfusion. Each transfusion of 400 ml of blood carries with it approximately 200 mg of iron, which cannot be excreted. Steady accumulation of body iron results, with similar consequences to those described above for hereditary haemochromatosis. The accumulation of iron in body stores is slowed appreciably by the administration of chelating agents such as desferrioxamine but, at present, these only delay the inevitable. Chronic iron chelation therapy is demanding as it requires a subcutaneous infusion lasting 8–12 hours per night, for five to seven nights a week, for as long as the patient continues to receive blood transfusions or has excess iron within the body. In 2005, an oral iron chelator called Exjade became available that is administered as a drink.

Dietary causes

Iron overload due to dietary causes was reported to be a serious problem in the Bantu people of southern Africa. The cause of this was reputed to be the local habit of cooking exclusively in iron pots, coupled with enthusiastic imbibing of strong home-brewed beer which had been brewed and illicitly stored in iron drums (see also *Box 4.13*). Further investigation of African iron overload, formerly known as Bantu siderosis, revealed a genetic polymorphism in the ferroportin gene (type 4 haemochromatosis) that is relatively common in people of African descent, and that predisposes to iron overload.

Acute iron poisoning due to ingestion of a large number of iron tablets intended for therapeutic use is one of the most common causes of fatal poisoning in young children. If discovered early, gastric lavage and desferrioxamine therapy may prevent serious toxicity. Chronic use of iron supplements in the absence of iron deficiency can lead to iron overload because the large quantities of iron present are absorbed by passive diffusion across the gut wall, regardless of the state of the body iron stores.

Box 4.13 Iron fortification

A Swedish study demonstrated the potential dangers of iron fortification of food in developed countries. The iron status of 350 subjects was assessed. About 1 in 20 men carried iron stores above reference limits and almost half of these had iron stores approaching those of early haemochromatosis! Iron fortification remains a useful public health measure in underdeveloped countries where the average diet is deficient in iron.

SUGGESTED FURTHER READING

Andrews, N.C. & Schmidt, P.J. (2007) Iron homeostasis. *Annu. Rev. Physiol.* **69:** 69–85.

Atanasiu, V., *et al.* (2007) Hepcidin – central regulator of iron metabolism. *Eur. J. Haematol.* **78:** 1–10.

Domellof, M. (2007) Iron requirements, absorption and metabolism in infancy and childhood. *Curr. Opin. Clin. Nutr. Metab. Care,* **10:** 329–335.

Dunn, L.L., *et al.* (2007) Iron uptake and metabolism in the new millennium. *Trends Cell Biol.* **17:** 93–100.

Ganz, T. (2007) Molecular control of iron transport. *J. Am. Soc. Nephrol.* **18:** 394–400.

Killip, S., *et al.* (2007) Iron deficiency anemia. *Am. Fam. Physician,* **75:** 671–678.

Pietrangelo, A. (2006) Hereditary hemochromatosis. *Biochim. Biophys. Acta,* **1763:** 700–710.

SELF-ASSESSMENT QUESTIONS

1. Where in the body is iron absorbed optimally?
2. Ascorbic acid is a reducing agent. Does it enhance or impair inorganic iron absorption? Why?
3. Where are the main body stores of iron?
4. Why might severe iron deficiency be associated with breathlessness on exertion?
5. What effect do you think that surgical removal of the stomach would have on iron absorption?
6. Differentiate between the terms negative iron balance, latent iron deficiency, iron-deficient erythropoiesis and iron deficiency anaemia.
7. List the three main causes of an increased iron requirement.
8. What are the main distinguishing features of an iron-deficient red cell?
9. Why are iron-deficient red cells microcytic?
10. Which of the sideroblastic anaemias is now considered to be a myelodysplastic syndrome?
11. Differentiate between the pathogenesis of haemochromatosis and haemosiderosis.

Megaloblastic anaemias

Learning objectives

After studying this chapter you should confidently be able to:

■ **Describe the importance of vitamin B_{12} and folate for optimal blood cell production**
Vitamin B_{12} and folate are essential for optimal DNA and RNA synthesis, so a ready supply is required to meet the needs of the rapidly dividing haemopoietic system.

■ **Describe the mechanisms that predispose to deficiency of vitamin B_{12} and folate**
Deficiency of folate is more likely if demand is increased, e.g. in haemolytic anaemia or pregnancy, or if the supply is reduced (perhaps due to poor diet or malabsorption). Vitamin B_{12} deficiency is most commonly a result of malabsorption, although poor diet or increased demand can play a role.

■ **List some causes of megaloblastic change other than haematinic deficiency**
Megaloblastic changes are also seen in association with cytotoxic chemotherapy, certain rare inborn errors of metabolism and haematological abnormalities such as acute erythroleukaemia.

■ **Describe the biochemical basis of the megaloblastic anaemias**
Vitamin B_{12} and/or folate deficiency impairs the rate of conversion of deoxyuridine-5′-mono-phosphate (dUMP) to deoxythymidine-5′-monophosphate (dTMP), the rate-limiting step in DNA synthesis, and results in asynchrony between DNA and RNA synthesis. This explains many of the morphological and biochemical features of megaloblastic anaemia.

Adequate nutrition is an essential requirement for the maintenance of normal bodily function, growth and repair. The nutritional requirements for optimal blood cell production are similar to those of the other cells of the body. Because of this, nutritional deficiencies seldom cause problems that are restricted to the blood. However, because of the relatively rapid turnover of blood cells, signs of deficiency often manifest early in the blood.

This chapter concentrates on vitamin B_{12} and folic acid metabolism and the megaloblastic anaemias that result from deficiency of these nutrients (see also *Box 5.1*).

Box 5.1 Vitamins

The existence of essential nutrients in certain foods was suspected long before their identification. For example, the importance of citrus fruits in the prevention of scurvy and of the inclusion of unpolished rice in a diet dominated by rice in the prevention of beriberi was well known. It was not until 1911, however, that the essential factor in unpolished rice was identified by the Polish chemist Casimir Funk as thiamine. It was he who coined the term 'vital amine', from which the name vitamin is derived.

5.1   VITAMIN B$_{12}$

Vitamin B$_{12}$ can exist in a variety of different chemical forms, which together constitute the family of cobalamins. The cobalamins are organometallic complexes comprising three major structures: a corrin nucleus and, bound at right angles to the nucleus, a nucleotide and a variable chemical group. The structure of the corrin nucleus is similar to that of haem in that it consists of four pyrrole rings with a Co$^+$ ion instead of an Fe^{2+} at the centre. The nucleotide comprises a base (5,6-dimethylbenzimidazole) bound to a phosphorylated sugar (ribose-3-phosphate).

The differences between the various cobalamins lie with the variable chemical group, which is bound to the central cobalt ion. In the physiologically active cobalamins, the variant chemical group is either a 5′-deoxyadenosyl group or a methyl group. 5′-deoxyadenosylcobalamin is the predominant form of the vitamin encountered in the liver while methylcobalamin predominates in the plasma. Both 5′-deoxyadenosylcobalamin and methylcobalamin are unstable compounds that, on exposure to light, rapidly denature to form hydroxocobalamin, which contains a Co^{3+} ion at its centre. Hydroxocobalamin is the main dietary form of the vitamin. Cyanocobalamin is a stable synthetic form that has been used therapeutically.

The role of vitamin B$_{12}$ within the body

In bacteria, vitamin B$_{12}$ is involved in a relatively large number of metabolic reactions but, in humans, it is required as co-enzyme for only two (see also *Box 5.2*):

- **conversion of L-methylmalonyl co-enzyme A to succinyl co-enzyme A.** 5′-deoxy-adenosylcobalamin is required as a co-enzyme in this isomerization reaction. A wide range of substances are catabolized via this reaction, e.g. cholesterol, odd chain fatty acids, the amino acids methionine and threonine, and the pyrimidines uracil and thymine.
- **methylation of homocysteine to methionine.** This reaction requires both methylcobalamin as a co-enzyme and *N*-5-methyltetrahydrofolate as the methyl donor, and is important in the intracellular synthesis of folate co-enzymes.

Box 5.2 Microbial assays

Certain micro-organisms are incapable of synthesizing vitamin B$_{12}$ or folate and so have an absolute requirement for exogenous supplies for growth. This fact has been exploited in the microbiological assay of vitamin B$_{12}$ and folate.

If suitable micro-organisms are maintained in a growth medium which contains all required nutrients except vitamin B$_{12}$ or folate, and a known volume of a test serum is added, then the rate of microbial growth is determined by the concentration of the missing nutrient in the test serum.

Examples of suitable test organisms include *Lactobacillus leichmanii* and *Euglena gracilis* for vitamin B$_{12}$ and *Lactobacillus casei* for folate. Although universally used in the past, this method of assay is technically demanding and subject to severe practical limitations and has been almost completely superseded by radio-isotopic and immunological methods. One great advantage of microbial assays is that they only measure forms of the vitamins that are biologically assimilable.

Daily vitamin B$_{12}$ requirements and body stores

Vitamin B$_{12}$ is synthesized exclusively by intestinal micro-organisms. In humans, certain colonic bacteria can synthesize vitamin B$_{12}$, but this is distal to the site of absorption of the vitamin so is unavailable for use by the body. The only source of vitamin B$_{12}$ available to humans is from dietary components of animal origin such as liver, kidney, red meat, eggs, shellfish and dairy products.

A typical mixed UK diet contains between 5 and 30 μg of vitamin B$_{12}$ per day, depending on the quantity of meat included. Diets that exclude all animal products contain no intrinsic vitamin B$_{12}$. However, even strict vegans obtain small amounts of vitamin B$_{12}$ from their diet because of bacterial contamination of their food. Vitamin B$_{12}$ is relatively heat-stable and so little loss occurs in cooking.

Typical daily losses of vitamin B$_{12}$ are 1–4 μg, primarily in the urine and faeces. Since there is no bodily consumption of vitamin B$_{12}$, the daily requirement matches daily losses. Thus, a typical UK mixed diet provides more than enough vitamin B$_{12}$ to meet requirements.

Normally, the body stores about 3–4 mg of vitamin B$_{12}$, primarily in the liver. This would be sufficient to meet the requirement for vitamin B$_{12}$ for about 3 years if dietary intake ceased or if the ability to absorb the vitamin was lost.

Vitamin B$_{12}$ absorption

Vitamin B$_{12}$ absorption is an active process that occurs optimally in the terminal ileum. Vitamin B$_{12}$ in food is liberated by gastric and duodenal proteolytic enzymes and rapidly complexes in a 1:1 ratio with a glycoprotein of molecular weight 45 000 called intrinsic factor (see also *Box 5.3*).

Intrinsic factor (IF) is synthesized and secreted by gastric parietal cells. The IF:B$_{12}$ complex then progresses to the ileum where it binds, via the intrinsic factor part of the complex, to an endocytic receptor complex called cubam. This receptor complex consists of two proteins: a receptor protein of molecular weight 460 000 called cubilin that binds the IF:B$_{12}$ complex, and amnionless which appears to direct uptake of the bound IF:B$_{12}$ complex into the cell. Both components are required for vitamin B$_{12}$ absorption. Within the mucosal cell, vitamin B$_{12}$ is released from its complex and, after a delay of about six hours, the newly absorbed vitamin is released into the portal circulation. Intrinsic factor is not recycled. Because of the finite number of cubam receptors, a maximum of about 2 μg of vitamin B$_{12}$ can be absorbed from each meal, regardless of its content. After each meal, cubam receptors are unresponsive to further IF:B$_{12}$ complex for up to six hours.

Although vitamin B$_{12}$ deficiency is typically treated by intramuscular injection of therapeutic doses of hydroxocobalamin, it is also possible to bypass the limitations of intestinal absorption mechanisms by administering large oral doses (1–2 mg) of vitamin B$_{12}$.

Excretion of vitamin B$_{12}$ occurs mainly via the biliary system. A proportion is reabsorbed from the bile during its passage through the gut. This salvage mechanism is known as the enterohepatic circulation of vitamin B$_{12}$.

Box 5.3 Key dates: vitamin B$_{12}$

1926 First demonstration by George Minot of Harvard University of the efficacy of eating raw beef liver in the treatment of pernicious anaemia.

1927 Identification by William Castle of Boston City Hospital that an 'extrinsic factor' in liver combines with an 'intrinsic factor' in gastric juice to produce this effect.

1930–47 Production of first clinically effective purified liver extract by Gänsslen in Germany. Identification of LLD factor, animal protein factor and ruminant factor, all of which turned out to be cobalamins.

1947 Demonstration by Mary Shorb that clinically effective liver extracts contained an essential growth factor for *Lactobacillus lactis*.

1948 Crystallization of cyanocobalamin by Karl Folkers and co-workers at the Merck laboratories in the USA and E.L. Smith and co-workers, a few months later, at the Glaxo laboratories in the UK.

Vitamin B$_{12}$ transport

Vitamin B$_{12}$ circulates in plasma bound to two carrier proteins called transcobalamin (TC) and haptocorrin (HC).

Transcobalamin

Transcobalamin is a protein of molecular weight 43 000 that is synthesized by enterocytes and several other organs. It used to be known as transcobalamin II. In contrast to haptocorrin, transcobalamin is not a glycoprotein. Vitamin B$_{12}$ is transferred from intrinsic factor to transcobalamin within the enterocytes of the terminal ileum. The bound vitamin then enters the bloodstream where it is transported to developing cells throughout the body. Transcobalamin is the physiologically important vitamin B$_{12}$ carrier protein. Vitamin B$_{12}$-saturated transcobalamin is known as holotranscobalamin (holoTC), and constitutes 6–20% of total plasma vitamin B$_{12}$. About 90% of circulating transcobalamin is unsaturated and is called apotranscobalamin (apoTC). Congenital absence of transcobalamin causes a severe megaloblastic anaemia within weeks of birth, despite normal vitamin B$_{12}$ absorption and a normal serum vitamin B$_{12}$ concentration.

Haptocorrin

Haptocorrin is the name given to a group of immunologically related glycoproteins that bind vitamin B$_{12}$, and used to be known as transcobalamins I and III, cobalophilins or R-binder. Haptocorrin is synthesized in many cells of the body, including leucocytes. The majority (about 80–94%) of circulating vitamin B$_{12}$ is bound to haptocorrin, but this is not readily released to developing cells, due to the firmness of binding. There is no known physiological function for haptocorrin. Congenital absence of haptocorrin causes no clinical disorder, despite a reduction in serum vitamin B$_{12}$ concentration. Haptocorrin levels in serum can rise dramatically in chronic myeloid leukaemia, leading to markedly raised serum vitamin B$_{12}$ levels, although this is physiologically unavailable.

5.2 FOLATES

The parent of the folate family of compounds is folic acid (pteroylglutamic acid). Humans are incapable of synthesizing folate: all requirements must be met by dietary intake. The most common forms of folate differ from the parent compound in three important respects:

- they exist in reduced form as dihydro- (DHF) or tetrahydrofolates (THF)
- they carry a single-carbon group (methyl – CH$_3$, formyl – CHO, formimino – CHNH, methenyl – CH=, or methylene – CH$_2$) bonded to the N5 and/or N10 nitrogen atom
- most are conjugated with a series of glutamate residues, and are known as folate polyglutamates; only folate monoglutamates can pass across cell membranes, so the extra glutamate residues must be stripped off before intestinal absorption can occur

The role of folate within the body

The various forms of folate function as single-carbon group donor–acceptors in a variety of linked biosynthetic reactions. Among them are:

- **synthesis of methionine** from homocysteine involves donation of the methyl group from *N*-5-methylTHF and requires methylcobalamin as a co-enzyme
- **pyrimidine synthesis** – the methylation of dUMP to dTMP is the rate-limiting step in DNA synthesis and requires *N*-5,10-methyleneTHF as a co-enzyme

- **purine synthesis** requires the presence of *N*-5,10-methyleneTHF or *N*-10-formylTHF as co-enzymes
- **conversion of serine into glycine** involves THF acting as *acceptor* of a single-carbon group, becoming *N*-5,10-methyleneTHF in the process
- **histidine catabolism** involves its conversion into *N*-formiminoglutamic acid (FIGLU) and subsequent conversion into glutamate by donation of the formimino group to THF.

Daily folate requirements and body stores

Losses of folate amount to about 100 μg per day, mainly via faeces, urine, sweat and desquamated skin cells. Faeces contain a relatively large amount of both vitamin B_{12} and folate but these represent the biosynthetic activities of the gut flora rather than losses from body stores. Thus, the normal adult daily requirement for folate is about 100 μg.

Folates are present to some extent in most foods but liver, eggs, some leafy vegetables, whole grains, some nuts and yeast are particularly rich sources. However, many common foods, including root vegetables, grains and muscle meat contain low levels of folate, which means that dietary choices are an important determinant of folate intake. A typical UK mixed diet may contain as much as 700 μg of folate per day. Folate in food is extremely sensitive to heat: cooking can reduce the folate content of food by as much as 95%.

Typical body stores of folate in a normal, healthy adult are about 10 mg and are located mainly in the liver. Thus, if dietary folate intake or intestinal absorption ceased, the body stores would become exhausted in less than four months.

Folate absorption and transport

Folates are absorbed maximally from the upper jejunum. Folate polyglutamates in food must be digested by the enzyme γ-glutamyl conjugase to form monoglutamates before they can be absorbed efficiently. Absorbed folates are converted within the jejunal mucosal cells into *N*-5-methyltetrahydrofolate monoglutamate and released into the portal bloodstream. Plasma folate circulates freely or loosely bound to a variety of plasma proteins. Once inside the developing blood cell, *N*-5-methyltetrahydrofolate is converted to tetrahydrofolate and reconjugated to the polyglutamate form. Conjugation facilitates the metabolic activities of folates and prevents leakage back into the plasma.

Role of vitamin B_{12} and folate in DNA and RNA synthesis

Synthesis of DNA and RNA requires a ready supply of the purines adenosine-5′-diphosphate (ADP) and guanosine-5′-diphosphate (GDP) and the pyrimidines cytidine-5′-diphosphate (CDP) and uridine-5′-diphosphate (UDP) as shown in *Figure 5.1*.

Folates are essential for optimal DNA and RNA synthesis: it is the cycling of folic acid between its various co-enzyme forms that unifies the seemingly disparate biochemical reactions in which vitamin B_{12} and folic acid are involved within the body (*Figure 5.2*; see also *Box 5.4*).

The folate taken up by dividing cells, *N*-5-methyltetrahydrofolate, cannot be conjugated with glutamate. First, it must donate its methyl group to homocysteine, a reaction that requires methylcobalamin as co-enzyme. In the absence of methylcobalamin, absorbed folate cannot be converted to a metabolically active form, a phenomenon known as the methyltetrahydrofolate trap. Further, in the absence of *N*-5,10-methylene THF the critical conversion step of dUMP to dTMP cannot take place. Thus, deficiency of vitamin B_{12} and/or folate results in failure of DNA synthesis and the development of megaloblastic anaemia.

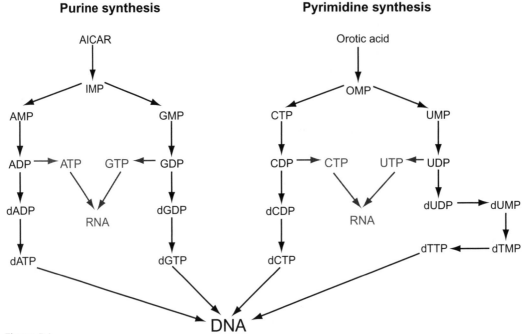

Figure 5.1
DNA and RNA synthesis.

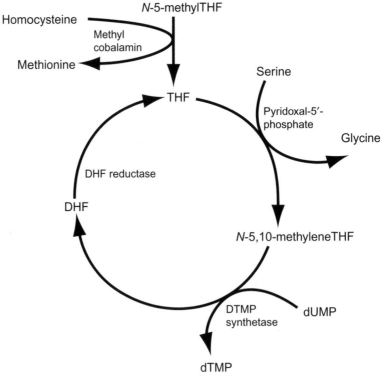

Figure 5.2
Cycling of folic acid between its various co-enzyme forms.

> **Box 5.4 Bases, nucleosides and nucleotides**
>
> Purines and pyrimidines such as adenine, guanine, cytosine, uracil, thymine and orotic acid are bases. The attachment of a sugar group (ribose or deoxyribose) to one of the nitrogen atoms of a base results in the formation of a nucleoside, e.g. adenine converts to adenosine and uracil converts to uridine. The addition of one or more phosphate groups to a nucleoside results in the formation of a nucleotide, e.g. adenosine diphosphate (ADP). The monophosphate form of a nucleotide can be designated as an *-ylic* acid, e.g. UMP is also known as uridylate. Nucleotides that contain a deoxyribose group are designated with a *d,* e.g. dTMP.

5.3   MEGALOBLASTIC ANAEMIAS

The term megaloblastic anaemia relates to a group of disorders of haemopoiesis characterized by retardation of DNA synthesis but a normal rate of RNA synthesis (see *Box 5.5*). These disorders show distinctive morphological and biochemical features that reflect the resulting asynchrony between nuclear and cytoplasmic maturation in developing cells. All dividing cells of the body are affected: anaemia is but one of a wide range of manifestations of the megaloblastic anaemias. Most megaloblastic anaemias are caused by a deficiency of vitamin B_{12} or folic acid.

> **Box 5.5 Megaloblasts**
>
> The term megaloblast means 'large immature cell' and is derived from the abnormally large erythroid precursor cells (megaloblasts) that are the hallmark of vitamin B_{12} and folate deficiency. The morphological abnormalities seen in these cells and the macrocytic red cells they produce are related to the fundamental biochemical abnormality of retarded DNA synthesis in the presence of normal RNA synthesis and function. This asynchrony results in the appearance of an immature nucleus in the presence of a relatively mature cytoplasm in terms of haemoglobinization. It also means that full haemoglobinization and nuclear condensation and loss occur in cells that have undergone fewer cell divisions and so are larger than normal, i.e. they are macrocytic and normochromic (see *Figure 3.3*).

Vitamin B_{12} deficiency

Deficiency of vitamin B_{12}, in common with deficiency of all nutrients, can result from inadequate dietary intake, intestinal malabsorption, increased requirements which cannot be met from the diet, or failure of utilization of absorbed vitamin (see also *Box 5.6*).

Inadequate dietary intake

Deficiency of vitamin B_{12} attributable solely to inadequate dietary intake is uncommon for three main reasons:

■   vitamin B_{12} is present in a wide range of readily available foodstuffs

> **Box 5.6 Diurnal variation**
>
> The value of many haematological parameters fluctuates in an individual during the course of the day. This phenomenon is entirely normal and is known as diurnal variation. The haemoglobin concentration and red cell count tend to be higher in the morning than in the evening. The platelet count and neutrophil count peak in the middle of the afternoon. The eosinophil count is at its lowest in the late morning and peaks just after midnight. Interestingly, these trends are reversed in night-shift workers.

- vitamin B_{12} is relatively heat-stable: cooking does not destroy it
- body stores of vitamin B_{12} are sufficient to meet the needs of the body for at least three years

Dietary deficiency of vitamin B_{12} is restricted to vegans, who eschew all animal and dairy products. Inadequate diet, however, frequently contributes to the development of vitamin B_{12} deficiency that is attributable mainly to other causes.

Malabsorption of vitamin B_{12}

Malabsorption of vitamin B_{12} is the most common cause of deficiency. A wide range of abnormalities exist that cause malabsorption of this vitamin:

- lack of intrinsic factor
- gastrointestinal disease
- drug-induced malabsorption

Lack of intrinsic factor. The most common cause of vitamin B_{12} deficiency in northern Europeans is pernicious anaemia (PA), which is characterized by achlorhydria and a failure of gastric parietal cells to synthesize intrinsic factor (see *Box 5.7*). The disease is uncommon below the age of 45 years, is more common in women than in men, and shows an association with blood group A and premature greying of the hair.

Cytotoxic IgG antibodies directed against gastric parietal cells or intrinsic factor are present in the serum of about 90% of people with PA. In about 75% of these cases, the antibody is also present in gastric juice. These anti-IF antibodies act in one of two ways:

- preventing binding of vitamin B_{12} to IF (type I antibody)
- inhibiting absorption of the IF:B_{12} complex (type II antibody); type II antibodies are only found in association with type I antibodies

About 30% of close relatives of people with PA also have anti-parietal cell antibodies in their serum but do not necessarily develop the disease. PA is associated with an increased incidence of other autoimmune diseases, both in the affected individual and in his/her family.

Congenital deficiency of IF or synthesis of a dysfunctional form of IF typically presents as a severe vitamin B_{12} deficiency. These conditions have sometimes, incorrectly, been called juvenile PA.

Gastrointestinal disease. Of this group of causes of vitamin B_{12} deficiency, the most obvious follows surgical removal of the source of intrinsic factor or the site of absorption of the vitamin.

- **Total gastrectomy** is associated with depletion of the vitamin B_{12} body stores. If vitamin B_{12} supplements are not given to these patients, megaloblastic anaemia develops within 5 years. The anaemia is frequently complicated by iron deficiency that also commonly follows gastrectomy.

Box 5.7 History of pernicious anaemia

In 1855, Thomas Addison first described a severe anaemia of unknown cause but uniformly fatal outcome and named it pernicious anaemia. The first real progress in the treatment of PA did not come for another 70 years when George Minot showed that the inclusion of 300 g of lightly cooked liver in the daily diet elicited a reticulocyte response and partial recovery of the haemoglobin concentration.

We now know that eating large amounts of liver provides massive doses of vitamin B_{12}, which are absorbed from the gut by passive diffusion. Modern therapy consists of regular injections of hydroxocobalamin.

■ **Partial gastrectomy** involves removal of part of the stomach and refashioning the junction with the gut, creating an afferent blind loop of gut, which becomes heavily colonized by bacteria. The vitamin B_{12} that these bacteria require for growth and metabolism is extracted from the gut, leading to reduced availability of the vitamin in the terminal ileum. This malabsorptive state is known as stagnant or blind loop syndrome. Bacterial overgrowth also occurs in ileal diverticulae, with similar results.

Because of advances in the pharmacological treatment of gastric, peptic and duodenal ulcers, total and partial gastrectomy are performed much less often than in the past.

Ileal resection or ileostomy involving removal or bypass of the terminal ileum (and so loss of the site of absorption) predisposes strongly to the development of vitamin B_{12} deficiency.

Generalized malabsorption of nutrients from the diet is a feature of intestinal disorders such as Crohn's disease (regional ileitis). Crohn's disease typically affects young adults in developed countries and leads to severe inflammation of the terminal ileum and ascending colon. Haematological complications of Crohn's disease include malabsorption of iron, folic acid and vitamin B_{12} leading to iron deficiency and megaloblastic anaemia. Chronic bleeding of the inflamed ileal mucosae frequently exacerbates the anaemia.

In contrast to the generalized malabsorptive states, Imerslund–Gräsbeck syndrome is characterized by selective malabsorption of the IF:B_{12} complex by the ileal mucosae due to deficiency of either cubilin or amnionless. The condition is inherited as an autosomal recessive trait and presents as the development of megaloblastic anaemia due to vitamin B_{12} deficiency once the body stores accumulated *in utero* are exhausted.

Infestation of the gut with the fish tapeworm *Diphyllobothrium latum* is acquired by eating infected raw fish. If the parasite lodges in the upper gastrointestinal tract, it is capable of extracting substantial quantities of vitamin B_{12}, both complexed with intrinsic factor and as free vitamin, from ingested food, thereby reducing the amount available for absorption.

Drug-induced malabsorption. A number of drugs have been reported to impair absorption of vitamin B_{12}, including the anticonvulsant phenytoin, the aminoglycoside antimicrobial agent neomycin, colchicine which is used in high doses in the treatment of gout and, most commonly, alcohol. Withdrawal of the drug usually reverses the malabsorption.

Increased requirements

The requirement for vitamin B_{12} is increased during pregnancy because of the expansion of the blood volume and the fetal requirement (see also *Box 5.8*). The increase is not sufficient to cause deficiency of vitamin B_{12} in a woman with normal stores prior to conception. It can, however, precipitate deficiency in a woman with previously borderline body stores of the vitamin. If a woman is severely vitamin B_{12} deficient throughout pregnancy, her baby is likely to have deficiency of the vitamin at birth, a situation seen most commonly in the Third World.

Box 5.8 Reference values

The reference ranges for vitamin B_{12} and folate are as follows:
Serum vitamin B_{12}
   170–1000 pg/ml
Serum folate
   3–25 ng/ml
Red cell folate
   145–600 ng/ml packed RBC

Failure of utilization

Failure of vitamin B$_{12}$ transport. Congenital deficiency of transcobalamin II is characterized by the development of severe megaloblastic anaemia in the first weeks of life, despite the presence of a normal serum concentration of vitamin B$_{12}$ and normal body stores of the vitamin. Early diagnosis is vital or severe neurological damage may result. Treatment requires very large doses of vitamin B$_{12}$ by intramuscular injection.

Failure of vitamin B$_{12}$ metabolism. A small number of examples of congenital failure to convert absorbed vitamin B$_{12}$ to its active co-enzyme forms have been described. Affected individuals fail to thrive and are mentally retarded. Only a minority of such cases develop megaloblastic anaemia, however.

Prolonged exposure to the anaesthetic nitrous oxide can induce megaloblastic change by inactivating vitamin B$_{12}$ co-enzymes due to oxidation of the central cobalt ion to the Co(II) state. Chronic exposure has been suggested as the cause of a mild neuropathy that has been described in dental surgeons, midwives and other professionals at risk of occupational exposure.

Folic acid deficiency

Deficiency of folic acid can result from an inadequate diet, intestinal malabsorption, increased requirements or failure of utilization of absorbed vitamin.

Inadequate dietary intake

Nutritional deficiency of folic acid is relatively common for four main reasons:

- the ideal UK diet contains about 700 μg of folate of which about half is absorbed; the daily requirement for folate is about 100 μg;
- folate is very heat-labile: cooking can destroy up to 90% of the folate present in food;
- body stores of folate are only sufficient to last about 3 months;
- many common (staple) foods are low in folate.

Folate deficiency can develop rapidly where dietary intake is suboptimal, either because folate-rich foods are lacking from the diet or because of losses during cooking. An inadequate diet is often a contributory factor in the development of folate deficiency due to malabsorption or where the requirement for folate is increased.

Intestinal malabsorption

Intestinal malabsorption is a common cause of folate deficiency. The most common cause of malabsorption of folate in the UK is coeliac disease, which has an incidence of about 1 in 2000. This disease is characterized by intolerance of gluten in the diet, atrophy of intestinal villi and malabsorption of iron and folate from the duodenum and jejunum. The cause of coeliac disease is autoimmune, but withdrawal of gluten from the diet reinstates jejunal absorption of iron and folate.

Tropical sprue is a similar condition to coeliac disease that is most common in the West Indies, the Indian subcontinent and in SE Asia. The cause of the disease is unknown but malabsorption of folate is commonly present. Crohn's disease commonly causes folate deficiency, especially where the jejunum and upper ileum are involved. Surgical causes of folate malabsorption include ileal resection where the site of maximal absorption of folate is removed.

Increased requirement

Deficiency of folic acid is especially common in pregnancy because dietary intake often fails to meet the increased demand for folate imposed by the growth of maternal blood volume and the developing fetus. The daily requirement for folate can rise to 500 μg in the third trimester of pregnancy. In the absence of folate supplementation, about 60% of pregnant women have subnormal plasma concentrations of folate. Folate deficiency is commonly accompanied by iron deficiency in pregnancy. Because of the recently demonstrated association between folate deficiency in pregnancy and fetal neural tube defects, folic acid supplementation starting several months before conception is widely recommended. Prophylactic iron therapy may be given at the same time.

As described in *Chapter 7*, the compensatory increase in the rate of haemopoiesis in chronic haemolytic conditions imposes a sustained excess demand for folate. The rate of haemopoiesis can be increased by up to a factor of ten in severe haemolytic conditions. When the increased demand for folate that this massively increased haemopoietic activity imposes exceeds the amount available from dietary sources, the development of folate deficiency is inevitable.

Drug-induced folate deficiency

A number of drugs have been reported to cause functional folate deficiency by interfering with folate absorption or metabolism (see *Box 5.9*). With some drugs, the antifolate effect is desired, while in others it is an unwanted side effect. For example, long-term therapy with the anticonvulsant drug phenytoin is associated with the development of folate deficiency due to impaired intestinal absorption of folate. Alcohol is also thought to inhibit folate absorption and metabolism, although the most common cause of folate deficiency in alcoholics is inadequate dietary intake.

The cytotoxic drug methotrexate is an example of a drug that is used specifically for its antifolate properties. It is a close structural analogue of folic acid and acts as a powerful competitive inhibitor of the enzyme dihydrofolate reductase. Ingestion of methotrexate rapidly causes intracellular deficiency of folate co-enzymes and depletion of thymidine and purine nucleotides. Methotrexate is used in the treatment of leukaemia.

Failure of utilization

Failure of folate metabolism. A number of rare enzyme deficiencies have been reported that cause impairment of folate metabolism. Most of these have been associated with megaloblastic anaemia and with some degree of mental retardation.

Box 5.9 Development of cytotoxic antifolates

The first cytotoxic drug to be effective in the treatment of leukaemia was a folate antagonist called *aminopterin*. In 1948, Sidney Farber reported that 10 of 16 children with acute leukaemia responded to treatment with this drug. These remissions were only temporary but represented an important step towards successful treatment of a hitherto intractable disease. Antimetabolites like methotrexate are still in common use in the treatment of leukaemia today.

5.4   CAUSES OF MEGALOBLASTIC ANAEMIA OTHER THAN HAEMATINIC DEFICIENCY

There are three main circumstances associated with megaloblastic change that are not attributable to deficiency of vitamin B_{12} or folic acid:

- ■ treatment with cytotoxic drugs
- ■ certain inborn errors of metabolism
- ■ association with other haematological disorders

Cytotoxic chemotherapy

Many of the cytotoxic drugs that are used in the treatment of malignant disease act by interfering with DNA synthesis. Four groups of cytotoxic drugs are associated with the induction of megaloblastic change of variable severity:

- inhibitors of pyrimidine synthesis such as 5-fluorouracil and 6-azauridine
- inhibitors of purine synthesis such as 6-mercaptopurine and 6-thioguanine
- inhibitors of enzymes required for DNA synthesis, e.g. hydroxyurea – this cytotoxic drug inhibits ribonucleotide reductase, an enzyme that controls the cellular concentration of deoxyribonucleotides
- folate antagonists such as methotrexate

Megaloblastic change secondary to inborn errors of metabolism

A small number of inborn enzyme disorders show megaloblastic change of varying severity along with other, more serious, clinical problems (see *Box 5.10*). Two examples, Lesch–Nyhan syndrome and hereditary orotic aciduria are described in *Box 5.10*.

Box 5.10 Inborn errors of metabolism

Deficiency of the purine salvage pathway enzyme HGPRTase (hypoxanthine–guanine phosphoribosyltransferase) causes Lesch–Nyhan syndrome, which is characterized by megaloblastic anaemia, hyperuricaemia, spasticity, mental retardation and self-mutilation. The disorder is very rare and shows an X-linked recessive pattern of inheritance.

Hereditary orotic aciduria results from a deficiency of either or both of the enzymes orotate phosphoribosyltransferase and orotidylate decarboxylase. This rare disorder of pyrimidine metabolism is associated with severe megaloblastic anaemia, growth retardation and excretion of large amounts of orotic acid in the urine. The anaemia is refractory to vitamin B_{12} or folic acid but responds well to the oral administration of uridine, which bypasses the enzyme block.

Megaloblastic change secondary to haematological disorders

Some degree of megaloblastic change is common in a wide range of malignant haematological disorders, e.g. in acute erythroleukaemia, the abnormal erythroblasts frequently show megaloblastic features in addition to the severe dysplasia which characterizes this disease.

Megaloblastic features are also common in pyridoxine-responsive sideroblastic anaemia. The biochemical basis for the megaloblastic change is unknown. One possible explanation lies with the fact that both pyridoxal-5′-phosphate and tetrahydrofolate are required as co-enzymes for the conversion of serine to glycine, an important step in haem synthesis.

Biochemical basis of megaloblastic change

An adequate supply of vitamin B_{12} and folate co-enzymes is essential for optimal DNA and RNA synthesis. The most significant effect of a deficiency of either of these vitamins is to reduce the rate of conversion of dUMP to dTMP, the rate-limiting step in DNA synthesis. The resulting asynchrony between DNA and RNA synthesis explains many of the morphological and biochemical features of megaloblastic anaemia.

Failure of dTTP synthesis results in an accumulation of dUTP relative to dTTP. DNA polymerases, the enzymes responsible for assembly of DNA from deoxynucleoside triphosphates, are unable to distinguish between dTTP and dUTP. The relative paucity of dTTP results in the misincorporation of uracil into DNA instead of thymine. An enzyme called uracil-DNA-glycosylase recognizes the aberrant uracils and excises them. Normally, a series of other enzymes mediate the repair of the mutilated DNA by incorporating thymine in place of the excised uracil. However, when thymine is in short supply, suboptimal repair of DNA leads to fragmentation of the helical structure, impaired mitosis and premature cell death.

Pathophysiology

Individuals with megaloblastic anaemia typically display the physiological changes that are common to all types of anaemia, i.e. pallor, weakness, shortness of breath on exertion, light-headedness, palpitations and congestive cardiac failure. In some cases, loss of appetite, weight loss and gastrointestinal disturbances are also present. In addition to these non-specific changes, a range of signs that are strongly suggestive of megaloblastic change may be noted. These typically affect the tissues that are most rapidly dividing and are attributable to impaired mitotic function. They can be grouped under three headings:

- general tissue manifestations
- neurological manifestations
- haematological manifestations

General tissue manifestations

The effects of a deficiency of vitamin B_{12} or folate are manifest most clearly in rapidly dividing tissues such as bone marrow and epithelial cells. Disturbances of epithelial cell turnover are responsible for oral symptoms such as angular stomatitis (lesions at the corners of the mouth) and glossitis (inflammation and depapillation of the tongue). Disturbed epidermal growth promotes widespread melanin hyperpigmentation. Sterility can occur. A variety of non-specific chromosomal changes such as random breaks are common in megaloblastic tissue, almost certainly due to uracil misincorporation as described above.

Neurological manifestations

Early neurological manifestations of vitamin B_{12} deficiency include a tingling sensation or loss of the sense of touch in the feet and fingers. This may progress to spasticity and degeneration of the spinal cord. Once established, neurological damage is irreversible. The mechanism of neurological damage is not fully understood but is probably due to secondary deficiency of *S*-adenosylmethionine and/or secondary up-regulation of neurotoxic cytokines and down-regulation of neurotrophic factors. Some workers also believe that the accumulation of methylmalonyl CoA that occurs in vitamin B_{12} deficiency promotes the incorporation of branched chain fatty acids into myelin and leads to disturbed neurological function. Folate deficiency may specifically affect central monoamine metabolism and aggravate depressive disorders. It is critically important that patients with suspected B_{12} deficiency are not treated with folate alone because this can precipitate or exacerbate neurological damage.

Folate deficiency in pregnancy is associated with an increased incidence of neural tube defects such as spina bifida and anencephaly in the fetus. For this reason, folate supplementation is recommended prior to conception and throughout pregnancy.

Haematological manifestations

Morphological changes. Typically, the megaloblastic bone marrow is hypercellular, with an increase in erythropoietic activity being especially prominent. There is an increased proportion of immature forms of all cell lines, reflecting the premature death of cells in the process of development. This combination of increased production of blood cells and increased intramedullary cell death is known as ineffective haemopoiesis, and is responsible for the pancytopenia that characterizes this condition.

The distinctive changes in blood and bone marrow cell morphology that accompany megaloblastic anaemia are the result of asynchrony between nuclear and cytoplasmic development. Megaloblastic red cell precursors typically display retarded maturation of the nucleus relative to the cytoplasm. This is exemplified by the appearance of the late megaloblast, which features an open, lace-like chromatin network and a fully haemoglobinized cytoplasm. Circulating red cells are typically macrocytic but there is a marked variation in size and shape of individual cells. Macrocytosis results from a decrease in the number of cell divisions prior to loss of the nucleus and release into the circulation. In contrast to the macrocytes that accompany alcoholic liver disease, megaloblastic macrocytes are typically oval. Absolute reticulocytopenia is invariably present.

The twin abnormalities of megaloblastic leucopoiesis are the appearance of bizarre, giant metamyelocytes in the bone marrow and an increase in the average number of nuclear lobes in circulating granulocytes (see *Box 5.11*). Nuclear hypersegmentation probably results from structural abnormalities in the nuclear chromatin.

Morphological changes in megaloblastic megakaryocytes include an increase in cell size and failure to develop the characteristic cytoplasmic granulation. However, these changes are often difficult to detect.

Biochemical changes. The increased marrow cell turnover results in alterations in the biochemistry of the blood such as an increase in the concentrations of unconjugated bilirubin, lactate dehydrogenase and lysozyme. Bilirubin is one of the products of haemoglobin catabolism and so its accumulation in the blood reflects ineffective erythropoiesis. Similarly, the enzymes lactate dehydrogenase and lysozyme reflect ineffective erythropoiesis and ineffective leucopoiesis, respectively. These changes in blood biochemistry are augmented by the shortened lifespan of circulating blood cells that is invariably present in megaloblastic anaemia.

Vitamin B_{12} deficiency is accompanied by specific biochemical changes in the blood, including a rise in the plasma concentration of homocysteine and methylmalonate and a fall in the plasma concentration of vitamin B_{12}. Alterations in the plasma concentration of homocysteine occur early in vitamin B_{12} deficiency, and can be used as a sensitive marker of the condition. Folate deficiency is accompanied by a fall in red cell and plasma folate concentration.

Box 5.11 Neutrophil hypersegmentation

Peripheral blood neutrophils normally have between one and five nuclear lobes, with an average of 2.8. A right shift is present when the average number of nuclear lobes is significantly increased. In practice, a rigorous lobe count (Cooke–Arneth count) is seldom performed. The presence of more than 3% of five-lobed neutrophils is used as a sensitive and readily discernible alternative indicator.

The presence of a right shift is not a reliable indicator of megaloblastic anaemia. This change is also seen in iron deficiency, uraemia, infection and even as an inherited abnormality (Undritz anomaly).

Diagnosis of megaloblastic anaemia

There are a great many potential causes of megaloblastic anaemia and a wide range of clinical and laboratory features. All of the laboratory tests have limitations. A full diagnosis relies on recognition of the clinical and haematological markers described and careful selection and interpretation of testing procedures.

The most useful initial screening tests remain a full blood count, examination of a blood film and assay of vitamin B_{12} and folate in serum and folate in red cells to determine the presence of deficiency. The microbiological assay methods described earlier in this chapter have largely been replaced by radioisotopic methods in routine practice. However, the results of vitamin assays must be interpreted with caution. Some cases of vitamin B_{12} deficiency have apparently normal serum vitamin B_{12} levels, do not demonstrate macrocytosis and may not be symptomatic.

In cases of doubt, supplementary tests can help in the diagnosis. For example, assay of serum or plasma metabolites such as methylmalonic acid (raised in vitamin B_{12} but not folate deficiency), total homocysteine (raised in both vitamin B_{12} and folate deficiency) or cystathione (raised in both vitamin B_{12} and folate deficiency) may help to confirm deficiency. Interpretation of these tests requires careful consideration of the full clinical picture. Measurement of serum holotranscobalamin is a particularly sensitive marker of early (subclinical) vitamin B_{12} deficiency.

The deoxyuridine suppression test is based on the ability of deoxyuridine to suppress the incorporation of thymidine into thymidylic acid and DNA, which is dependent on the presence of metabolically active folate and vitamin B_{12}. Thymidine incorporation is impaired by vitamin B_{12} and/or folate deficiency. The test is performed using incubated marrow cells. If an abnormal result is obtained, the nature of the deficiency is determined by adding folate or cobalamin compounds *in vitro*, to determine if they will correct an abnormal result. The deoxyuridine suppression test is very sensitive, but obviously invasive and expensive to perform.

Discovery of the presence of vitamin B_{12} and/or folate deficiency is only part of the diagnosis: determination and treatment of the underlying cause is required to prevent recurrence or deterioration. Where PA is suspected, investigations may include tests for the presence of PA (measurement of the absorption of a test dose of radiolabelled vitamin B_{12} in the presence and absence of added intrinsic factor, assay of intrinsic factor levels in gastric juice, or immunological screening for antibodies against parietal cells or intrinsic factor). Gastrointestinal investigations such as duodenal and jejunal biopsy, barium meal, endoscopy, etc. are required where intestinal malabsorption is suspected. Specialized enzyme assays may be required in cases of congenital megaloblastic anaemia. In all cases, recording of dietary habits should be part of the investigation, because poor diet is commonly a contributory factor.

Other causes of macrocytic anaemia should form part of the differential diagnosis of megaloblastic anaemia including liver disease, alcoholism, thyroid deficiency, haemopoietic disorders such as myelodysplastic syndrome or aplastic anaemia, and pregnancy. Folate and/or vitamin B_{12} deficiency can often coexist with these conditions. Moderate reticulocytosis can lead to mistaken reporting of macrocytosis because reticulocytes are normally larger than mature red blood cells. Similarly, the red blood cells of neonates are normally larger than those of adults.

SUGGESTED FURTHER READING

Andres, E., *et al.* (2007) B_{12} deficiency: a look beyond pernicious anemia. *J. Fam. Pract.* **56:** 537–542.

Carmel, R. (2009) Megaloblastic anemias: disorders of impaired DNA synthesis. In: *Wintobe's Clinical Hematology* (Greer, J.P., *et al.*, eds), Vol. 1, pp. 1143–1172. Lippincott Williams and Wilkins, Philadelphia.

Kaferle, J. and Strzoda, C.E. (2009) Evaluation of macrocytosis. *Am. Fam. Physician,* **79:** 203–208.

Tamura, T. and Picciano, M.F. (2006) Folate and human reproduction. *Am. J. Clin. Nutr.* **83:** 993–1016.

Wickramasinghe, S.N. (2006) Diagnosis of megaloblastic anaemias. *Blood Rev.* **20:** 299–318.

SELF-ASSESSMENT QUESTIONS

1. Where are vitamin B_{12} and folate absorbed optimally?
2. Where are the main body stores of vitamin B_{12} and folate?
3. Why might severe folate deficiency be associated with breathlessness on exertion?
4. What effect do you think that surgical removal of the stomach would have on vitamin B_{12} absorption?
5. What effect does severe vitamin B_{12} deficiency have on folate utilization within the body?
6. Why is vitamin B_{12} deficiency in pregnancy uncommon in the developed world even when the daily requirement exceeds supply?
7. Why is folate deficiency common in pregnancy?
8. Why does assay of red cell folate give a better guide to folate status than assay of serum folate?
9. Which of the following statements are true?
   a. Dietary deficiency of vitamin B_{12} is common in the UK.
   b. Folate deficiency inhibits RNA synthesis.
   c. PA is an autoimmune condition.
   d. Methotrexate is an inhibitor of folate absorption.
10. Why does the plasma concentration of homocysteine rise in vitamin B_{12} deficiency?
11. Why are chromosomal breaks common in megaloblastic tissue?

CHAPTER	
6	

Inherited disorders of haemoglobin

Learning objectives

After studying this chapter you should confidently be able to:

■ **Outline the structure and biosynthesis of haemoglobin**
Although haem and globin syntheses occur separately within developing red cell precursors, their rates of synthesis are carefully coordinated to ensure optimal efficiency of haemoglobin assembly. Haem is synthesized to some extent in virtually all human tissues but the most important sites are the liver (for incorporation into cytochromes), muscle (for incorporation into myoglobin) and red cell precursors. Globins are all single chain polypeptides and their synthesis is under genetic control. Humans normally synthesize six different types of globin chains (α, β, γ, δ, ζ and ε) at different stages of life.

■ **Discuss the relationship between structures and function of haemoglobin**
The structure of haemoglobin is intimately related to its function as a transporter of oxygen and carbon dioxide. Each haemoglobin molecule is capable of carrying four oxygen molecules, one for each haem group. Among the most important facets of the structure:function relationship are the haem:haem interaction, the maintenance of iron in the Fe^{2+} state, the impact of pH, and the binding of 2,3-DPG to β-globin chains.

■ **Differentiate clearly between the thalassaemias and structural haemoglobinopathies**
The thalassaemias are inherited disorders of the *rate* of globin synthesis whereas structural haemoglobinopathies are disorders of globin structure. In practice, there is overlap between these because some structurally abnormal globins are synthesized at a reduced rate.

■ **Outline the pathophysiology of α and β thalassaemia**
The thalassaemias are among the most common single gene disorders in the world and are most common in malarial areas, demonstrating balanced polymorphism. They are characterized by reduced, or absent, synthesis of one or more globin chain type. The resultant imbalance in globin chain synthesis leads to ineffective erythropoiesis and a shortened red cell lifespan. The spectrum of clinical severity of the thalassaemias is very wide.

■ **Outline the classification of the structural haemoglobinopathies**
The alteration in molecular function induced by structural abnormality is dependent upon the position of the mutation and on the properties of the amino acids involved. Alterations to the amino acid sequence within areas important for normal function typically lead to predictable alterations in molecular behaviour. In general terms, the structural haemoglobinopathies can be classified according to the impact of their altered function as, for example, unstable or thalassaemia-like.

■ **Describe the pathophysiology of sickle cell disease**
The clinical consequences of haemoglobin S stem from its tendency to polymerize, forming long, rigid structures called 'tactoids', which cause contortion of the red cell into elongated and poorly deformable sickle shapes. Typically, heterozygotes are clinically normal but homozygotes can experience vaso-occlusive sickling crises, aplastic crises, acute splenic sequestration and are susceptible to bacterial infection. Co-inheritance of other haemoglobinopathies can influence the clinical course of this disease.

The haemoglobins are red globular proteins which have a molecular weight of about 64 500 and comprise almost one-third of the weight of a red cell. Their primary function is the carriage of oxygen from the lungs to the tissues. A vital secondary role is the facilitation of the reverse transportation of carbon dioxide. They also play a role in blood buffering. Over 400 different variants of haemoglobin have been described but all share the same basic structure of four globin polypeptide chains, each with a single prosthetic haem group.

6.1 HAEMOGLOBIN SYNTHESIS

Although haem and globin syntheses occur separately within developing red cell precursors, their rates of synthesis are carefully coordinated to ensure optimal efficiency of haemoglobin assembly.

Haem synthesis

Haem belongs to the class of pigments known as porphyrins. It is composed of four pyrroles linked by methene bridges, with each pyrrole being bound to a central ferrous ion (Fe^{2+}) as shown in *Figure 6.1* (see also *Box 6.1*). Haem is synthesized to some extent in virtually all human tissues but the most important sites are the liver (for incorporation into cytochromes), muscle (for incorporation into myoglobin) and red cell precursors.

The first step of haem synthesis is the rate-limiting reaction for the whole process and involves the combination of glycine and the succinic acid derivative succinyl Co-A to produce δ-aminolaevulinic acid (δ-ALA). The reaction is energy-dependent and occurs within the mitochondria. The catalyst for δ-ALA synthesis is the enzyme δ-ALA synthetase. The presence of free globin chains stimulates δ-ALA synthesis while the presence of free haem groups is inhibitory, thus providing a control mechanism for the rate of haem synthesis and its coordination with globin synthesis. Several co-factors are required for δ-ALA synthesis, including the vitamin B_6 derivative pyridoxal phosphate and the presence of free ferrous and copper ions. Synthesis of the enzyme δ-ALA synthetase is also inhibited by the presence of free haem, providing a further feedback inhibition mechanism.

Two molecules of δ-ALA condense asymmetrically to form a pyrrole called porphobilinogen (PBG) under the influence of the enzyme δ-ALA dehydrogenase and glutathione. This and subsequent reactions occur in the cytoplasm of the cell (see also *Box 6.2*).

The next step requires the synthesis of the porphyrin ring. The reactions involved in this process are extremely complex but can be summarized as the condensation of four PBG molecules to form the asymmetric cyclic tetrapyrrole uroporphyrinogen III (UPG III). Synthesis of UPG III requires the presence of two enzymes (uroporphyrinogen I synthetase and uroporphyrinogen III co-synthetase) and involves the formation of several short-lived intermediates.

UPG III is converted to co-proporphyrinogen III (CPG III) by decarboxylation of the acetate side chains under the influence of the enzyme uroporphyrinogen decarboxylase. CPG III

Box 6.1 Importance of cyclic tetrapyrroles

Cyclic tetrapyrroles are extremely important structures in the maintenance of life in all of its myriad forms. For example, haem is an essential component of the oxygen transporting proteins of animals (haemoglobin and myoglobin); chlorophyll is central to photosynthesis, which maintains plant life and acts as an important source of atmospheric oxygen; and vitamin B_{12} is essential for DNA synthesis.

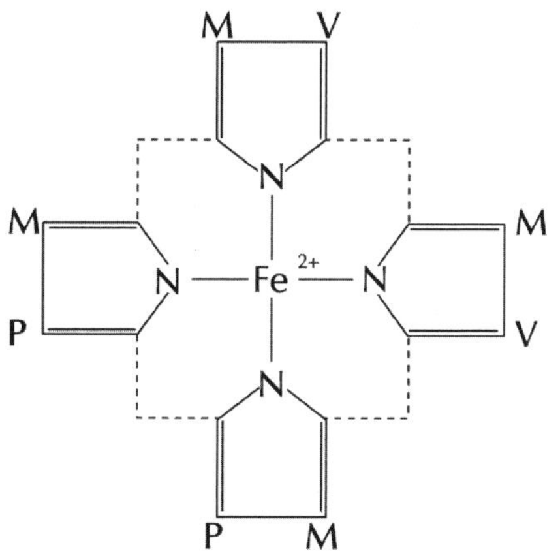

Figure 6.1
The structure of haem. M is a methyl group, V is a vinyl group, and P is a propionyl group.

Box 6.2 Porphyrias

The porphyrias are a group of inherited abnormalities of haem metabolism and are characterized by accumulation of intermediates of haem synthesis. One of the rarest forms, congenital erythropoietic porphyria, is associated with severe photosensitivity (exposure to sunlight must be avoided), scarring, excessive hair growth, deformity of the fingers and fingernails, reddish discoloration of the teeth and chronic haemolysis, and is associated with psychiatric disorder. The teeth and urine fluoresce under UV light. Some workers believe that the physical appearance and nocturnal habits of these unfortunate people could explain the popular legend of the werewolf, particularly since one of the best studied families, although from South Africa, can trace their ancestry to Transylvania! Alan Bennett's renowned play 'The Madness of George III', subsequently made into a memorable film, is based on the widely held belief that King George III of England was a sufferer. There have also been suggestions that porphyria may have been the cause of some of the aberrations of King James V of Scotland, and of his relative Mary, Queen of Scots.

---

enters mitochondria where it is converted to protoporphyrinogen IX (PPG IX) by an unknown mechanism. This reaction is catalysed by the enzyme co-proporphyrinogen oxidase. PPG IX is further converted within the mitochondria to protoporphyrin IX. It only remains for the central ferrous ion to be inserted to complete the synthesis of haem. This reaction is catalysed by the enzyme ferrochelatase and requires the presence of reducing agents. The synthesis of haem is depicted schematically in *Figure 6.2*.

Globin synthesis

The various globins that combine with haem to form haemoglobins are all single chain polypeptides and, in common with all other proteins, their synthesis is under genetic control. Humans normally carry eight functional globin genes, arranged in two duplicated gene clusters: the β-like cluster (β-, ^{G}γ-, ^{A}γ-, δ- and ε-globin genes) on the short arm of chromosome 11 and the α-like cluster (α1-, α2- and ζ-globin genes) on the short arm of chromosome 16 (see *Figure 6.3*). These genes code for seven different types of globin chains: α-, β-, ^{G}γ-, ^{A}γ-, δ-, ζ- and ε-globin. The genes in both clusters are arranged in the order of their expression during development. Functional haemoglobins all contain two α-like and two β-like globin chains.

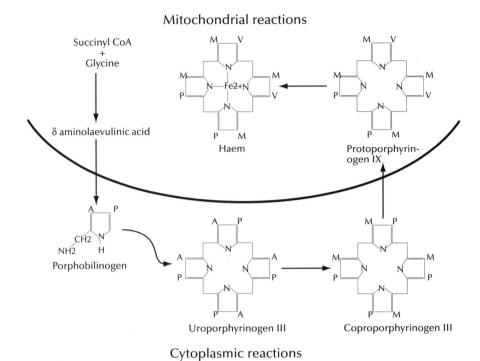

Figure 6.2
The synthesis of haem.

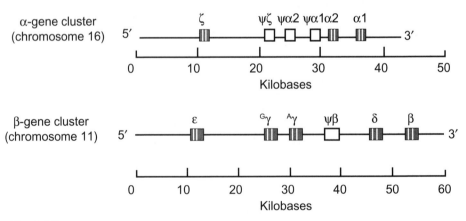

Figure 6.3
The α- and β-globin gene clusters.

Ontogeny of globin synthesis

Globin synthesis is first detectable in the primitive erythroid precursor of the yolk sac at about three weeks gestation. At this stage of development, the embryonic globin genes ζ and ε are synthesized, resulting in the formation of haemoglobin Gower I ($\zeta_2\varepsilon_2$). Activation of the α and γ genes occurs at about five weeks gestation when haemoglobin Portland ($\zeta_2\gamma_2$) and haemoglobin Gower II ($\alpha_2\varepsilon_2$) are synthesized. These three embryonic haemoglobins are undetectable by routine methods after about 10 weeks gestation. This is coincident with the end of the yolk sac phase of erythropoiesis.

As the rate of synthesis of ζ- and ε-globins decreases, that of α- and γ-globins increases sharply. Thus, the predominant haemoglobin for the remainder of fetal life is haemoglobin F ($\alpha_2\gamma_2$). The predominant form of γ-globin during fetal life is $^G\gamma$. At birth, approximately 50–80% of the haemoglobin content is haemoglobin F, although the rate of synthesis of γ-globin is by this time markedly reduced. Maximal synthesis of γ-globin coincides with the hepatic phase of fetal erythropoiesis.

Synthesis of β-globin begins at about the same time as α- and γ-globin but it remains a minor component until well into the third trimester of pregnancy. The sharp increase in synthesis of β-globin coincides with the establishment of the bone marrow as the main site of erythropoiesis. After birth, β-globin synthesis rapidly replaces γ-globin synthesis and by around six months 97% of the haemoglobin present is haemoglobin A ($\alpha_2\beta_2$) and haemoglobin F accounts for less than 1%. The predominant form of γ-globin during adult life is normally $^A\gamma$. There is no known physiological reason for the change from $^G\gamma$ to $^A\gamma$. The remaining 2–3% of haemoglobin consists of haemoglobin A_2 ($\alpha_2\delta_2$). δ-globin synthesis begins at about 30 weeks gestation but remains a minor component throughout life. The mechanism of switching from embryonic to fetal to adult globin chain synthesis is extremely complex and appears to involve a region known as the locus control region (LCR) and as yet incompletely understood epigenetic mechanisms. The relative rates of synthesis of the different globins throughout life are depicted in *Figure 6.4*.

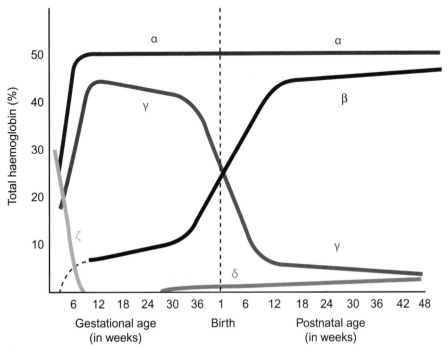

Figure 6.4
Changes in globin concentrations at different stages of life.

6.2 HAEMOGLOBIN STRUCTURE

Primary structure of globin

The primary structure of globin refers to the amino acid sequence of the various chain types. The position of individual amino acids is identified by numbering from the N-terminal end. Thus, the sixth amino acid from the N-terminal end of the β-globin chain is designated β^6. However, certain amino acids perform the same essential role in all normal globin chains. The identity and position of these amino acids cannot be changed without causing gross impairment to molecular function. Numbering according to primary sequence does not reveal the positional similarities of these so-called 'invariant amino acids', however.

Secondary structure of globin

The secondary structure of all globin chain types comprises nine non-helical sections joined by eight helical sections as shown in *Figure 6.5*. The helical sections are identified by the letters A–H while the non-helical sections are identified by a pair of letters corresponding to the adjacent helices, e.g. NA (N-terminal end to the start of A helix), AB (joins the A helix to the B helix), etc.

One complete turn of the helix requires between three and four amino acid residues. The amino acid side chains point outwards from the axis of the helix. This means that the side chains of amino acids which are in closest apposition, and therefore most likely to interact with each other, are not those of sequentially adjacent amino acids but of amino acids which are one turn of the helix apart. Individual amino acids can be identified according to their position in the secondary structure. This is a useful notation because invariant amino acids often appear in the same positions in all types of globin chain. For example, the α^{58} and β^{63} amino acids are both histidine residues, but their position in the primary structure provides no clue that their function may be related. However, both residues occupy the position E7 in the secondary structure of their respective globin chains. A histidine residue must always occupy this position because it is one of the two sites to which the haem group is bound (see also *Box 6.3*).

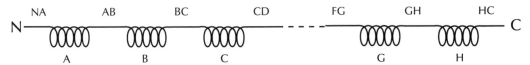

Figure 6.5
The secondary structure of globin.

Tertiary structure of globin

The tertiary folding of each globin chain forms an approximate sphere. The intra-molecular bonds that give rise to the helical parts of the chain impart considerable structural rigidity, causing chain folding to occur in the non-helical parts. Tertiary folding gives rise to at least three functionally important characteristics of the haemoglobin molecule, as follows:

■ Polar or charged side chains tend to be directed to the outside surface of the subunit and, conversely, non-polar structures tend to be directed inwards. The effect of this is to make the surface of the molecule hydrophilic and the interior hydrophobic.

Box 6.3 Key dates

1660	Air recognized as absolute requirement for life by Boyle
1777	Oxygen identified as vital component of air by Lavoisier
1848	Guinea pig haemoglobin crystallized
1864	Name haemoglobin coined and oxygen binding capacity demonstrated by Hoppe–Seyler
1894	Hüfner demonstrated haemoglobin oxygen capacity of 1.34 ml O_2/g Hb
1913	Suggestion that haem is a cyclic tetrapyrrole
1929	Synthesis of protoporphyrin by Fischer
1946–60	Elucidation of haem biosynthetic pathway
1960	Elucidation of structure of haemoglobin by Perutz using X-ray crystallography
1978	β-globin gene cloned
1978–present	Rapid advances in understanding of molecular biology of globin synthesis and abnormal haemoglobins

■ An open-topped cleft in the surface of the subunit known as the haem pocket is created. Each globin subunit has one haem pocket in which a single haem group is bound. Within this hydrophobic cleft, the ferrous ion of the haem group is protected from the oxidative effects of water, which would destroy its oxygen-binding capability.

■ The amino acids that form the inter-subunit bonds responsible for maintaining the quaternary structure, and thus the function, of the haemoglobin molecule are brought into the correct spatial orientation to permit these bonds to form.

Quaternary structure of haemoglobin

The quaternary structure of haemoglobin has four subunits arranged tetrahedrally as shown in *Figure 6.6*. The structure of haemoglobin is often written as '$\alpha_2\beta_2$', but this is misleading because the structure is that of a double dimer, so the more correct formula should be '$(\alpha\beta)_2$'. Each dimer is held together very firmly and inflexibly by strong inter-subunit bonds involving over 30 amino acid residues, which impart stability. The area of contact is known as the $\alpha_1\beta_1$ or $\alpha_2\beta_2$ junction. $\alpha\beta$ dimers have a limited ability to exist separately and a small proportion of all normal haemoglobin exists in this dissociated form.

The $\alpha_1\beta_2$ and $\alpha_2\beta_1$ contact areas that hold the tetramer together are much less tight than the $\alpha_1\beta_1$ and $\alpha_2\beta_2$ contact areas. The $\alpha_1\beta_2$ and $\alpha_2\beta_1$ contact areas involve less than 20 amino acid residues each, and it is across these junctions that the sliding, rotational molecular movements that accompany oxygen uptake and release occur.

There are two other areas of contact between globin subunits in the haemoglobin tetramer, i.e. the $\alpha_1\alpha_2$ and the $\beta_1\beta_2$ contact areas. Bonding at these contact areas is, of necessity,

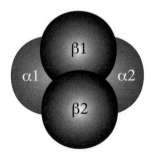

Figure 6.6
The quaternary structure of haemoglobin.

considerably weaker than at the other contact areas. In deoxyhaemoglobin, the two β chains are too far apart for bonding to occur, and a functionally significant area, the β cleft, is created. It is in this cleft that 2,3-DPG binds. On oxygenation, however, the whole molecule contracts and the β cleft disappears as the two chains move very close together, and 2,3-DPG is ejected. Weak interaction between the β chains is possible in this state. Strong bonding would interfere with oxygen release because deoxygenation involves the two β chains separating again. Conversely, the two α chains are some distance apart in the oxygenated state and move closer together on deoxygenation when weak interaction is possible; strong bonding between α chains would inhibit oxygenation.

6.3   HAEMOGLOBIN FUNCTION

Haemoglobin oxygen binding

Each haemoglobin molecule is capable of carrying four oxygen molecules, one for each haem group. The ferrous (Fe^{2+}) ions at the centre of each haem molecule are capable of forming six covalent bonds using electrons in their outer shell (see *Box 6.4*). Four of these bonds bind to the nitrogen atoms of the four pyrrole groups and the remaining two bind to invariant histidine residues in the attached globin chain. The distal histidine (E7) residue binds closely, but the distance between the proximal histidine (F8) and the ferrous ion is large enough to permit the insertion of a single oxygen molecule. It is important that the iron in the haem is maintained in the ferrous state. If it is oxidized to the ferric (Fe^{3+}) form, the ion can only form five bonds and oxygen cannot be bound. This form is known as methaemoglobin.

Oxygenation of haemoglobin is associated with considerable movement within the molecule. In the deoxygenated state, the central ferrous ions of the four haem groups are too large to fit into the plane of their porphyrin rings without causing severe distortion of the optimal ring structure. Oxygenation of the first haem group causes distortion of the electron cloud of the ferrous ion and facilitates the assumption of a truly planar configuration. Movement of the ferrous ion into the plane of the porphyrin ring pulls the attached α-globin chain inwards, thereby reducing the width of the haem pocket and allowing the haem group to tilt from its upright, deoxygenated position.

Movement of the first α-globin chain pulls on the other globin chains and causes a conformational change in the whole haemoglobin molecule, which results in increased oxygen affinity. As each haem group is oxygenated, reduction in the size of its haem pocket induces further conformational change, which further increases the oxygen affinity of the molecule. This process, whereby the sequential oxygenation of haem groups has an effect on the subsequent oxygenation of the others is known as haem–haem interaction, and is an important feature of normal haemoglobin function.

Box 6.4 Iron chemistry

Iron is a transition metal with atomic number 26. The electrons in an atom of iron are arranged as $1s^2\ 2s^2\ 2p^6\ 3s^2\ 3p^6\ 3d^6\ 4s^2$. The ferrous ion ($Fe^{2+}$) is formed by the loss of the two $4s$ electrons. This leaves six electrons in the outer shell that can form covalent bonds. Thus the ferrous ion in haem can bond as described in the text and is capable of binding oxygen. Ferric ions (Fe^{3+}) are formed by loss of one of the $3d$ electrons, leaving only five electrons available for covalent bonding. Thus the ferric ions in methaemoglobin bond with the four pyrrole nitrogen atoms and the distal histidine residue at E7. It cannot bind to the proximal histidine at F8 or to oxygen.

In the process of complete oxygenation, the diameter of the haemoglobin molecule is reduced by about 10%. Molecular compaction makes the binding of an oxygen molecule to the fourth haem group difficult despite the high oxygen affinity of this binding site. The 'effort' required to oxygenate the four haem groups of a typical haemoglobin molecule is depicted graphically in *Figure 6.7a*. Oxygenation of the first haem group requires the greatest effort but haem–haem interaction ensures that oxygenation of the second and third haem groups is made progressively easier. Steric hindrance caused by molecular compaction makes oxygenation of the last haem group more difficult than expected.

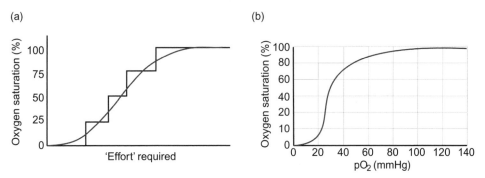

Figure 6.7
(a) 'Effort' required to sequentially oxygenate the four haem groups of a single molecule of haemoglobin.
(b) The haemoglobin:oxygen dissociation curve.

The derivation of *Figure 6.7a* is clearly hypothetical and simplistic. Oxygenation is an integrated process, involving all four subunits acting in concert. It is the whole molecule that oxygenates or releases oxygen, not the individual subunits. For this reason, each haemoglobin molecule exists only in the fully oxygenated or fully deoxygenated states. Based on the free energy required or generated as the transition between them occurs, the fully deoxygenated and fully oxygenated conformations are known as 'tense' (T) and 'relaxed' (R) forms of haemoglobin respectively.

Exposure of a haemoglobin solution to increasing partial pressures of oxygen results in an increasing proportion of haemoglobin molecules that exist in the fully oxygenated (R) form. The relationship between partial pressure of oxygen and the degree of oxygen saturation it causes is shown graphically in *Figure 6.7b*. This curve is known as the haemoglobin:oxygen dissociation curve and characteristically is sigmoidal in shape (see also *Box 6.5*). The shape of the curve for a range of saturation from around 5% to 95% can be represented mathematically by a complex equation known as the Hill equation, but at either extremity the curve can only be defined empirically.

Box 6.5 Myoglobin

The oxygen-carrying protein of muscle, myoglobin, consists of a single polypeptide chain with a single prosthetic haem group. Because it has no haem–haem interaction, the oxygen dissociation curve of myoglobin is hyperbolic rather than sigmoidal.

Oxygen delivery

The haemoglobin:oxygen dissociation curve shown in *Figure 6.7b* is of limited value as drawn because it is difficult to interpret in terms of oxygen carriage and delivery. The y-axis can be recalibrated to show the volume of oxygen carried per 100 ml of blood. Under physiological conditions, 100 ml of normal adult blood is capable of carrying a theoretical maximum of about 20 ml of oxygen (see *Box 6.6*).

Although the mean alveolar pO_2 of 100 mmHg is sufficient to saturate the oxygen-binding capacity of haemoglobin, for various physiological reasons, blood that enters the aorta typically carries only about 97% of the theoretical maximum quantity of oxygen, i.e. about 19.5 ml of oxygen per 100 ml of blood. When this oxygenated blood reaches the systemic capillaries where the pO_2 is typically about 40 mmHg, it is no longer in equilibrium with its environment and so releases about 4.5 ml of oxygen per 100 ml of blood to the tissues. This reduces the oxygen saturation of the haemoglobin to 75%. The partially deoxygenated blood is then transported back to the lungs where it will, again, encounter a mean pO_2 of 100 mmHg and start the cycle all over again with 19.5 ml of oxygen per 100 ml of blood. This chain of events is shown in *Figure 6.8a*.

The extra oxygen, which is apparently needlessly carried, acts as an instantly available reserve when oxygen demand increases. For example, when a muscle contracts oxygen utilization increases, causing a localized fall in pO_2. When blood arrives at the capillaries supplying that muscle, it encounters a pO_2 of, for example, 30 mmHg and is forced to give up more oxygen as it equilibrates. Because of the sigmoidal shape of the haemoglobin:oxygen dissociation curve, a small drop in partial pressure of oxygen causes a disproportionately large increase in oxygen donation. This chain of events is shown in *Figure 6.8b*.

Box 6.6 Oxygen binding capacity

The theoretical maximum oxygen binding capacity of 'normal blood' assumes a haemoglobin concentration of 14.6 g/dl. Since 1 g of haemoglobin can bind up to 1.34 ml of oxygen, it follows that 100 ml of normal blood can bind up to (1.34 x 14.6) ml of oxygen, i.e. about 20 ml. Obviously, if the haemoglobin concentration is higher or lower, the maximum oxygen binding capacity alters proportionately.

(a)

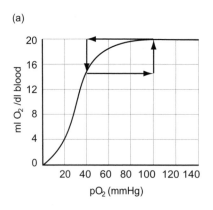

(b)

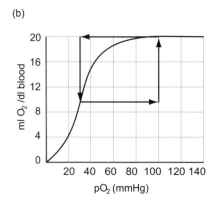

Figure 6.8
(a) Delivery of oxygen under normal physiological conditions.
(b) Increased delivery of oxygen in response to decreased tissue pO_2.

As shown in *Figure 6.8*, a reduced alveolar pO_2 of 70 mmHg would still result in about 90% haemoglobin saturation (around 18 ml O_2/dl blood). It is therefore extremely unlikely that, under normal atmospheric conditions, a sufficiently low alveolar pO_2 could ever arise which would reduce significantly the oxygen saturation of blood leaving the lungs. Indeed, breathing could cease altogether for a considerable time before an alveolar pO_2 of 70 mmHg was reached and, even then, the oxygen saturation of the arterial blood would be sufficient to meet the demands of the tissues for several minutes. Even when oxygen saturation reduces markedly, the maximum hypoxic effect on ventilation is less than double (see also *Box 6.7*). This means that oxygen saturation cannot be the driver for ventilation. The true principal driver is the pH of cerebrospinal fluid (CSF), which sensitively reflects systemic pH. Thus it could be said that the function of ventilation is the maintenance of brain pH; take care of that and, at sea level at least, oxygen will look after itself!

At rest, the typical cardiac output is about 5 litres of blood per minute. This is the minimum blood flow that meets the resting oxygen demand of the body. Since each 100 ml of blood delivers about 4.5 ml of oxygen, the resting, or basal, oxygen requirement is about 225 ml of oxygen per minute. Oxygen demand increases rapidly when activity exceeds the basal level. Failure to meet this increased demand by an appropriate increase in oxygen delivery severely limits performance. The necessary increase in oxygen delivery can be achieved by increased release of oxygen per 100 ml of blood, by increasing cardiac output, or both. In normal individuals these and other mechanisms ensure that oxygen delivery to the tissues is adequate over a wide range of activity levels.

When severe anaemia is present, increases in oxygen demand may be difficult to meet. The value of 20 ml of oxygen carried per 100 ml of blood assumes a normal haemoglobin concentration of 14.6 g/dl. If the haemoglobin concentration falls to, for example, 7 g/dl, maximal oxygen carriage falls to less than 10 ml per 100 ml of blood. Greater proportional donation of oxygen by the mechanism described above can still meet basal oxygen demands in this case, but a greatly increased cardiac output and respiration rate is required when activity levels rise. This is manifest as a normal heart rate at rest, but an exaggerated cardiorespiratory response to exercise: the degree of exaggeration is directly related to the severity of the anaemia. This gives rise to the classical signs of anaemia: shortness of breath on exertion and palpitations.

Box 6.7 Hypoxia and sport

Long distance runners often train at high altitude before an important race. Running in a reduced partial pressure of oxygen stimulates erythropoiesis which increases their oxygen carrying capacity and triggers a rise in red cell 2,3-DPG concentration which improves oxygen delivery to the tissues. These changes favour the prolonged effort required of distance runners, for a short time after they return to lower altitudes.

Carbon dioxide transport

Carbon dioxide is excreted via the lungs in exhaled air. It is transported from the tissues to the lungs in the blood in three forms, as follows.

- Approximately 78% is transported in the form of bicarbonate ions (HCO_3^-), formed by the ionization of carbonic acid (H_2CO_3). Carbonic acid is formed by the reaction of carbon dioxide and water, a reaction catalysed by the red cell enzyme carbonic anhydrase. Haemoglobin, acting as a buffer, is an important acceptor of the H^+ ions that are produced along with the HCO_3^- ions.

- Approximately 13% is transported bound to proteins as carbaminoproteins. About half of the total is bound to plasma proteins, principally as carbaminoalbumin, and the other half is bound intracellularly to globin chains as carbaminoglobins. The mechanism of carbon dioxide binding to globin is completely different to that of oxygen binding to haem. Carbon dioxide is acidic and therefore binds to the basic groups that are present on all proteins at physiological pH.
- Approximately 9% is transported in solution in plasma and cell water.

Haemoglobin oxygen affinity

The haemoglobin molecule must achieve two apparently contradictory functions, i.e. it must have a high enough affinity for oxygen to load up fully in the lungs, but have a low enough affinity to deoxygenate in the tissues (see also *Box 6.8*). A number of substances help to solve this dilemma by modulating the oxygen affinity of haemoglobin, e.g. carbon dioxide, bicarbonate ions (HCO_3^-), H^+ and 2,3-DPG.

The oxygen affinity of haemoglobin is affected by the presence of carbon dioxide in two ways:

- H^+ ions formed by the ionization of carbonic acid within the red cell bind preferentially to deoxyhaemoglobin, thereby favouring the deoxygenated form of haemoglobin
- carbon dioxide binds to basic amino groups at the N-terminal ends of deoxygenated α-and β-globin chains, again favouring the deoxygenated form; the effect of pH on haemoglobin oxygen affinity is much more important and is known as the Bohr effect.

This is a physiologically appropriate response because the pCO_2 and H^+ concentrations are relatively high in the tissues where pO_2 is relatively low, thereby maximizing oxygen donation to the tissues. In the lungs, pO_2 is high and pCO_2 and H^+ concentration are relatively low, thereby promoting expulsion of CO_2 from the haemoglobin and uptake of oxygen as shown in *Figure 6.9*.

One of the products of red cell glycolysis is 2,3-diphosphoglyceric acid (2,3-DPG), which binds to the β-globin chains of deoxygenated haemoglobin A (($\alpha\beta)_2$). One molecule of 2,3-DPG occupies the β cleft, and must be ejected before oxygenation can occur. Thus, the relatively high concentration of 2,3-DPG found in red cells decreases the oxygen affinity of haemoglobin A and improves oxygen delivery to the tissues. It is important to realize that, as far as 2,3-DPG is

---

Box 6.8 Adaptation

Animals that live only at high altitude such as Andean llamas typically have haemoglobins that have a high affinity for oxygen. This adaptation ensures maximum uptake of oxygen in the lungs, even at the low partial pressures of oxygen found at altitude. Llamas do not develop the raised red cell count that typifies the physiological response of humans at altitude.

Humans can meet the challenge of high-altitude life in three different ways as exemplified by indigenous Andean, Tibetan and Ethiopian high-altitude populations. Andean highlanders respond to the chronic hypobaric hypoxia at altitude by increasing the red cell count and [Hb]. This represents the normal physiological response to hypoxia. Ethiopian highlanders and Tibetans who live below 4000 m above sea level do not respond to hypoxia with an erythrocytosis. Tibetans typically have profoundly low oxygen saturation, and an arterial oxygen content about 10% lower than sea-level reference values. There is evidence for a genetically determined physiological adaptation that means Tibetans experience less physiological hypoxic stress under these conditions. Ethiopian highlanders typically have [Hb], oxygen saturation, and arterial oxygen content comparable to those of healthy sea-level populations. The mechanism underlying this observation has not been determined.

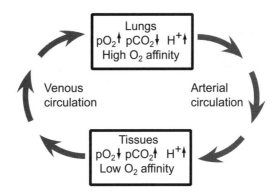

Figure 6.9
How physiological conditions in the lungs and tissues promote oxygen and carbon dioxide transport.

concerned, only two states can exist: either a molecule is bound to β-globin or it is not. Thus, there are only two physiological oxygenation states in which the haemoglobin A molecule is stable, either 100% saturated (no 2,3-DPG bound) or 0% saturated (2,3-DPG bound), all three intermediate states being unstable and, physiologically, extremely transient.

2,3-DPG binds avidly to β-globin, but not to other non-α-globins, since only β-globin chains have the required amino acids in the right position to bind 2,3-DPG. This means that haemoglobins that lack β-globin chains, such as haemoglobin F ($(\alpha\gamma)_2$) do not have to eject 2,3-DPG before oxygenating and thus have a higher oxygen affinity than haemoglobin A in the presence of 2,3-DPG. This increased oxygen affinity of haemoglobin F confers its ability to extract oxygen from maternal haemoglobin A at the placental barrier. However, the high oxygen affinity also means oxygen is released to the tissues somewhat less readily than in the adult. This does not present a problem because fetal activity levels are necessarily restricted and the excess oxygen demand that accompanies strenuous physical exercise does not arise.

6.4 INHERITED HAEMOGLOBIN DISORDERS

Haemoglobin disorders, or haemoglobinopathies, fall into two main types:

- the thalassaemias are disorders of the *rate* of globin synthesis; globin structure is normal in thalassaemia
- the structural haemoglobinopathies where globin *structure* is abnormal

Classification is not always straightforward, however, since many structurally abnormal globins are synthesized at a reduced rate and so do not fit clearly into either category.

The thalassaemias

The thalassaemias are characterized by reduced, or absent synthesis of one or more globin chain type (see also *Box 6.9*). The resultant imbalance of globin chain synthesis leads to formation of A or B tetramers rather than exclusively αβ dimers which causes ineffective erythropoiesis and a shortened red cell lifespan.

Box 6.9 Naming thalassaemia

The eminent haematologist George Whipple coined the name thalassaemia in 1932 as an alternative to the eponymous 'Cooley's anaemia'. He wanted a name that would convey the sense of an anaemia that is prevalent in the region of the Mediterranean Sea, since most of the early cases originated there. Thalassaemia is derived by contraction of thalassic anaemia (from the Greek *thalassa* - sea, *an* - none and *haima* - blood).

Classification

The thalassaemias are classified according to three criteria:

- the affected globin gene(s) e.g. α, β, $\delta\beta$, etc.
- whether the reduction in the rate of synthesis of the affected globin is partial (designated by a + superscript after the affected gene, e.g. β^+) or absolute (designated by a 0 superscript after the affected gene e.g. β^0)
- the genotype, i.e. homozygous, heterozygous or compound heterozygous, e.g. homozygous β^0

Incidence and distribution

The thalassaemias are among the most common single gene disorders in the world. They are most common in parts of the world where malaria is endemic because the heterozygous state affords some protection against malaria (see *Figure 6.10*). This phenomenon, where an apparently severely detrimental genetic abnormality persists because it confers a survival advantage is known as a 'balanced polymorphism'. The incidence of thalassaemia is also high in immigrant populations that originate in these parts of the world. The distribution of the different forms of thalassaemia is not uniform.

- β thalassaemia is most common in people from the Mediterranean, Africa, India, SE Asia and Indonesia. The incidence of β thalassaemia mutations is almost 10% in some parts of Greece.

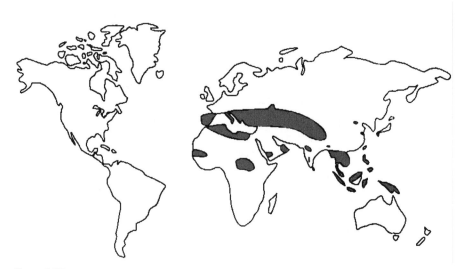

Figure 6.10
The worldwide distribution of the thalassaemias. The shaded area represents areas where the disease is most common, but it is found in most populations of the world.

■ α⁺ thalassaemia is most common in African-Americans and in people from Indonesia, SE Asia, the Middle East, India, the Mediterranean and the S. Pacific islands. 30% of African-Americans are 'silent' carriers of α⁺ thalassaemia, while about 3% are homozygous. Homozygotes express minimal symptoms of disease.

■ α⁰ thalassaemia is most common in people from the Philippines, SE Asia and southern China. The population incidence of deletions that lead to this form of α thalassaemia reaches 25% in some parts of Thailand.

α thalassaemia. Normal individuals carry four α-globin genes, two tandem pairs on the short arm of each chromosome 16. More than 95% of α thalassaemias result from the deletion of one or both of the tandem α-globin genes. This gives rise to six possible genotypes (see *Figure 6.11*):

Type	Genotype
Normal	αα/αα
α⁺ heterozygote (silent carrier)	α–/αα
α⁺ homozygote (α thalassaemia trait)	α–/α–
α⁰ heterozygote (α thalassaemia trait)	αα/––
α⁰ homozygote (Barts hydrops fetalis)	––/––
α⁰α⁺ double heterozygote (haemoglobin H disease)	––/α–

The frequencies of the different deletions that give rise to α thalassaemia vary widely in different races. Deletion of both α-globin genes on one chromosome 16 is relatively common in SE Asia and the Philippines, leading to a high incidence of haemoglobin H disease and haemoglobin Barts hydrops fetalis (see also *Box 6.10*). Conversely, the most common deletion in African-Americans is of only one α-globin gene: haemoglobin H disease is rare in this population and haemoglobin Barts hydrops fetalis exceedingly so.

β thalassaemia. Normal individuals carry two β-globin genes, one on the short arm of each chromosome 11. Most β thalassaemias result from a point mutation within or close to the

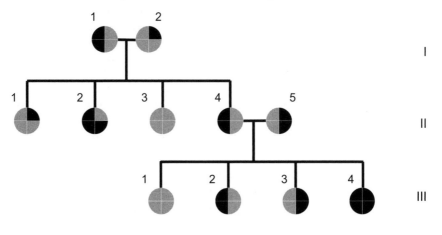

α thalassaemia gene

Normal α-globin gene

Figure 6.11
Pedigree chart of a typical family with α thalassaemia. The investigation was prompted by the stillbirth of baby III4.

Box 6.10 Classifying α thalassaemia

Because there are two α-globin genes on each chromosome 16, classification of the α thalassaemias relies on applying the synthesis rules to each *pair* of genes rather than each individual gene, e.g. deletion of one gene reduces but does not abolish α-globin synthesis by that pair of genes so α^+ thalassaemia results. The picture is complicated, however, by the fact that the two genes in each pair are not expressed equally. Normally, the α2 gene encodes most of the α-globin present. This means that identical mutations in the α2 and α1 genes would have differing impacts on total α-globin synthesis and so different clinical impact.

β-globin gene complex. Each mutation can result in a reduction or abolition of β-globin gene function and so to β^+ or β^0 thalassaemia. Therefore, the classification of β thalassaemia is similar to that for α thalassaemia:

Type	Genotype
Normal	$\beta\,/\beta$
β^+ heterozygote	β^+/β
β^+ homozygote	β^+/β^+
β^0 heterozygote	β^0/β
β^0 homozygote	β^0/β^0

Molecular basis

The classification scheme outlined above, although useful, greatly underestimates the complex nature of the relationship between genotype and phenotype in the thalassaemia syndromes. More than 100 different gene defects which cause thalassaemia have been described.

Gene deletion form – α thalassaemia. Most α thalassaemias result from gross deletions within the α-globin gene complex. At least nine deletions that result in complete abolition of α-globin synthesis have been described. Each is most closely associated with a particular population. For example, the most common deletions found in SE Asia are designated $--^{\text{SEA}}$, $--^{\text{FIL}}$ (Philippines) and $--^{\text{THAI}}$ (Thailand). Two deletions are common in the Mediterranean region and these are designated $--^{\text{MED}}$ and $--^{20.5}$ (see *Figure 6.12*). All of these deletions remove both α-globin genes on one chromosome and so result in an α^0 haplotype. Haemoglobin Barts hydrops fetalis is most common in those parts of the world where such deletions are prevalent. Deletions of only one α-globin gene have been described in many populations and are the most common deletions in α thalassaemia. Such deletions are denoted according to the size of the deleted region as shown in *Figure 6.13*. These deletions arise from unequal crossing-over of two chromosome 16s within the homologous α-globin gene complexes as shown in *Figure 6.14* (see also *Box 6.11*).

Box 6.11 Crossing-over

Crossing-over describes the reciprocal exchange of chromosomal material between homologous chromosome pairs during prophase I of meiosis. The exchange occurs when two chromatids align, break at corresponding locations, swap sides and rejoin. Unequal crossing-over occurs when the material swapped is of different length, and results in gene deletion on one chromosome and the acquisition of an extra gene on the other. As will be seen later in this chapter, the same mechanism is an important cause of some structurally abnormal haemoglobins.

Chromosomes with three α genes are relatively common in the populations in which these deletions are found. These represent the reciprocal $\alpha\alpha\alpha^{\text{anti3.7}}$ and the $\alpha\alpha\alpha^{\text{anti4.2}}$ formed during the process of unequal crossing-over. The extra α-globin gene in these cases is usually functional.

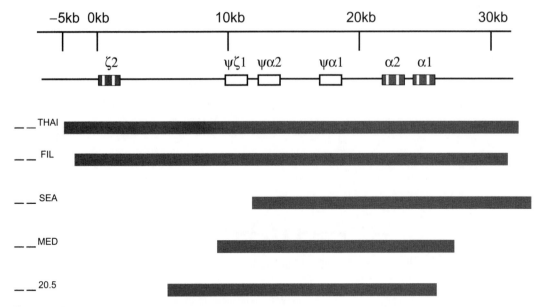

Figure 6.12
Gene deletions that result in α⁰ thalassaemia. The solid bars correspond to the extent of the deleted area for each type of deletion.

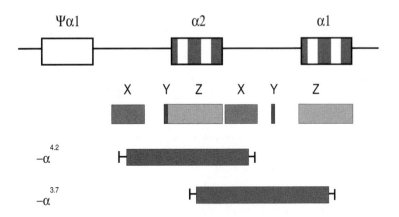

Figure 6.13
Gene deletions that result in α⁺ thalassaemia. The solid bars represent the extent of the deleted area for each type of deletion. The regions labelled X, Y and Z denote areas of homology that are hot spots for recombination events.

Gene deletion form – β thalassaemia. Several deletions that affect only the β-globin gene and result in β thalassaemia have been described, but all except one are extremely rare. About one-third of β thalassaemias from the Indian subcontinent result from deletion of a large part of the 3′ end of the β-globin gene. This mutation is most common in the Gujarati and Sind peoples.

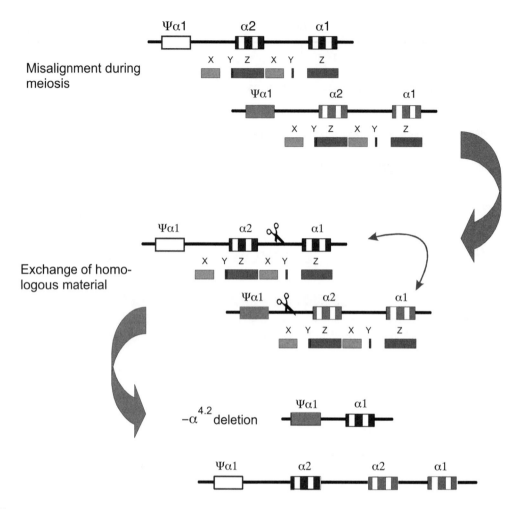

Figure 6.14
The process of unequal crossing-over that results in $-\alpha^{4.2}$ deletion.

Non-deletion forms. In contrast to α thalassaemia, most cases of β thalassaemia result from point mutations within or close to the β-globin gene. More than 200 different such mutations have been described. As well as mutations within the exons that code directly for β-globin, mutations of the promoter region, mRNA cap site, the 5′ untranslated region, the intron splice sites, the polyadenylation region, as well as within the introns themselves, have all been described as causing β thalassaemia. However, the distribution of mutations is non-random, with certain mutations having distinct geographic associations.

Mutations that do not lie within the β-globin introns can cause a thalassaemic phenotype in several ways, for example:

- they may impair gene transcription, resulting in reduced β-globin synthesis.
- mutations within the mRNA cap site or the polyadenylation region can lead to defective stabilization of transcribed β-globin mRNA, with consequent failure of β-globin synthesis.

■ defective splicing of the mRNA transcript due to mutations at the splice sites or within the intron means that functional β-globin cannot be synthesized.

Point mutations that result in an α thalassaemia phenotype are rare. Examples include:

■ a point mutation within the stop codon of the α2-globin gene (α2 codon 142 TAA→CAA) that leads to synthesis of a long chain unstable α-globin variant called Haemoglobin Constant Spring. This is one of a small family of similar chain extension abnormalities, all of which have an identical extra 31 amino acids, but which differ in the point mutation at 142.
■ mutation of α2 codon 125 (CTG→CCG) results in proline instead of leucine at this point in the α-globin and results in an extremely unstable variant called Haemoglobin Quong Sze.

Two rare forms of α thalassaemia exist that are associated with severe mental retardation and other characteristic clinical findings. These are caused by mutations of ATR genes on chromosome 16 or chromosome X. ATR-16 encodes the SOX8 transcription factor, while ATR-X encodes a protein that is involved in chromatin remodelling (see also *Box 6.12*).

Box 6.12 Key dates

1925	First clinical description by Cooley and Lee
1932	Name thalassaemia first coined by Whipple and Bradford; first published suggestion that thalassaemia is an inherited disease
1946	Demonstration of raised HbF level in β thalassaemia
1955	Demonstration of raised HbA₂ level in β thalassaemia; first description of HbH disease by Rigas
1958	First description of Hb Barts hydrops fetalis
1964	First use of α:β globin synthetic ratio by Weatherall
1970	First description of Hb Constant Spring
1978	β-globin gene cloned
1982–present	Rapid advances in knowledge of molecular genetics
1980	First antenatal diagnosis using linked RFLP
1982	Concept of haplotype analysis introduced
1987	First use of polymerase chain reaction in diagnosis of thalassaemia

---

Pathophysiology

The thalassaemia syndromes encompass a wide spectrum of clinical severity. The heterogeneity is further increased by the frequency of coincident inheritance of a structural haemoglobinopathy such as haemoglobin S (see also *Box 6.13*).

The myriad manifestations of this complex group of disorders can all be traced to a single cause, the imbalance of the synthesis of α-like and non-α-like globin chains. All normal mammalian haemoglobins are composed of two α-like and two non-α-like globin chains. Under normal circumstances, the rate of α-globin synthesis is matched by the total synthesis of β-, δ- and γ-globin chains. Impaired synthesis of α-globin results in the accumulation of unpaired non-α-globins within the developing erythroblast and vice versa. Unpaired globin chains are short-lived; they form aggregates and precipitate within the cell, causing membrane damage and selective removal of the damaged cell by the spleen.

Red cells possess mechanisms that block a moderate imbalance in globin chain synthesis through the action of the α haemoglobin stabilizing protein (AHSP), an abundant erythroid-specific protein that is induced by the transcription factor GATA-1 and forms a stable complex with free β-globin chains (see also *Box 6.14*). This mechanism of protection of erythroid cells,

---

Box 6.13 Malaria and inherited disease

The geographic distribution of the thalassaemias overlaps with that of sickle cell disease and G6PD deficiency. This is because carriage of these abnormal genes affords some protection against malaria. Thus, being heterozygous for one of these conditions offers a selective survival advantage and increases the opportunity for these genes to be passed on, another example of balanced polymorphism.

Box 6.14 Unpaired globin chains

Unpaired α-globin chains are extremely insoluble and cause severe damage to developing erythroblasts. Unpaired β-globin chains, on the other hand, form haemoglobin H, which is relatively stable and only precipitates as the red cell ages. Thus moderate impairment of β-globin synthesis is associated with a greater degree of ineffective erythropoiesis and haemolysis than an equivalent impairment of α-globin synthesis.

---

however, is insufficient to protect the cells when the globin chain synthesis is greatly unbalanced, as occurs in thalassemia.

α thalassaemia. Although α thalassaemia encompasses the complete spectrum of disease severity, affected individuals are considered to belong to one of four groups, according to the increasing severity of their symptoms:

- 'silent' carriers
- α thalassaemia trait
- haemoglobin H disease
- haemoglobin Barts hydrops fetalis

The groups correspond approximately to the *functional equivalent* of the deletion of 1, 2, 3 or 4 α-globin genes respectively. Thus, if a point mutation completely prevents expression of an α-globin gene, the result is equivalent to deletion of that gene. Similarly, the presence of two point mutations, which reduce the output of their respective genes to about 50% of normal, approximates to deletion of a single gene.

Silent carriers. Deletion of a single α-globin gene (heterozygous α^+ thalassaemia) has no significant effect on the well-being of the affected individual. In adults, no haematological abnormality can be demonstrated using standard laboratory techniques (i.e. excluding DNA analysis; see also *Box 6.15*). Blood drawn from the umbilical cord of newborns contains 1% of haemoglobin Barts (γ_4). Such individuals are usually identified by deduction from a pedigree chart in the course of a family study. They can only be defined with complete reliability by DNA analysis.

Box 6.15 Haemoglobin electrophoresis

Different forms of haemoglobin can often be separated from each other by electrophoresis. This method involves application of a blood lysate to a carrier such as a cellulose acetate strip soaked in buffer at pH 8.4. When a current is applied across the strip, the haemoglobins present migrate towards the cathode at a rate proportional to the charges present on the haemoglobin molecule, i.e. changes in the amino acid structure affect electrophoretic mobility and permit identification of abnormal forms. Not all haemoglobins are separated by this method, however. Supplementary tests are required to confirm the identity of any abnormal haemoglobins.

α thalassaemia trait. Individuals with the equivalent of two α-globin genes deleted may be α$^+$ homozygotes (α–/α–) or α^0 heterozygotes (––/αα). It is important to know to which group a given individual belongs so that accurate genetic counselling may be offered, in particular about the risk of bearing a child with HbH disease or Hb Barts hydrops fetalis (see *Box 6.16*). The two groups are clinically indistinguishable and present identical laboratory profiles using standard laboratory techniques.

Affected individuals show a mild microcytic, hypochromic anaemia but exhibit no significant symptoms of disease. Precipitated haemoglobin H (β$_4$) can be demonstrated by supravital staining in a small minority of red cells. Blood drawn from the umbilical cord can be shown to contain up to 10% of haemoglobin Barts.

Haemoglobin H disease arises from the deletion of three α-globin genes or the equivalent and is seen most commonly in SE Asian populations. The most common genotype is that of a compound heterozygote for α$^+$ and α^0 thalassaemia (α-/--). Haemoglobin H disease is characterized by a moderately severe anaemia and hepatosplenomegaly. Typically, the haemoglobin level is maintained at around 8 g/dl and transfusion support is unnecessary. Characteristic findings on the peripheral blood film include microcytosis, hypochromasia, fragmented red cells, poikilocytosis, polychromasia and target cells. Multiple haemoglobin H inclusions are demonstrable in most of the red cells and are the main cause of the haemolytic anaemia that characterizes the condition. Adult blood contains between 5 and 35% of haemoglobin H and traces of haemoglobin Barts. Umbilical cord blood contains up to 40% haemoglobin Barts. The α:β globin chain synthesis ratio is typically reduced to between 0.2 and 0.4. Haemoglobin molecules that are composed of four identical globin chains such as haemoglobin H and haemoglobin Barts do not carry oxygen effectively.

Haemoglobin Barts hydrops fetalis. The most severe form of α thalassaemia results from the deletion of all four α-globin genes and is seen most commonly in SE Asia and the Mediterranean region. Because of the absence of α-globin synthesis, no functionally normal haemoglobins are formed after the cessation of ζ-globin synthesis at about 10 weeks gestation. Instead, functionally useless tetrameric molecules such as haemoglobin Barts (γ$_4$) and haemoglobin H (β$_4$) are synthesized (see also *Box 6.17*). Thus, although the haemoglobin concentration at delivery is typically about 6 g/dl, the *functional* anaemia is much more severe. The severity of the anaemia causes gross oedema secondary to congestive cardiac failure and massive hepatosplenomegaly. Pregnancy usually terminates in a third trimester stillbirth, often after a difficult delivery. The peripheral blood smear shows marked microcytosis, hypochromasia, poikilocytosis, fragmentation and numerous nucleated red cells. Haemoglobin electrophoresis confirms the presence of haemoglobin Barts and haemoglobin H.

Box 6.16 Haemoglobin H

Haemoglobin H within red cells is demonstrated by incubation in a redox dye such as 1% Brilliant Cresyl Blue at 37°C for 1 hour, followed by microscopic examination. Precipitated HbH appears as multiple blue inclusions, giving a 'golf ball' appearance. This method can also be used, with a much shorter incubation time, to demonstrate reticulocytes.

Box 6.17 Naming haemoglobin Barts

An abnormal haemoglobin which travelled faster than haemoglobin A on electrophoresis was identified in the blood of a baby with haemoglobin H disease in 1958 by Ager and Lehmann. Since the letters of the alphabet had been exhausted by then, the new variant was called after the hospital where the baby was a patient – St Bartholomew's Hospital in London. Haemoglobin Barts was subsequently shown to be a γ-globin tetramer.

β *thalassaemia*. Because β thalassaemia usually results from point mutations within the β-globin gene cluster, the relationship between genotype and phenotype is less straightforward than for α thalassaemia. It is still convenient, however, to group affected individuals according to the severity of their symptoms. Three groups are recognized:

■ β thalassaemia minor (or trait)
■ β thalassaemia major
■ β thalassaemia intermedia

β thalassaemia minor. The mildest form of β thalassaemia arises from the inheritance of a single abnormal β-globin gene. Affected individuals exhibit no significant signs of disease, and may be unaware of their condition. Laboratory analysis reveals a mild microcytic, hypochromic anaemia, with target cells a prominent feature on the peripheral blood film. In most cases, the red cell count appears to be inappropriately high given the degree of anaemia. Most cases can be demonstrated to have raised levels of one or both of the minor haemoglobins A$_2$ and F. It is important to differentiate β thalassaemia minor from iron deficiency anaemia, which produces superficially similar results. Iron deficiency causes a greater decrease in the level of Hb A$_2$ than Hb A, which may obscure the diagnosis of β thalassaemia minor when iron deficiency is also present (see also *Box 6.18*).

β thalassaemia major results from the inheritance of two β thalassaemia genes. Affected individuals are thus either homozygous for a particular gene defect or doubly heterozygous for two distinct mutations. In the absence of treatment, the condition is characterized by severe anaemia, gross hepatosplenomegaly, failure to thrive and skeletal deformities such as bossing of the skull and maxillary prominence. The skeletal deformities are the result of marked erythroid hyperplasia with consequent expansion of the bone marrow volume, which causes outward pressure and marked thinning of the bones.

The peripheral blood film shows marked microcytosis, hypochromasia, numerous target cells and nucleated red cells. The prominent haemolytic component of the anaemia is manifest as teardrop poikilocytes, fragmented red cells and microspherocytes. Analysis of the haemoglobins present reveals a marked increase in the proportion of haemoglobin F, the precise value of which is dependent on the genetic defect(s) present. In homozygous β⁰ thalassaemia, for example, Hb F accounts for up to 98% of the total. Marked reduction in the synthesis of β-globin is reflected in an α:β globin synthetic ratio of greater than 2.5.

Bone marrow examination reveals extreme erythroid hyperplasia with marked ineffective erythropoiesis. The presence of precipitated aggregates of excess α-globin chains promotes intramedullary death of developing erythroblasts and a reduced lifespan of circulating red cells.

The mainstay of current treatment is regular blood transfusion, aimed at maintaining the haemoglobin level above about 10–12 g/dl, thereby effectively suppressing erythropoiesis and preventing skeletal changes and extramedullary haemopoiesis. However, such a programme of regular, lifelong transfusion leads to the accumulation of large amounts of iron within the body, which is severely toxic. Treatment of iron overload involves chelation therapy, which binds excess iron so that it can be excreted in urine or faeces. At best, this treatment is currently only partially effective.

Box 6.18 Discriminant function

One approach to the discrimination between thalassaemia and iron deficiency anaemia is the use of a mathematical formula known as the discriminant function: $DF = MCV - ([5 \times Hb] - RBC - k)$

where MCV is mean cell volume, [Hb] is haemoglobin concentration, RBC is red cell count, and k is a locally determined constant. Using this formula, positive values of DF indicate iron deficiency and negative values suggest thalassaemia. A number of other variants of discriminant function exist.

β thalassaemia intermedia. Not all cases of homozygous or doubly heterozygous β thalassaemia have severe disease. Because of the diversity and high frequency of thalassaemic mutations, a complete spectrum of disease severity exists. Thalassaemia intermedia encompasses all cases of β thalassaemia with significant symptoms of disease which do not require regular transfusion to maintain their haemoglobin level above about 7 g/dl. Typically, thalassaemia intermedia arises from one of three circumstances:

- inheritance of 'mild' β thalassaemia mutation(s);
- co-inheritance of a gene which increases the rate of γ-globin synthesis;
- co-inheritance of α thalassaemia; reduction in α-globin synthesis reduces the imbalance in the α:non-α globin synthetic ratio.

The laboratory and clinical features of thalassaemia intermedia mirror those of the more severe phenotype. Paradoxically, despite the absence of regular transfusion, iron overloading remains a major cause of morbidity.

The structural haemoglobinopathies

The structural haemoglobinopathies are characterized by the synthesis of structurally abnormal globin chains. These abnormal globins can exert a wide range of effects on the behaviour of the haemoglobin molecule. More than 1000 different structurally abnormal haemoglobins have been described, but most are rare and clinically silent. In some respects, the scientific importance of the structural haemoglobinopathies lies in what they tell us about the structure–function relationship of the normal haemoglobin molecule. The four most common examples are, in order of decreasing incidence, haemoglobins S, C, D and E. Haemoglobin S is by far the most common structural haemoglobinopathy and is most prevalent in Afro-Caribbeans but it also is relatively common in central India, the eastern Arabian peninsula and the southern Mediterranean (see also *Box 6.19*). About 30% of live births in Nigeria carry the abnormal gene. In common with thalassaemia, the carrier state for haemoglobin S confers selective resistance to the malarial parasite *Plasmodium falciparum*. Haemoglobin C is most common in West and central Africa, particularly in Ghana. It is frequently co-inherited with haemoglobin S. Haemoglobin D is most common in the Punjab but is seen in a wide range of populations. Haemoglobin E is most common in SE Asia.

Classification

The alteration in molecular function induced by structural abnormality is dependent upon the position of the mutation and on the properties of the amino acids involved. Functionally, the haemoglobin molecule can be considered to have a number of important areas:

- the exterior surface of the molecule, which confers water solubility.
- the $\alpha_1\beta_1$ and $\alpha_2\beta_2$ contact areas, which confer stability on the molecule.
- the $\alpha_1\beta_2$ and $\alpha_2\beta_1$ contact areas, which confer flexibility during oxygenation and deoxygenation.
- the $\alpha_1\alpha_2$ and $\beta_1\beta_2$ contact areas.

Box 6.19 Naming haemoglobins

In 1953 a standard nomenclature for haemoglobins was proposed. It was decided that normal **A**dult haemoglobin should be designated HbA, **F**etal haemoglobin as HbF and **S**ickle haemoglobin HbS. The two abnormal haemoglobins discovered by Itano in 1950 and 1953 were designated HbC and HbD, respectively. There is no haemoglobin B because some workers had used this term to describe sickle haemoglobin. When the term HbS was adopted HbB was permanently abandoned.

- the 2,3-DPG binding site, which affects the oxygen affinity of the molecule.
- the hydrophobic haem pockets, which protect the haem groups from oxidation.
- the C-terminal histidines of the β chains, which contribute to the Bohr effect.

Alterations to the amino acid sequence within these areas typically lead to predictable alterations in molecular behaviour. For example, changes in the $\alpha_1\beta_1$ and $\alpha_2\beta_2$ contact areas are likely to affect molecular stability, while changes in the $\alpha_1\beta_2$ and $\alpha_2\beta_1$ contact areas are likely to affect oxygen affinity.

In general terms, the phenomena resulting from the presence of an abnormal haemoglobin will fall under one or more of the following headings:

- clinically silent.
- thalassaemia-like syndrome.
- methaemoglobinaemia.
- molecular instability.
- altered oxygen affinity.
- miscellaneous atypical effects, e.g. haemoglobin S.

Clinically silent haemoglobinopathies

Most structurally abnormal haemoglobins have no apparent effect. Over 300 such 'silent' abnormal haemoglobins have been described. Almost all are caused by alterations to amino acids on the external surface of the haemoglobin molecule, a position where change is readily tolerated; many involve the so-called 'variable' amino acid residues. Most of these silent haemoglobinopathies have been discovered by chance and are mainly of interest to population geneticists.

The thalassaemia-like syndromes

Any abnormality of globin that leads to mRNA instability is likely to lead to a thalassaemia-like syndrome. Abnormalities of this type are more common in β-globin than in α-globin, probably because severe abnormalities of α-globin synthesis are more likely to be incompatible with life. Important examples of thalassaemic haemoglobinopathies include haemoglobin E and the chain fusion haemoglobins such as haemoglobin Lepore and haemoglobin anti-Lepore, which are δ–β and β–δ fusions respectively, and haemoglobin Kenya which is a $^A\gamma$–β fusion. These haemoglobins result from unequal crossing-over during meiosis with the formation of hybrid globin genes.

Haemoglobin Constant Spring arises as a result of a mutation in the α-globin gene stop codon, which results in chain extension (the α-globin chain is 172 residues long instead of the normal 141). The resulting mRNA is unstable and is partially degraded prior to protein synthesis. Furthermore, the mutant α-globin is itself unstable. The result is a thalassaemic phenotype.

Haemoglobin Wayne arises as a result of a deletion of the third nucleotide of codon 139 of the $\alpha2$-globin gene, resulting in a frameshift mutation that causes the carboxyl-terminal tripeptide sequence, Lys-Tyr-Arg to be replaced by the octapeptide sequence Asx-Thr-Val-Lys-Leu-Glu-Pro-Arg. In affected patients, two abnormal haemoglobins are present; Hb Wayne I which is as described above, and Hb Wayne II which is formed by a post-translational deamidation of the new asparagine residue. Haemoglobin Wayne is a relatively stable variant.

Haemoglobin Tak results from an insertion of the dinucleotide CA into codon 147 of the β-globin gene, which abolishes the normal stop codon (TAA) at position 147, leading to an abnormal elongation of the beta chain by 11 amino acids – (147)THR Lys-Leu-Ala-Phe-Leu-Leu-Ser-Asn-Phe-(157)Tyr-COOH. The resulting haemoglobin molecule is unstable and has a high oxygen affinity. In contrast to the α-globin chain extension variants, which are typically expressed as α thalassaemias, the haematological effect of HbTak is a mild polycythaemia caused by the increased oxygen affinity.

Methaemoglobinaemia

Methaemoglobinaemia is the result of irreversible oxidation of the ferrous (Fe^{2+}) ion in haem to the ferric (Fe^{3+}) state. In all instances where this occurs, molecular instability also results. Similarly, in many cases where an amino acid change causes the formation of an unstable haemoglobin, there is an increase in methaemoglobin formation. Whether the abnormal haemoglobin is classified as unstable or as a methaemoglobinaemia is to some extent arbitrary, but as a general rule it is classified according to which of the results predominates.

The four members of the haemoglobin M group are the most important of the abnormal haemoglobins that cause methaemoglobinaemia (see also *Box 6.20*). All result from the substitution of the haem-binding histidine by tyrosine as shown in *Table 6.1*.

Table 6.1 The M haemoglobins

Haemoglobin	Mutation
Hb M Saskatoon	b63 (E7) distal His Tyr
Hb M Hyde Park	b92 (F8) proximal His Tyr
Hb M Boston	a58 (E7) distal His Tyr
Hb M Iwate	a87 (E7) proximal His Tyr

Haemoglobin Milwaukee was originally also classified as a haemoglobin M but the substitution involved is not of a haem-binding histidine, but of β67 (E11) valine by glutamic acid. Being four amino acids away, the highly active glutamic acid is spatially adjacent to the haem binding histidine with which it interacts, resulting in methaemoglobin formation. Similarly, haemoglobin Zürich (β63 (E7) distal His → Arg) was originally classified as a haemoglobin M because of the methaemoglobinaemia which results. However, the predominant effect of this substitution is molecular instability and haemoglobin Zürich is now classified as an unstable haemoglobin.

Box 6.20 Haemoglobin M

Medical workers in northern Japan had been puzzled for some time about the origin of a familial disease, which they called *kuchikuru* or 'black mouth'. The mystery was solved when the abnormality was linked to haemoglobin M. The black discoloration of the mouth was due to the peripheral cyanosis that accompanies methaemoglobinaemia.

Unstable haemoglobins

More than 60 haemoglobin variants have been described where the principal defect is instability (see also *Box 6.21*). Frequently the amino acid substitution involves the invariant amino acids. The reasons for the instability can be grouped under three main headings:

- weakened haem–globin contact.
- weakened tetrameric structure.
- disruption of normal or helical structure.

Weakened haem–globin contact. The abnormalities leading to weak haem–globin contact usually involve amino acids in the haem pocket. The most common unstable variant, haemoglobin Köln, results from a Val→Met substitution at β98, which destabilizes the haem pocket. In haemoglobin Hammersmith, the invariant β42 (CD1) phenylalanine is substituted by serine. Serine is a much smaller molecule than phenylalanine so the distance between the globin chain and the haem at this point is greater. The consequent weakening of the haem-β-

---

Box 6.21 Unstable haemoglobins

The earliest description of an unstable haemoglobin was made in 1952. It concerned a young boy with congenital haemolytic anaemia of unknown aetiology for whom splenectomy in early childhood had no beneficial effect. The presence of Heinz bodies in his red cells suggested to the investigators that chemical poisoning was the most likely cause of the haemolysis, but no culprit could be identified. It was not until 1970 that the presence of an unstable haemoglobin, Hb Bristol (β67 (E11) val→asp), was demonstrated.

The first unstable haemoglobin to be definitively identified was haemoglobin Zürich, which was identified in a young girl who developed acute haemolysis after ingestion of sulphonamide drugs, which are known to exert oxidative stress on red cells.

---

globin binding at this important position results in molecular instability. In addition, serine is hydrophilic and so encourages water to enter the haem pocket, leading to oxidation of the haem iron and methaemoglobinaemia.

Haemoglobin Gun Hill arises as a result of a 15 BP deletion in the β-globin gene that results in the expression of an abnormal β-globin that is missing amino acid residues 93–97. This region includes the haem-binding proximal histidine at position 92 so the β-globins of haemoglobin Gun Hill lack haem groups. The resulting molecule is unstable, has a high oxygen affinity and an absence of the Bohr effect. Haemoglobin Gun Hill is synthesized at a greater rate than haemoglobin A but the instability of the molecule means that its concentration in circulating red blood cells remains low. The clinical consequences of haemoglobin Gun Hill are relatively minor; most reported cases have shown evidence of a mild, compensated chronic haemolysis.

Weakened tetrameric structure. The substitution of the β35 (C1) tyrosine by phenylalanine (which has no polar OH group) in haemoglobin Philly results in weakened $\alpha_1\beta_1$ bonding, monomer formation and precipitation of the haemoglobin as Heinz bodies (see also *Box 6.22*).

Disruption of helical structure. Haemoglobin Genova results from substitution of the β28 (B10) leucine by the imino acid proline. The introduction of proline causes a 'kink' and, occurring within the B helix, it cannot be tolerated, resulting in molecular instability (see also *Box 6.23*). The substitution of an amino acid by proline inevitably leads to a 'kink', and such a change within any helix other than in the first or last three amino acids of the helix produces the same effect.

Insertion of a polar amino acid into the interior of the haemoglobin molecule also causes molecular instability. In haemoglobin Wien, substitution of the tyrosine at β130 (H8) by aspartic acid causes the NA2 histidine to move closer to the –COO⁻ of the aspartic acid, thereby disrupting the alignment of the A helix and leading to instability.

Box 6.22 Impact of polarity

The R groups of phenylalanine and tyrosine are identical apart from the tyrosine OH group. Phenylalanine is a non-polar (hydrophobic) amino acid while tyrosine is polar (hydrophilic).

Box 6.23 Proline is an imino acid

Proline is designated an imino acid rather than an amino acid because it contains a secondary, not a primary, α amine group.

Altered oxygen affinity

Several mechanisms exist that result in altered oxygen affinity:

- direct interference with oxygen binding, especially of α haem.
- abnormality of the $\alpha_1\beta_2$ ($\alpha_2\beta_1$) contact area.
- alteration of $\alpha_1\alpha_2$ or $\beta_1\beta_2$ interaction.
- changes in 2,3-DPG binding.
- changes in Bohr effect H^+ binding.

Interference with oxygen binding. The unstable haemoglobin Hammersmith also has a reduced oxygen affinity because the CD1 phenylalanine helps to maintain the correct orientation of the haem group and is responsible for the tilt of the haem on oxygenation. In the absence of phenylalanine, the haem group remains in the upright, deoxygenated position, which lowers its oxygen affinity. In addition, haemoglobins M Boston and Iwate have lowered oxygen affinity since they involve α chains, whereas in haemoglobins M Saskatoon and Hyde Park the oxygen affinity is normal because they involve β chains.

Abnormality of the $\alpha_1\beta_2$ ($\alpha_2\beta_1$) contact. Interference with the $\alpha_1\beta_2$ ($\alpha_2\beta_1$) contact is a common cause of altered oxygen affinity. For example, in haemoglobin Chesapeake the α92 (FG4) arginine is substituted by leucine. The α92 arginine is normally in Van der Waals' contact with the arginine at β35 (C2), stabilizing the deoxygenated conformation of haemoglobin. In haemoglobin Chesapeake, this interaction is absent and the deoxygenated conformation is no longer favoured thereby causing increased oxygen affinity.

Conversely, the oxygenated conformation is normally stabilized by a bond between the β102 (G4) asparagine and α94 (G1) aspartic acid. In haemoglobin Kansas, formation of this stabilizing bond is precluded by the substitution of threonine for the β102 (G4) asparagine. This mutation therefore reduces the stability of the oxygenated conformation and results in reduced oxygen affinity.

Alteration of $\alpha_1\alpha_2$ and $\beta_1\beta_2$ interaction. Abnormalities affecting $\alpha_1\alpha_2$ are very rare. No mutations affecting $\beta_1\beta_2$ interaction have yet been reported. In theory, stabilizing $\beta_1\beta_2$ interactions should increase oxygen affinity; conversely stabilizing $\alpha_1\alpha_2$ substitutions should reduce oxygen affinity.

In the deoxygenated form, the N-terminal (α1) valine of each α chain bonds with C-terminal arginine (α141) and aspartic acid (α126) on the opposite α chain. These bonds stabilize the deoxygenated conformation, since they must be broken during oxygenation. In haemoglobin Suresnes the α141 arginine is replaced by histidine, which precludes bonding with the α1 valine on the opposite α chain and results in increased oxygen affinity.

Changes in 2,3-DPG binding. There are three amino acid residues on the β-globin chain which are responsible for the binding of 2,3-DPG; the β1 (NA1) valine, the β82 (EF6) lysine and the β143 (H21) histidine. One of the sequence differences between β- and γ-globin is at (H21) where the histidine is replaced by serine. This explains the inability of γ-globin to bind 2,3-DPG and the resultant elevated oxygen affinity of haemoglobin F ($\alpha_2\gamma_2$).

The β82 lysine is involved in at least three abnormal haemoglobins, Helsinki ($\rightarrow$Met), Rahere ($\rightarrow$Thr) and Providence ($\rightarrow$Asn/Asp). In all three the positive charge is lost, resulting in weakened DPG binding and increased affinity.

Altered H^+ binding. Hydrogen ions (H^+) are bound in the process of deoxygenation, but must be released for association of oxygen to occur. The shift in the position of the haemoglobin–oxygen dissociation curve that results from changes in pH is called the Bohr effect. Half of the

H$^+$ binding is due to the interaction of the C-terminal histidines of the β chains (β146, HC3), via their side chains, to the aspartic acid at β94 (FG1) of their own chains. Mutations that remove the β146 (HC3) histidine therefore affect H$^+$ binding and the oxygen affinity of the molecule. For example, the increased oxygen affinity of haemoglobin York is explained by the substitution of the β146 (HC3) histidine by proline.

Miscellaneous effects

Polymerization. By far the most clinically significant structural haemoglobinopathy is haemoglobin S. The clinical consequences of the presence of this abnormal haemoglobin all stem from its tendency to polymerize in hypoxic conditions, forming long, rigid structures called 'tactoids', causing contortion of the red cell into elongated and poorly deformable sickle shapes.

Haemoglobin S results from a substitution of the glutamic acid in the external position β6 (A3) by valine. Genetic analysis of HbS mutations has identified five different disease haplotypes. The HbS gene is always the same in these haplotypes, but there is co-inherited variation in the surrounding (non-coding) DNA. These haplotypes are each associated with a particular geographic region and are named to reflect this: HbS (Benin), HbS (Senegal), HbS (Central African Republic), HbS (Cameroon), HbS (Asian). In general, the Asian and Senegal haplotypes tend to be less clinically severe than the Central African Republic haplotype (see also *Box 6.24*).

Sickle cell anaemia follows a highly variable clinical course; some patients die in infancy from the disabling effects of recurrent crises or overwhelming infection; others may live for a normal lifespan. The precise causes of this variability are incompletely understood but the physical and social environment plays a large part. Symptoms of sickle cell anaemia are seldom manifest before the age of about 6 months when the level of circulating fetal haemoglobin falls to the adult level. Between crises, the condition is characterized by a chronic haemolytic state with jaundice and a relatively constant haemoglobin level of 7–8 g/dl. The anaemia may be exacerbated by the presence of folate deficiency. This quiescent state is punctuated by crises of four main types:

- **vaso-occlusive sickling crises** are the most common manifestation and occur when poorly deformable sickle cells occlude small blood vessels, e.g. in the spleen, leading to downstream tissue hypoxia and infarction. Repeated sickling crises cause cumulative tissue damage (see also *Box 6.25*).
- **aplastic crises** are manifest as a sudden fall in haemoglobin concentration with no compensatory reticulocytosis and are usually secondary to infection, most commonly with parvovirus.
- **acute splenic sequestration**, where a large proportion of the circulating red cell mass is suddenly sequestered by the spleen, is a major cause of infant mortality in sickle cell anaemia.

Box 6.24 Sickle cell anaemia

James Herrick published the first description of a case of sickle cell anaemia in 1910. The patient described was a young West Indian student who demonstrated many of the classical clinical features of this condition recognized today (*Archives of Internal Medicine*, **6**: 517–521).

Box 6.25 Autosplenectomy

Repeated sickling crises within the microcirculation of the spleen cause cumulative damage, which can ultimately lead to the loss of a functional spleen. This condition is relatively common in adults with sickle cell disease and is known as autosplenectomy.

■ **susceptibility to bacterial infection** is a hallmark of sickle cell anaemia, and a common cause of infant mortality. The most common infections are pneumococcal and staphylococcal.

There are several known risk factors that may trigger a sickling crisis:

■ hypoxia due to cigarette smoke, high altitude or flying in an unpressurized aircraft;
■ exposure to cold air, wind or water;
■ dehydration with slowing of blood flow;
■ infection;
■ stress;
■ strenuous exercise.

Heterozygotes for haemoglobin S are said to have sickle cell trait, while homozygotes have sickle cell anaemia. Typically, individuals with sickle cell trait are clinically normal and may be unaware of their condition. Laboratory analysis reveals the presence of about 40% HbS. Sickle cell crises are extremely rare in heterozygotes but affected individuals should be warned of the potential dangers of severe hypothermia or hypoxia.

Co-inheritance of other haemoglobinopathies can influence the clinical course of sickle cell trait or anaemia. For example, HbS homozygotes that also inherit α thalassaemia trait typically have higher haemoglobin levels and a less severe clinical picture. On the other hand, compound heterozygotes for HbS and β^0 thalassaemia have relatively severe disease. One particularly important example of such an interaction is where sickle cell anaemia is co-inherited with the benign condition hereditary persistence of fetal haemoglobin (HPFH) in which levels of haemoglobin F do not fall. The presence of significant amounts of haemoglobin F has a protective effect against sickling and such individuals have relatively mild disease.

Substitution of the β6 glutamic acid (the same amino acid as HbS) by lysine gives rise to haemoglobin C, the second most common of the structural haemoglobinopathies. This mutation is most closely associated with West Africa. Haemoglobin C is associated with decreased solubility and crystallization and dehydration and poor deformability of red cells. Homozygotes and HbC–β^0 thalassaemia compound heterozygotes have a chronic haemolytic anaemia.

Investigation of suspected haemoglobinopathy

The laboratory diagnosis of a haemoglobinopathy usually requires a combination of different tests, with results being assessed in relation to clinical features, the ethnic origin of the patient, and the blood count and blood film. Serum ferritin is also performed in those patients who present with microcytosis, because iron status may affect some test results (including HbA_2 estimation).

The basic laboratory screening tests aim to readily detect the most common forms of haemoglobinopathy and include measurement of the red blood cell indices (RBC, MCV, MCH in particular), quantification of HbA_2 and HbF levels, detecting the reduced solubility of HbS, and haemoglobin electrophoresis or equivalent technique to detect structural haemoglobinopathy. The results of these tests, interpreted together with any evidence of family history and ethnic origin, will identify the vast majority of abnormalities. It is important that all of the components of this screen are performed because of the common inheritance of more than one abnormality, e.g. HbS and β thalassaemia. If HPLC is used to determine HbF and HbA_2 levels, the most clinically important structural variants will be determined simultaneously (see also *Box 6.26*).

The results of this screen can be divided into five groups:

■ **reduced MCH (<27 pg) and raised HbA_2 (>3.5%)** is typical of heterozygous β thalassaemia. The HbF level is also raised (1–3%) in about one-third of cases. Because of the huge

---

Box 6.26 HPLC

Charge-dependent HPLC has largely replaced standard alkaline cellulose acetate electrophoresis for haemoglobinopathy screening, because it can simultaneously detect the most clinically important structural haemoglobinopathies and quantitate HbA_2 and HbF with greater accuracy.

---

variety of mutations and the possible co-inheritance of other abnormalities, the range of possible results in this category is wide.

- **normal HbA_2 (<3.5%) and reduced MCH (<27 pg)** is most commonly explained by iron deficiency. If this has been excluded, the most likely explanations are heterozygous α^0 thalassaemia, homozygous α^+ thalassaemia, mild β thalassaemia trait, and rarer forms of thalassaemia such as $\delta\beta$ thalassaemia or $\epsilon\gamma\delta\beta$ thalassaemia. Genetic testing may be required to differentiate between these.

- **normal HbA_2 (<3.5%), reduced MCH (<27 pg) and raised HbF (>1%)** raises the suspicion of $\delta\beta$ thalassaemia trait or HPFH. Genetic testing is required for definitive diagnosis here.

- **normal HbA_2 (<3.5%) and normal MCH (>27 pg)** is most likely normal but may be explained by the uncommon silent β thalassaemia trait. Where a family history is positive for thalassaemia intermedia, the only way to exclude silent β thalassaemia trait is by genetic testing.

- **abnormal haemoglobin present**. The most common clinically relevant abnormal haemoglobins (HbS, C, D-Punjab, O-Arab and E) can all be identified using haemoglobin electrophoresis or HPLC. Identification of less common abnormalities requires genetic testing or amino acid analysis. Identification of an abnormal band on haemoglobin electrophoresis should trigger a sickle solubility test to identify the presence of HbS. Using alkaline cellulose acetate electrophoresis, HbS co-migrates with HbD and HbC co-migrates with HbA_2, HbE and HbO^{Arab}. In cases of doubt, acid agar gel electrophoresis permits resolution of these subtypes (see also *Box 6.27*).

Box 6.27 Isoelectric focusing

Isoelectric focusing (IEF) is an alternative form of haemoglobin electrophoresis. Although it is more technically demanding than cellulose acetate electrophoresis, the resolution of minor haemoglobin fractions is better.

SUGGESTED FURTHER READING

Giardina, B., Messana, I., Scatena, R. and Castagnola, M. (1995) The multiple functions of hemoglobin. *Crit. Rev. Biochem. Mol. Biol.* **30**: 165–196.

Hazelwood, L. (2003) *Can't Live Without It: the story of hemoglobin in sickness and in health*. New York: Nova Biomedical.

Perutz, M.F. (1998) *Science Is Not a Quiet Life: Unravelling the Atomic Mechanism of Haemoglobin (Series in 20th Century Biology)*. Singapore: World Scientific Publishing.

Steinberg, M.H., Forget, B.G., Higgs, D.R. and Nagel, R.L. (eds) (2009). *Disorders of Haemoglobin: genetics, pathophysiology and clinical management*. Cambridge: Cambridge University Press.

SELF-ASSESSMENT QUESTIONS

1. What is the rate-limiting step in haem synthesis?
2. Where in the cell does haem synthesis occur?
3. Name three embryonic haemoglobins and define their globin content.
4. Why is it important that haem does not come into contact with water?
5. What is the normal alveolar pO_2?
6. Why is anaemia associated with shortness of breath on exertion?
7. Why is anaemia associated with pallor?
8. Do you think that δ^0 thalassaemia would be a severe disease?
9. Why is haemoglobin Barts hydrops fetalis rare in African-Americans?
10. What effect might coincident inheritance of heterozygous α^0 thalassaemia have on the severity of a moderately severe β thalassaemia?
11. Why are the haemoglobins M associated with peripheral cyanosis?
12. Why should patients with sickle cell disease avoid flying in unpressurized aircraft?

Disorders of red cell survival

Learning objectives
After studying this chapter you should confidently be able to:

■ **Differentiate between the terms haemolytic disorder, haemolytic anaemia and haemolytic component**
Any condition, other than haemorrhage, that leads to a reduction in the mean lifespan of the red cell is a haemolytic disorder. Where the rate of haemolysis cannot be balanced by increased erythropoiesis, haemolytic anaemia is present. Conditions such as thalassaemia, where anaemia is caused partly by haemolysis but mainly by the underlying condition, are said to have a haemolytic component.

■ **Outline the difficulties associated with the classification of haemolytic disorders**
There is no single, overarching classification scheme that satisfactorily encompasses all haemolytic disorders. Instead, haemolytic disorders are categorized by the site of haemolysis (intravascular or extravascular), as intrinsic or extrinsic to the red cell, by the nature of the defect and whether they are inherited or acquired.

■ **Describe the structure and function of the normal red cell membrane**
The red cell membrane consists of a phospholipid bilayer with free cholesterol sandwiched between the layers. This structure rests upon and is anchored to a protein cytoskeleton. Together, these structures confer the essential features of deformability and biconcave shape to the cell. Numerous proteins rest within the membrane and regulate transport of essential substances into and out of the cell.

■ **Demonstrate a detailed knowledge of the pathogenesis of hereditary spherocytosis and hereditary elliptocytosis**
Both of these relatively common inherited disorders result from a deficiency or defect of cytoskeletal protein(s) that causes membrane instability. There are many different genetic mutations responsible, but most are linked to deficiency or defect of spectrin, AE1 (band 3), band 4.2 or ankyrin.

■ **Outline the autoimmune and alloimmune haemolytic disorders**
The autoimmune haemolytic anaemias are caused by the presence of an antibody that attacks red cell antigen or a drug that triggers a haemolytic immune response. Alloimmune haemolysis results from a host antibody attacking transfused red cells or maternal antibody attacking fetal red cells (HDN).

■ **List the mechanisms that underpin the haemolytic disorders**
Broadly, haemolysis results from inherited or acquired intrinsic or extrinsic defects. Among the intrinsic defects are red cell membrane abnormalities, enzyme deficiencies and haemoglobinopathies. Extrinsic factors include immune-mediated haemolysis, physical factors such as trauma or burns, and the action of chemicals, drugs or toxins.

A normal, mature red cell survives in the circulation for about 120 days. The ageing process within red cells is associated with a reduction in glycolytic activity, reduced concentrations of 2,3-DPG and ATP, accumulation of Na^+ and Ca^{2+} ions, and increased rigidity due to loss of membrane lipid and changes in the cytoskeleton. These changes promote the sequestration and destruction of senescent cells in the spleen. Normally, the rate of destruction of senescent cells is balanced by the rate of synthesis and release of juvenile cells from the bone marrow (see *Box 7.1*).

Any condition, other than haemorrhage, that leads to a reduction in the mean lifespan of the red cell within the circulation is a haemolytic disorder. A reduction in red cell lifespan requires a balancing increase in the rate of erythropoiesis if anaemia is to be avoided. The reserve erythropoietic capacity of normal bone marrow is usually sufficient to prevent the development of anaemia until the mean red cell lifespan falls to about 20 days, when haemolytic anaemia ensues. The onset of anaemia is often accelerated by the presence of a haematinic deficiency, particularly folate, or by another complicating pathological condition. Such conditions are said to have a haemolytic component in their pathogenesis but are typically not considered to be haemolytic disorders (see also *Box 7.2*).

The haemolytic disorders can be classified in several different ways.

- **Site of haemolysis**. Most haemolytic disorders result from the premature destruction of red cells by the macrophages of the reticuloendothelial system. These are **extravascular haemolytic disorders**. Conversely, where haemolysis occurs mainly within the circulatory system, an **intravascular haemolytic disorder** is said to exist. The problem with this scheme is that it groups together some highly disparate disorders and says little about the pathogenesis of particular disorders.
- **Intrinsic or extrinsic** to the red cell. Haemolytic disorders can be divided into those caused by a structural or functional defect within the red cell (i.e. an intrinsic defect) and those caused by an abnormality in the red cell environment (i.e. an extrinsic defect). Knowledge of the site of the defect is useful in that transfused blood survives normally where the defect is intrinsic but may be rapidly destroyed in the presence of an extrinsic defect. Even here there can be difficulties of classification, since some intrinsically defective red cells may need extrinsic triggers to precipitate haemolysis (e.g. glucose-6-phosphate dehydrogenase (G-6-PD) deficiency, see *Chapter 8*), or where initially intrinsically sound cells may be altered to become inherently liable to lysis (e.g. paroxysmal nocturnal haemoglobinuria (PNH; see *Chapter 17*).

Box 7.1 The life of a red cell

During its 120 days in the circulation, the average red cell travels about 300 miles around the body. The senescent red cells that are destroyed within the spleen are constantly replaced by juvenile cells synthesized and released by the bone marrow. An average 70 kg adult male produces about 2.3×10^6 red cells every second!

Box 7.2 Red cell lifespan

Hawkins and Whipple performed the earliest reliable determination of red cell lifespan in 1938. They created an opening in the bile ducts of dogs to enable the measurement of the amount of bile excreted daily. A number of experimental animals were rendered acutely anaemic by the administration of acetyl-phenylhydrazine, thereby eliciting a marked reticulocytosis. About 120 days after the reticulocyte response was noted, a peak of bile pigment production was observed. This was interpreted to be due to the destruction of the reticulocyte response cohort, suggesting that newly released red cells survive in the circulation for 120 days.

- **Nature of the defect**. Grouping haemolytic disorders according to the mechanism involved can aid understanding of underlying processes, but can lead to confusion between hereditary and acquired types and unnecessary investigation of blood relations.
- **Inherited or acquired**. Typically, inherited haemolytic disorders are caused by an intrinsic defect whereas acquired haemolytic disorders are caused by an extrinsic defect. However, there are several exceptions to this rule, e.g. PNH is an acquired intrinsic defect and hereditary G-6-PD deficiency typically requires the presence of an extrinsic trigger such as an antimalarial drug to precipitate acute haemolysis. Recognition that a disorder is hereditary can facilitate diagnosis in blood relations.

None of these classification schemes is universally applicable and, in practice, an amalgam of all four schemes is used.

7.1 INHERITED INTRINSIC HAEMOLYTIC DISORDERS

The inherited intrinsic haemolytic disorders can be sub-classified into three main groups, according to the nature of the defect:

- disorders of globin synthesis and/or structure;
- enzyme disorders;
- primary membrane disorders.

The disorders of globin synthesis and/or structure are described in *Chapter 6* and disorders of red cell metabolism are described in *Chapter 8*. The inherited membrane defects are described below.

Composition of the red cell membrane

The approximate composition of the red cell membrane is shown in *Table 7.1*.

Table 7.1 Composition of the red cell membrane

50% Protein
10% Carbohydrate (glycoproteins and glycolipids)
40% Lipid ⌐ 30% free unesterified cholesterol
└ 10% glycerides and free fatty acids
60% phospholipid ⌐ 30% phosphatidyl choline (lecithin)
└ 30% phosphatidyl ethanolamine
25% sphingomyelin
15% phosphatidyl serine

Lipids

All of the lipid associated with red cells is present in the cell membrane. The mature red cell has no capacity to synthesize lipid: alterations in membrane lipid content can only occur by exchange with plasma lipids.

As shown in *Table 7.1*, about 60% of the red cell membrane lipid is composed of one of four different phospholipids: phosphatidyl choline, phosphatidyl ethanolamine, sphingomyelin and phosphatidyl serine. Phospholipid molecules are characterized by a polar head group attached to a non-polar fatty acid tail. The polar head group is hydrophilic (water-loving) while the fatty acid tail is hydrophobic (water-fearing) or lipophilic (fat-loving). Thus, the phospholipid molecules in the cell membrane tend to arrange themselves in a bilayer with their hydrophilic heads pointing towards the inner and outer aqueous phases (the cytoplasm and plasma respectively) while the hydrophobic tails point towards each other as shown in *Figure 7.1*. Small amounts of phosphatidic acid, phosphatidyl inositol, lysophosphatidyl choline and glycolipids are also present.

The distribution of the different phospholipids between the two leaflets of the bilayer is not symmetrical. The choline phospholipids phosphatidyl choline and sphingomyelin are mainly present in the plasma layer while the amino phospholipids phosphatidyl ethanolamine, phosphatidyl serine and phosphatidyl inositol are restricted to the cytoplasmic layer.

The membrane cholesterol is unesterified and lies between the two layers of the lipid bilayer as shown in *Figure 7.1*. The concentration of cholesterol in the membrane is an important determinant of membrane surface area and fluidity: an increase in membrane cholesterol leads to an increased surface area and decreased deformability. Red cell membrane cholesterol is in rapid exchange with the unesterified cholesterol of plasma lipoproteins. Red cell lysophosphatidyl choline, phosphatidyl choline and sphingomyelin are also in exchange with their plasma lipoprotein counterparts.

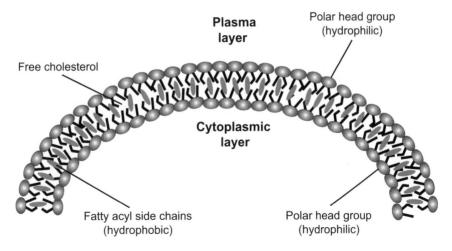

Figure 7.1
Structure of the red cell membrane lipids.

Proteins

Most red cell membrane proteins are tightly associated with the lipid bilayer and require treatment with powerful detergents such as sodium dodecyl sulphate (SDS) to extract them for analysis by polyacrylamide gel electrophoresis (PAGE). This technique separates substances according to their molecular weight, the lightest travelling the furthest from the origin. Red cell membrane proteins have been named according to their relative positions on SDS–PAGE electrophoresis, as shown in *Figure 7.2*. Some of the better-characterized proteins also have trivial names, e.g. bands 1 and 2 are more commonly known as spectrin.

Red cell membrane proteins can be grouped into two types:

- **integral proteins**, which penetrate the lipid bilayer and are firmly anchored within it via interactions with the hydrophobic core. Only a relatively small portion of an integral protein molecule is exposed to the inner and outer aqueous phases, the majority being

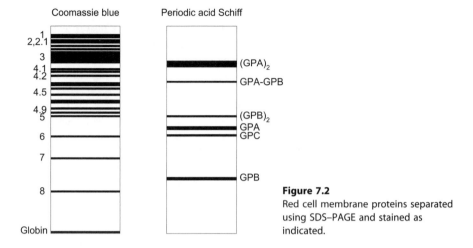

Figure 7.2
Red cell membrane proteins separated using SDS–PAGE and stained as indicated.

contained within the lipid bilayer. About 60–80% of red cell membrane proteins are of this type. Examples of important integral proteins include AE1 (band 3) and the glycophorins. AE1 acts as the anion transport channel while the glycophorins are associated with the MNSs blood group system. Both of these integral proteins are bound tightly to the protein cytoskeleton.

■ **peripheral proteins**, which are in contact with the inner aspect of the lipid bilayer but are not strongly attached to it. About 20–40% of red cell membrane proteins are peripheral proteins. Examples of important peripheral proteins include haemoglobin, the enzyme glyceraldehyde-3-phosphate dehydrogenase and the cytoskeletal proteins spectrin and actin.

Red cell membrane integral proteins. AE1 is a single chain molecule with a molecular weight of about 95–105 000. It accounts for close to 25% of the total protein content of the red cell membrane. AE1 has two major functions within the red cell membrane, each associated with a distinct functional domain. Its primary function is to facilitate anion transport across the membrane but it also acts as an important binding site for cytoskeletal and other red cell proteins.

The central portion of the band 3 molecule consists of a series of hydrophobic helices that traverse the lipid bilayer 12 times, forming a roughly cylindrical channel. These helices are linked by short hydrophilic sequences, which are exposed to the inner and outer aqueous phases. This arrangement forms a transmembrane channel that facilitates the rapid transport of Cl^- and HCO_3^- anions. A large carbohydrate side chain that carries the Ii blood group antigens is attached to one of the external hydrophilic linking sequences.

The N-terminal portion of AE1 is hydrophilic and projects into the cytoplasm of the cell. This functional domain has a molecular weight of about 43 000 and contains binding sites for haemoglobin, the glycolytic enzymes glyceraldehyde-3-phosphate dehydrogenase, aldolase, and phosphoglycerate kinase, and the cytoskeletal proteins ankyrin, band 4.1 and band 4.2.

Glycophorins are sialoglycoproteins that carry the blood group antigens for the MNSs and Gerbich systems and also act as binding sites for viruses, bacteria and parasites. The five members of the red cell glycophorin family are most commonly known as glycophorins A, B, C, D and E, although several other classification schemes exist.

Glycophorin A accounts for close to 2% of the mass of the red cell membrane. It is encoded by the *GYPA* gene on 4q31. The genes for glycophorins B (*GYPB*) and E (*GYPE*) are highly homologous to *GYPA* and also reside in this chromosomal region. It is thought that these genes arose from a common ancestral gene. The glycophorin A molecule has been shown to consist of three distinct domains: a receptor domain that projects into the outer aqueous phase, a transmembrane domain that spans the lipid bilayer and an interior domain that projects into the cytoplasm of the cell. The receptor domain is very hydrophilic and contains large amounts of carbohydrate and sialic acid. The MN blood group antigens are located on this portion of the molecule. The transmembrane domain is hydrophobic and therefore serves to anchor the molecule in the membrane. Red cell membrane glycophorin A is thought to exist as a dimer, coupled at the transmembrane domain. The interior domain is hydrophilic and contains an assemblage of cationic amino acid residues near to the C-terminal end. This portion of the molecule binds to anionic phospholipids and to certain cytoskeletal proteins. Glycophorin A has been shown to act as a receptor for several pathogens, including the malarial parasite *Plasmodium falciparum*.

Glycophorin B is structurally closely related to glycophorin A and carries the Ss blood group antigens. Glycophorin E is also structurally homologous and may carry the M antigen.

Glycophorins C and D are structurally distinct from glycophorins A, B and E. They are both encoded by the same gene at 2q14–21. Glycophorin D is a truncated form of glycophorin C. These glycophorins carry the Gerbich blood group antigens.

Glycophorin C has three domains, a glycosylated N-terminal domain that is extracellular, a hydrophobic membrane spanning domain and a C-terminal cytoplasmic domain that interacts with the cytoskeleton. Glycophorin D is identical except that it lacks the N-terminal 21 residues of glycophorin C. The function of these proteins appears to be related to the structural integrity of the red cell membrane because Gerbich-deficient red cells (known as the Leach phenotype) are elliptocytic. Glycophorin C also serves as an attachment site for the *Plasmodium falciparum* malarial parasite.

Na$^+$/K$^+$ ATPase is an enzyme that probably exists in the membrane as an oligomer containing three subunits, designated α, β and γ. The α subunit has a molecular weight of about 112 500, while the β subunit has a molecular weight of about 45 000. Both are integral proteins. The bulk of the extramembranous portion of the α subunit projects into the cytoplasm, while that of the β subunit projects into the outer aqueous phase. The γ subunit has a molecular weight of 10 000 and is not required for ATPase activity. As its name suggests, this enzyme catalyses the hydrolysis of ATP to ADP, liberating energy in the process. The action of the Na$^+$/K$^+$ ATPase is mediated by phosphorylation and dephosphorylation of a specific aspartic acid residue on the α subunit. Phosphorylation of the aspartic acid requires the presence of Na$^+$ and Mg^{2+} ions, but not K$^+$ ions, while dephosphorylation requires K$^+$, but not Na$^+$ or Mg^{2+} ions. Each ATP molecule hydrolysed via this system results in the ejection of three Na$^+$ ions from the cell and the transport of two K$^+$ ions into the cell. This mechanism is present in all mammalian cells and accounts for about one-third of all ATP hydrolysis at rest. The action of the red cell cation pump is shown schematically in *Figure 7.3*.

Glucose transport protein has a molecular weight of 45–75 000 and is an integral protein with 12 transmembrane domains. It is encoded by the gene *GLUT1* and is a member of a family of glucose transporters, designated GLUT1–7. The red cell membrane concentration of the transporter appears to increase in the presence of a low plasma glucose concentration and to decrease in the presence of increased plasma glucose. GLUT1 is widely distributed in fetal tissues but, in adults, is expressed most strongly in red cells and also in the endothelial cells of the blood–brain barrier. Glucose transport in red cells is ATP-dependent and Na$^+$-independent.

Rh proteins are integral membrane proteins and are important blood group antigens from the point of view of blood transfusion and pregnancy. The proteins are associated in the membrane in a multimeric complex that is suspected to be involved in ammonia and/or carbon dioxide transport and to interact with the cytoskeleton, influencing cell shape and deformability. A complete absence of Rh proteins (Rh$_{null}$) is associated with red cell shape changes and a

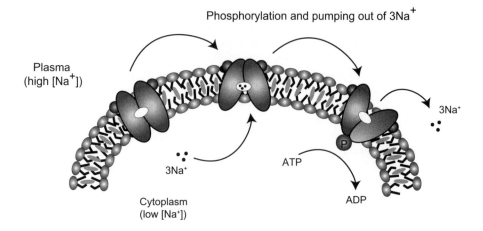

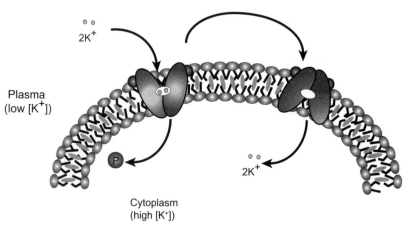

Figure 7.3
Function of the red cell Na+/K+ ATPase.

shortened red cell lifespan. The Rh proteins are encoded by two homologous genes (*RHD* and *RHCE*) that are located close to each other in a 'tail to tail' configuration (5 RHD3 –3 RHCE5) on chromosome 1. One gene encodes the RhD antigen and the other encodes the RhCcEe antigens. However, the RH genes are highly polymorphic and are susceptible to recombination events, resulting in the generation of abnormal or hybrid proteins, giving rise to more than 50 Rh antigens.

Within the red cell membrane, the Rh proteins are associated with a glycoprotein known as Rh-associated glycoprotein, RhAG, which is encoded by the *RHAG* gene on chromosome 6. This glycoprotein does not carry any Rh antigen, but its presence is essential for Rh antigen expression. In the absence of RhAG, no Rh antigens are expressed.

Individuals that have a complete deletion of the *RHD* gene or a mutation that renders it completely inactive are said to be 'rhesus negative'. About 15–17% of Caucasians are rhesus negative, mostly due to gene deletion. About 5% of black Africans and 3% of Asians are rhesus negative, but in these cases the genetic basis is more variable and can lead to problems in blood typing for transfusion. More than 100 mutations of the *RHD* gene have been identified that result in a reduced quantity of RhD on the red cell membrane, altered spatial arrangement of the RhD protein, or a hybrid protein. Accurate determination of RhD status is critical for blood transfusion and the avoidance of haemolytic disease of the newborn.

The red cell membrane carries numerous surface receptors, including the physiologically vital surface transferrin receptors TfR1 and TfR2 (see *Chapter 4*). A large variety of other surface receptors have been demonstrated on the red cell membrane, including those for insulin, parathyroid hormone, vitamin E, the complement components C3b and C4b, opiates and oestradiol. In most cases, the function of these receptors in the context of red cells remains obscure.

Red cell membrane peripheral proteins. The red cell membrane peripheral proteins interact to form a cytoskeleton, which acts as a tough supporting framework for the lipid bilayer. Four proteins play a key role in the structure of the red cell cytoskeleton: spectrin, ankyrin, band 4.1 and actin, although many others play ancillary roles in this complex structure.

Spectrin (bands 1 and 2) constitutes about two-thirds of the total weight of the cytoskeleton. This protein is a heterodimer composed of two subunits designated α and β that have molecular weights of 240 000 and 220 000 and are encoded by genes on chromosomes 1 and 14 respectively. These subunits are bound together in an antiparallel, i.e. 'head to tail' configuration. Further, the two subunits are twisted around one another as shown in *Figure 7.4*. Spectrin heterodimers can associate head to head to form heterotetramers or can form higher oligomers in a branching, radial structure. *In vivo*, red cell membrane spectrin is thought to be composed of a mixture of these three forms, with the heterotetrameric form predominating. Spectrin also associates with ankyrin, band 4.1, actin and anionic phospholipids.

Ankyrin (bands 2.1–2.3 and 2.6) occurs in two forms within the red cell membrane of molecular weight 206 000 and 190 000, respectively. Both forms serve to anchor assembled spectrin molecules to the lipid bilayer. This is accomplished by binding simultaneously to spectrin tetramers and to the interior domain of the integral protein, AE1.

Actin (band 5) is synthesized as a globular protein of molecular weight 45 000, but readily polymerizes to form filaments. These filaments bind weakly to the tail end of both α and β

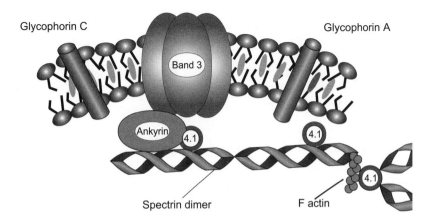

Figure 7.4
Structure of the red cell cytoskeleton.

spectrin. The result is a two-dimensional lattice of spectrin tetramers held together by actin filaments. The lipid bilayer is attached to this lattice via AE1.

Band 4.1 is a globular protein of molecular weight 78 000 that serves two distinct functions in the red cell membrane. It binds to spectrin close to the actin binding site, thereby strengthening and stabilizing the cytoskeletal lattice. It also binds directly to glycophorins A and C, AE1 and phosphatidyl serine, and therefore strengthens the links between the lipid bilayer and the protein cytoskeleton.

The currently accepted model of the structure of the red cell membrane is shown in *Figure 7.4*.

Primary membrane disorders

Membrane disorders fall into two groups, namely those that are inherited ('primary') and those that are secondary to some other factor or disorder. The secondary ones will be dealt with later. The primary red cell membrane disorders are associated with alterations of cell shape and are classified according to the shape of the abnormal red cells.

Hereditary spherocytosis

Hereditary spherocytosis (HS) is the most common of the inherited primary red cell membrane abnormalities in northern Europeans, with an incidence of at least 1 in 5000. The condition is transmitted as an autosomal dominant characteristic although a less common autosomal recessive variant exists. No homozygotes for the autosomal dominant form have been described, suggesting that this state is incompatible with life. HS is caused by a genetic defect that results in a deficiency or defect of the cytoskeletal proteins spectrin, AE1 (band 3), band 4.2 or ankyrin.

The most common abnormality associated with HS is spectrin deficiency. Spectrin monomers exist in two forms: α spectrin is encoded by a gene at 1q22–23 and β spectrin is encoded by a gene at 14q23–24. Normally, α spectrin is synthesized at around 3–4 times the rate of β spectrin. Therefore, β spectrin synthesis is the rate limiting factor for cytoskeletal spectrin assembly. Because of this, in many heterozygous α spectrin abnormalities the appropriate balance between α and β spectrin that is required for a normal cytoskeleton can still be retained and the defect is clinically silent or mild. In other words, α spectrin deficiency is often seen as an autosomal recessive condition, whereas β spectrin abnormalities are autosomal dominant.

Whereas the spectrin defects produce membrane instability through an absolute quantitative defect, the other causes of HS produce membrane instability through an inability to bind normal levels of spectrin. Ankyrin defects are associated with a translocation or deletion of the short arm of chromosome 8 where the gene is located (8p11.2). A considerable majority of all autosomal dominant HS patients (70–80%) demonstrate a co-deficiency of ankyrin and spectrin, the deficiencies being in proportion. Some 10–20% of patients with the mild to moderate form of autosomal dominant HS demonstrate AE1 deficiency. Some band 4.2 deficiencies, which are rare and to some extent population-specific, produce some of the most clinically severe HS cases (see also *Box 7.3*).

Box 7.3 History of HS

The earliest description of a case of HS was published in 1871 by two Belgian physicians, Vanlair and Masius. The index case presented with the classical symptoms of an aplastic crisis, jaundice, splenomegaly, abdominal pain and collapse. Microscopic evaluation of the blood of this patient revealed numerous microspherocytes which remained after the apparent remission of the crisis. Similar symptoms were noted in her sister and mother. Vanlair and Masius, who named this hitherto unknown condition microcythemie, thought it was caused by an overproduction of the spherocytes by the spleen coupled with a deficiency in their removal by the liver.

The clinical presentation of HS is very variable, ranging from essentially asymptomatic through to a severe haemolytic anaemia. The principal features include congenital haemolytic anaemia with variable spherocytosis, increased red cell osmotic fragility, episodic jaundice and variable splenomegaly. The haemolysis in HS is episodic and highly variable: it is not uncommon for the diagnosis to be missed until adulthood. Less common manifestations of HS include pigment gallstones (cholelithiasis), often at an unusually young age, and aplastic crises in which erythropoiesis is almost completely suppressed for up to 72 hours, leading to severe but self-limiting anaemia. Aplastic crises commonly follow infection with human parvovirus type B19.

The major site of haemolysis in HS is the spleen. Two routes through the spleen exist; the faster, open circulation and the slower and more challenging closed circulation. Red cells that take the closed route face an inhospitable environment, which tests to the limit the deformability and metabolic competence of the cell. The defective red cells in HS have an increased flux of Na^+ ions into the cell leading to greatly increased activity of the cation pump and necessitating an increased rate of glycolysis. Because of this, HS red cells find passage through the spleen particularly hazardous. Detention in the glucose-poor environment of the splenic cords rapidly leads to metabolic exhaustion in HS red cells and causes the loss of intact portions of membrane. The cell that results has a reduced surface area : volume ratio and so is less readily deformable. Reduced deformability of the cell causes an increase in subsequent splenic transit times. HS reticulocytes have a normal biconcave discoid shape and normal deformability but, with each passage through the spleen, they become progressively spherocytic and rigid. This vicious circle leads inevitably to the early death of the spherocyte within the splenic circulation.

The clinical severity of HS is highly variable. In mild cases, which constitute some 20–30% of cases, increased erythropoiesis compensates for the shortened red cell lifespan and the haemoglobin concentration remains within normal limits. A common consequence of chronic erythroid hyperplasia such as this is depletion of body folate stores. Oral folate supplementation may be required to prevent the development of megaloblastic anaemia. Where haemolysis is troublesome, in approximately the most severe 5% of cases, the only effective treatment is splenectomy. Although this procedure does not affect the red cell defect, removal of the main site of haemolysis effectively 'cures' the condition and returns the mean red cell lifespan to normal. Some 65–70% of cases fall between these two extremes, with intermittent jaundice, mild splenomegaly and mild to moderate anaemia.

Hereditary elliptocytosis

Hereditary elliptocytosis (HE) encompasses a disparate group of primary red cell membrane disorders, characterized by the presence of a large proportion of oval or elliptical red cells. The frequency of HE may be as high as 1 in 1000. The condition is typically transmitted as an autosomal dominant characteristic, although less common autosomal recessive forms exist. Homozygous HE presents as severe, transfusion-dependent haemolytic anaemia (see also *Box 7.4*).

The clinical severity of HE ranges from clinical silence (some estimates suggest that up to 90% of cases fall into this category) to severe, life-threatening haemolysis. In some forms, the severity can vary within an individual over time. Broadly, HE can be divided into five major forms:

Box 7.4 History of HE

The earliest published description of hereditary elliptocytosis is attributed to M. Dresbach, a physiology lecturer at Ohio State University. The abnormality first came to his attention during a student practical class in which students were examining their own blood. The hereditary nature of the condition was not established until 1929 when W.C. Hunter demonstrated transmission of HE through three generations of a US family.

- **common HE** has been described in virtually all races of the world and is, at worst, a mild, compensated haemolytic disorder. Elliptocytes represent 15–90% of all erythrocytes. There is no splenomegaly, and the osmotic fragility test is normal. The inheritance pattern is autosomal dominant. A variant known as HE with infantile poikilocytosis presents as a moderately severe congenital haemolytic disorder with neonatal jaundice, elliptocytosis, marked poikilocytosis, red cell fragmentation and susceptibility of the red cells to heat damage. This condition progressively moderates until, by the age of one year, it is indistinguishable from common HE.
- **haemolytic HE** is a recessive trait. Homozygotes have a severe, transfusion-dependent haemolytic anaemia, which is characterized by marked poikilocytosis, micro-elliptocytosis and red cell fragmentation. Heterozygotes are less severely affected. Splenomegaly is usually present and the osmotic fragility test may show normal or increased haemolysis. Depending on the severity, elliptocytes, poikilocytes and cell fragments may be seen in the peripheral blood.
- **hereditary pyropoikilocytosis** (HPP) is now usually classed as a variant of HE. It is characterized by moderately severe haemolysis, microspherocytosis, micropoikilocytosis and an unusual susceptibility of the red cells to heat damage. Unlike most examples of 'classical' HE, the condition is inherited as an autosomal recessive characteristic, and is most common in people of African descent. Splenectomy ameliorates the haemolysis in most cases of HPP but does not provide the 'cure' seen in HS or HE with haemolysis.
- **HE with spherocytosis**, also known as spherocytic elliptocytosis, has mainly been described in Caucasians and is characterized by rounded elliptocytes, microspherocytes, micro-elliptocytes and a mild, incompletely compensated haemolytic state. The osmotic fragility test shows increased red cell fragility. About one in five cases of HE in Caucasians is of this type. The inheritance is autosomal dominant.
- **HE with stomatocytosis** is characterized by elliptocytes, which show slit-like areas of pallor, an autosomal dominant mode of inheritance, the absence of splenomegaly, and mild or absent haemolysis. The osmotic fragility test shows normal or decreased red cell fragility. The condition is most common in south-east Asians (Malaysia, New Guinea, Indonesia, and the Philippines). This form of HE does give some protection from malaria. A single mutation of AE1 is responsible for the defect.

A wide range of cytoskeletal defects has been described in association with HE, but the most common are structural abnormalities of spectrin. Tetramers of correctly formed α and β spectrin are critical for normal red cell membrane stability, shape and function. HE heterozygotes synthesize an abnormal spectrin, which forms heterodimers but cannot self-associate to form tetramers and higher oligomers, resulting in a clinically mild form of HE. In 65% of cases the defect is with α spectrin, and in 30% of cases it is in β spectrin; the majority of the remainder are defects in band 4.1.

Deficiency of band 4.1 is a common cause of HE in southern France and northern Africa, accounting for more than one-third of cases in these areas. Heterozygotes have a partial deficiency of band 4.1 and mild HE with spherocytosis, whereas homozygotes have a complete absence of this protein and severe haemolytic anaemia.

Abnormal binding of the integral protein AE1 to ankyrin has been described in association with HE with moderately severe haemolysis. The molecular basis for this abnormality remains obscure.

AE1 is not a cytoskeletal protein, rather it lies in the membrane itself, bound to ankyrin. In HE with stomatocytosis, the bonding is firmer than normal, and causes rigidity and a restriction of movement of AE1. In order for malaria to enter the cell, it induces an aggregation of AE1 proteins, which act as a receptor, forming a channel through which the parasite gains entry. It is thought that the increased rigidity in this variant prevents the aggregation, hence preventing parasite entry.

HE reticulocytes are initially normal in shape but become progressively elliptocytic with age.

Box 7.5 Naming membrane disorders

Primary red cell membrane disorders caused by deficiency of a known cytoskeletal protein are denoted by the abbreviation for the disease state followed by the name of the affected protein in brackets. A complete deficiency is denoted by a ^{0} superscript while a partial deficiency is denoted by a $^+$ superscript, e.g. HE[4.1^0] denotes hereditary elliptocytosis caused by a complete lack of band 4.1 in the red cell membrane.

Where a primary membrane disorder is caused by a defect in a cytoskeletal protein, rather than a deficiency, the affected protein is underlined, e.g. HS[Sp-4.1] denotes hereditary spherocytosis caused by a defective spectrin molecule which cannot bind to band 4.1.

Elliptocytes are poorly deformable and so are sequestered in the spleen. In most cases of HE, haemolysis is so mild that clinical intervention is unnecessary. Where haemolysis is troublesome, splenectomy typically provides a functional cure (see also *Box 7.5*).

Hereditary stomatocytosis and hereditary xerocytosis

Hereditary stomatocytosis (HSt) and hereditary xerocytosis (HX) are the extreme ends of a spectrum of membrane disorders related to ion and water transport across the red cell membrane, and all of which display stomatocytes in the peripheral blood film. In addition, other morphological abnormalities may be seen, ranging from spherocytes to target cells. There is a variable range of clinical severity across the spectrum from severe haemolysis to clinical silence (see also *Box 7.6*).

Stomatocytes can be produced *in vitro* as an artefact due to inappropriate processing and by means of drugs. Drugs that intercalate the inner surface of the membrane can cause it to expand, leading to stomatocyte formation (whilst those that intercalate the outer layer cause that layer to expand, leading to echinocyte formation). Stomatocytes can also be seen as an acquired disorder in association with several conditions including acute alcoholism, hepatobiliary disease, vinca alkaloid administration, various neoplasms and cardiovascular disease (see also *Box 7.7*).

Box 7.6 History of HSt

Hereditary stomatocytosis was first described in 1961 by Lock, Sephton-Smith and Hardisty. The index cases were a mother and daughter with chronic haemolytic anaemia, which had failed to respond to splenectomy. The name is derived from the Greek στομα (*stoma*), meaning mouth, and refers to the slit-like area of central pallor that characterizes this condition.

Box 7.7 Acanthocytes and echinocytes

Several acquired conditions, including liver disease, malnutrition (including anorexia nervosa), hypothyroidism, and sometimes post-splenectomy, are associated with the appearance of abnormally shaped red cells known as acanthocytes or spur cells. These appear as dense, contracted cells lacking central pallor but with variable spiky projections from their surface. The mechanism of acanthocyte formation appears to be an excess deposition of material in the outer leaflet of the red cell membrane, causing buckling and deformity. Acanthocytes may also be present in the rare congenital disorders, abetalipoproteinemia, the McLeod phenotype, and the neuro-acanthocytosis syndromes.

By contrast, echinocytes display uniform, fine spicules projecting from the membrane. The cause is frequently artefactual, but can also be associated with uraemia, hypophosphataemia or pyruvate kinase deficiency. It is thought that acanthocytes result from expansion of the outer lipid layer more markedly than the inner one.

HSt is characterized by the presence of red cells that, on dried blood films, have a slit-like area of central pallor. These stomatocytes result from increased sodium transport (15–40 times normal) into the cell, which cannot be compensated for by increased cation pump activity, resulting in the ingress of water and cellular deformation, in that they become uniconcave and bowl-shaped rather than the normal biconcave shape. HSt is inherited in an autosomal dominant fashion and presents as congenital haemolytic anaemia of variable severity, which is incompletely resolved by splenectomy. The molecular defect responsible for this disorder remains obscure, although it appears to be linked to the absence of stomatin (band 7.2b), a membrane protein of unknown function.

By contrast, the red cells of hereditary xerocytosis (HX) are characterized by excessive leakage of K^+ from the cell, leading to progressive water depletion. Xerocytes are thus dehydrated cells, which are irregularly contracted and have an abnormally high MCHC. Haemolysis is usually mild and compensated. Splenectomy has no clinical effect. Hereditary xerocytosis is inherited as an autosomal dominant characteristic. The molecular defect that causes this condition remains obscure.

The spectrum of conditions (from 'wet' to 'dry') include severe HSt, moderate/mild HSt, cryohydrocytosis, stomatocytic xerocytosis, xerocytosis with high phosphatidyl choline, and HX. The osmotic fragility test shows a decrease from the 'wet' end to the 'dry' end of the spectrum. This parallels a fall in Na^+ content and an increase in K^+ content. The inheritance pattern of all appears to be autosomal dominant. The severity of anaemia varies and the molecular mechanisms that underlie these conditions remain unclear.

Rh null disease

Rh null disease includes a genetically heterogeneous group of disorders that share the serological characteristic of the absence of red cell Rh antigens. The condition is manifest as mild to moderate normocytic, normochromic haemolytic anaemia with stomatocytes and occasional spherocytes in the peripheral blood film. Rh proteins are required to stabilize the red cell membrane through its linkage with ankyrin (see also *Box 7.8*).

Box 7.8 Target cells

An interesting and somewhat puzzling phenomenon is that of target cell (codocyte) formation. These cells have the appearance of an archery target because of their central dark area, surrounded by annular light and dark areas. Target cells have a disproportionate increase in the surface membrane area:volume ratio, resulting from either an increase in membrane surface area or a decrease in haemoglobin content. Among the conditions associated with target cell formation are liver disease, thalassaemia, haemoglobin C disease, and familial lecithin-cholesterol acyltransferase (LCAT) deficiency.

7.2 ACQUIRED (EXTRINSIC) HAEMOLYTIC DISORDERS

The acquired haemolytic disorders can be sub-classified into four groups, according to the nature of the defect as haemolysis secondary to:

- immune mechanisms;
- the action of chemicals, drugs or toxins;
- infection;
- physical damage.

Haemolysis secondary to immune mechanisms

Immune haemolysis results from the binding of antibodies to the red cell surface with consequent complement activation. The antibodies concerned may be synthesized by the host immune system and be directed against host red cell antigens leading to **autoimmune haemolysis,** or they may be derived from exogenous sources or be directed against foreign antigens leading to **alloimmune haemolysis**. Therapy with certain drugs can also stimulate immune haemolysis.

Autoimmune haemolysis

The autoimmune haemolytic anaemias (AIHA) can be divided into three types:

- **warm-reactive antibody AIHA,** where the offending autoantibody reacts most strongly above 32°C;
- **cold-reactive antibody AIHA,** where the offending autoantibody reacts most strongly below 32°C;
- **drug-induced AIHA,** where immune haemolysis is triggered by the presence of a drug.

Warm-reactive antibody AIHA

Warm-reactive antibody AIHA is a relatively common condition responsible for around 50–75% of all AIHA cases. It affects all ages and races, and women are more commonly affected than men. It occurs commonly in association with viral infections, lymphoproliferative disorders, immunodeficiency states or autoimmune disorders such as systemic lupus erythematosus (SLE), but it has been described in association with a huge range of disparate diseases. Typically, the autoantibody in warm-reactive antibody AIHA is a polyclonal IgG_1 panagglutinin, which activates complement via the classical pathway and triggers extravascular haemolysis. Treatment of this condition involves immunosuppressive drug therapy or splenectomy to remove the major site of red cell destruction.

Cold-reactive antibody AIHA

Cold-reactive antibody AIHA can be divided into two main types: cold agglutinin syndrome and paroxysmal cold haemoglobinuria (PCH). Cold agglutinin syndrome is a disease of old age with a peak incidence over the age of 70 years. It is associated with *Mycoplasma pneumoniae*, Epstein–Barr virus and cytomegalovirus infection where the autoantibody is polyclonal, and also with lymphoproliferative disorders where monoclonal antibodies are produced. The autoantibody is an IgM immunoglobulin with anti-I, anti-i or anti-Pr specificity. The temperature of capillary blood in the body extremities can be as low as 25°C, allowing the cold-reactive antibody to agglutinate red cells and activate complement, leading to intravascular haemolysis and obstruction of capillary blood flow. Capillary obstruction is reversible on warming but, over a period of time, necrotic tissue damage and even gangrene can result. The most important measure in the treatment of cold agglutinin syndrome is the avoidance of cold. Immunosuppressive therapy is usually ineffective (see also *Box 7.9*).

Classically, PCH is a chronic haemolytic condition, which is characterized by intravascular haemolysis following exposure to cold, and is found in association with syphilis and viral illnesses such as measles or mumps. It is caused by a unique haemolytic IgG antibody called the Donath–Landsteiner antibody, which has anti-P blood group specificity. Haemolysis in PCH is

---

Box 7.9 History of AIHA

The earliest clear description of a cold-reactive antibody AIHA was published in 1873 by R. Druitt. In this paper, he described two cases of haematinuria, one of which was a fellow doctor who had suffered for several years from acrocyanosis with haematinuria and loss of sensation in the hands and feet. Apparently miraculously, these distressing symptoms disappeared completely when the patient moved to the warmer climate of India.

Box 7.10 History of PCH

PCH has been well recognized for over a century. The first description of this condition was published in 1854 and involved a young boy who probably had congenital syphilis. In the years that followed, several reports appeared of an association between inclement weather and haemoglobinuria. The relationship between cold and haemolysis in affected individuals was clearly demonstrated by Ehrlich 27 years later. His experiment involved the isolation of blood flow in a single finger of an affected individual by tightly tying a cord around its base. The finger was then held in iced water for some time. Serum obtained from the chilled finger was tinged red due to haemolysis whereas serum from a similarly isolated but unchilled finger remained unchanged.

---

biphasic, requiring both exposure to cold and subsequent warming. The Donath–Landsteiner antibody binds to red cells most strongly at temperatures below 15°C, so exposure to cold triggers antibody binding but no haemolysis because complement is inactive at these temperatures. However, following warming, rapid complement-mediated intravascular haemolysis ensues (see also *Box 7.10*).

Drug-induced immune haemolytic anaemia (DI-IHA)

Once a relatively common cause of haemolysis, DI-IHA has markedly reduced with greater awareness of which drugs are commonly implicated and improved regulatory surveillance. The current incidence has been estimated to be around 1 in 1 000 000. Treatment with a wide range of drugs has the potential to stimulate immune haemolysis by one of four mechanisms, although some drugs appear to act through more than one mechanism, sometimes simultaneously. The four are:

- **penicillin-type immune haemolysis** in which the drug binds non-specifically to the red cell surface, coating it, where it acts like a foreign antigen (as a hapten or hapten-like phenomenon), stimulating the production of IgG antibodies directed against the drug. These antibodies bind to the surface-bound drug, leading to the selective removal of affected cells by the reticulo-endothelial system. The cell itself is unchanged, and the antibody is not directed to any membrane component. This type of immune haemolysis is most commonly associated with high dose intravenous penicillin therapy, and, because the use of such therapy has declined with the introduction of newer drugs, this form of DI-IHA has reduced dramatically. Other drugs that have been associated with this mechanism include some cephalosporins, tetracycline and tolbutamide.

- **neo-antigen or immune complex formation**. In this case it is the combination of the drug with the red cell membrane that creates a compound antigen. Implicated drugs include quinidine and stibophen. The drugs bind loosely to specific sites on the red cell, and only small doses are required to induce haemolysis, which is usually sudden and severe.

- **α-methyldopa-type immune response**. Long-term treatment with this centrally acting anti-hypertensive drug frequently produces a warm-reactive autoantibody; this is thought to be through direct stimulation of the immune system, which may have anti-Rh specificity. These are true autoimmune disorders in that the antibody is directed against a present red cell antigen. The binding of the antibodies to the red cell is, however, often very weak, with the result that it tends to be stripped from the cell by the RE system without haemolysis occurring. A positive direct anti-globulin test (Coombs' test) is nonetheless invariably noted. For these reasons α-methyldopa is now seldom used. Other drugs implicated in this form of immune response include levodopa and mefenamic acid, but in all cases associated haemolysis is rare.

- **rifampicin-type immune haemolysis**, in which the drug forms a stable complex with plasma protein and induces the synthesis of IgG and IgM anti-drug antibodies. Large immune complexes are formed and these are adsorbed onto the surface of red cells, triggering complement-mediated intravascular haemolysis. Because the red cells are not directly the subject of the antibody attack, this mechanism is sometimes known as 'innocent bystander' immune haemolysis. Withdrawal of the drug typically resolves the problem.

Alloimmune haemolysis

Alloimmune haemolysis results from the immunization of the host to transplanted foreign antigen, or the action of foreign antibody to normal host antigen. Broadly, there are two circumstances where this can occur:

- haemolytic transfusion reactions;
- haemolytic disease of the newborn (HDNB).

Haemolytic transfusion reactions

Transfusion of blood from one individual to another is fraught with dangers. Aside from infection, chief among these is the risk of antibody-mediated haemolysis of donor or recipient red cells, a condition that can be life threatening. The most severe haemolytic transfusion reactions are seen when ABO-incompatible blood is transfused. For example, if group A blood cells are transfused into a group O individual the IgM anti-A in the recipient plasma will immediately bind to the donor cells and activate the complement cascade. The resultant acute intravascular destruction of the donor cells can cause renal failure, hypotension and disseminated intravascular coagulation, and may be fatal. Transfusion of red cells that carry an antigen to which the recipient has previously been sensitized also causes an immediate haemolytic transfusion reaction (see section on HDNB, below).

Less commonly, haemolytic transfusion reactions can be delayed, often for several days following transfusion. In these cases, the recipient usually has previously been sensitized to donor red cell antigen, but the titre of the immune antibody is very low. Transfusion of red cells that carry the offending antigen stimulates a vigorous synthesis of antibody and, after a variable delay of up to several days, haemolysis ensues.

The levels of anti-A or anti-B antibody in the plasma of some group O blood donors can sometimes be very high. If whole blood from such donors is transfused to a blood group A or B recipient, there can be a risk of a haemolytic transfusion reaction, which can be severe. The haemolysis in these cases is self-limited because the offending antibody is exogenous and is not replaced.

Haemolytic disease of the newborn (HDNB)

During pregnancy, the mother supplies nutrients to the developing fetus via the placenta and umbilical cord, and fetal waste products are transported in the opposite direction for excretion by the mother. In the placenta, the fetal and maternal circulations are separated by a single layer of endothelium. Given this, it is inevitable that minor bleeds occur, even in normal pregnancy, allowing small amounts of fetal blood to enter the maternal circulation. Most of these do not trigger a maternal antibody, possibly because of the immune tolerance associated with pregnancy which ceases at, or shortly after, parturition. Towards the end of pregnancy and at delivery, compression of the placenta can result in the injection of much larger amounts of fetal blood into the maternal circulation. If these fetal red cells carry paternal antigens that are foreign to the mother, she may respond by producing antibody directed against the offending antigen. For example, a Rh-negative mother carrying a Rh-positive fetus is likely to respond to the presence of fetal red cells in her circulation by synthesizing an antibody with anti-D specificity. In subsequent pregnancies, further stimulation by fetal red cells can provoke the synthesis of a high-titre IgG anti-D, which can cross the placental barrier and trigger the premature destruction of fetal red cells (see also *Box 7.11*).

Box 7.11 History of HDNB

Although P. Levine is credited with the first unequivocal demonstration that most cases of HDNB could be attributed to maternal immunization against a shared feto-paternal Rh factor, a less well known figure deserves much of the credit. In 1938, a year before Levine's seminal observation, R. Darrow published a theoretical account of the pathogenesis of HDNB in which she speculated that the most likely cause was maternal immunization against a hitherto unrecognized fetal antigen.

In severe cases (where maternal antibody titre and/or avidity is high), acute haemolysis in the fetus results in profound anaemia, hepatosplenomegaly, oedema secondary to cardiac failure, and portal hypertension. This full-blown manifestation of HDNB is known as hydrops fetalis, and was a relatively common cause of stillbirth in the first half of the twentieth century. In less severe cases, the baby is born alive but haemolysis continues after birth, causing progressive anaemia and hyperbilirubinaemia as a result of haemoglobin catabolism. Unless treated by exchange transfusion, the hyperbilirubinaemia may cause severe neurological damage leading to spasticity, deafness and mental retardation. This condition is known as bilirubin encephalopathy or kernicterus and is irreversible once established.

Prior to 1970, the most common cause of severe HDNB was maternal antibodies with anti-D specificity. The incidence of this form of HDNB was initially greatly reduced by the routine injection of IgG anti-D into all Rh-negative mothers immediately following delivery. This has now been extended to mothers who do not come to term, and current (2008) NICE guidelines extend the practice to the administration of prophylactic anti-D in weeks 28 and 34 of pregnancy, or as a single large dose between weeks 28 and 34. This procedure elicits the rapid destruction of any Rh-positive fetal red cells that may be present, thereby minimizing the risk of maternal sensitization.

The most common cause of HDNB today is ABO incompatibility of maternal and fetal blood. This form of HDNB is almost always associated with group O mothers and group A or B babies. It is caused by the presence in maternal plasma of naturally occurring IgG antibodies with anti-A or anti-B specificity, crossing the placental barrier and eliciting the destruction of fetal red cells which carry the A or B antigen. Typically, ABO-incompatibility produces mild, self-limiting HDNB, which frequently occurs a few days after birth rather than immediately: kernicterus and hydrops fetalis are rarely observed.

Haemolysis secondary to the action of chemicals, drugs or toxins

Immune-mediated haemolysis is not the only mechanism whereby drug therapy can promote premature destruction of red cells. Free oxygen radicals and peroxides generated by the action or metabolism of a wide range of drugs can inflict severe oxidative damage on haemoglobin and red cell membrane components and can lead to early cell death. Some drugs are powerful oxidizing agents in their own right, and directly inflict oxidative damage to the red cell. The drugs which are most commonly associated with haemolysis are shown in *Table 7.2*.

The bite of a number of venomous spiders and snakes, e.g. bites of the brown recluse spider *Loxosceles reclusa*, the king cobra *Ophiophagus hannah*, the Indian cobra *Naja naja*, and the Egyptian cobra *Naja haje*, can cause acute intravascular haemolysis. In extreme cases, even multiple honeybee (*Apis mellifera*) stings have caused acute haemolysis in children.

Haemolysis secondary to infection

A wide range of infections are associated with secondary haemolysis. By far the most common culprits are the *Plasmodia* parasites that cause malaria. Other parasitic diseases are also associated with haemolysis, e.g. toxoplasmosis, trypanosomiasis, leishmaniasis and babesiosis.

Oroya fever is caused by infection with *Bartonella bacilliformis*. The infection is transmitted

Table 7.2 Drugs and chemicals commonly implicated as triggers of non-immune haemolysis

Substance	Comment
Sulphonamides and sulphones Sulphadiazine Sulphanilamide Sulphapyridine	Antimicrobial drugs less used nowadays because of bacterial resistance and side effects
Antimalarials Chloroquine Primaquine Quinine Maloprim	Used in the treatment and prevention of malaria
Nitrofurans Nitrofurantoin	Antimicrobials used for urinary tract infections
Others Salazopyrin p-aminosalicylic acid	Used in treament of Crohn's disease and ulcerative colitis
Vitamin K derivatives	Used for treatment of vitamin K deficiency (especially in neonates)
Chemicals Potassium chlorate	Widely used as a weedkiller
Naphthalene	Used in mothballs
Arsine	AsH3 encountered in extraction and refining of metal ores

by the bite of the *Phlebotomus* sandfly and is found most commonly in Peru and surrounding countries. The acute phase of the disease is frequently accompanied by severe, acute extravascular haemolysis.

Infections with the anaerobic bacterium *Clostridium perfringens* are most commonly seen in poorly treated or contaminated wounds. This organism secretes a substance called phospholipase C that causes severe, acute intravascular haemolysis, which commonly results in death.

A common misconception is that haemolytic streptococci cause their pathogenic effects in man, at least in part, through haemolysis. This is not the case. They gain their name through their ability to lyse the blood in the blood agar plates used for their culture, not through their ability to induce haemolysis in man!

Haemolysis secondary to physical damage

Haemolysis secondary to physical damage to red cells is characterized by the presence of fragmented red cells (schistocytes) in the peripheral blood. Physical damage may be inflicted by abnormalities within the circulatory system or by external changes such as thermal injury or repeated physical trauma.

The classical cause of haemolysis secondary to physical damage to red cells occurs in a minority of patients who have undergone surgery to replace diseased aortic or mitral valves. In most cases, haemolysis is associated with extreme turbulence due to regurgitation of blood around an improperly fitted or faulty prosthesis. Local shear stresses in such circumstances may be sufficient to tear the red cell apart, resulting in intravascular haemolysis. The presence of non-physiological material in the prosthesis is almost certainly an important contributor to the promotion of red cell fragmentation. Recent improvements in surgical technique and the design of implants have made this form of haemolysis much less common.

Disorders of the microvasculature are frequently associated with intravascular deposition of fibrin, thrombocytopenia and intravascular haemolysis secondary to physical trauma. This clinical syndrome is termed micro-angiopathic haemolytic anaemia and encompasses a number of important disease states, including haemolytic uraemic syndrome (HUS), thrombotic thrombocytopenic purpura (TTP), disseminated intravascular coagulation (DIC), and eclampsia of pregnancy. These disorders are described in *Chapter 19*. All are characterized by the deposition of fibrin within the microvasculature, which acts like a cheese-wire, 'slicing' passing red cells to form schistocytes.

Prolonged and repeated physical trauma, especially to the hands and feet, can cause transient intravascular haemolysis. This condition was first described following prolonged marching and was termed march haemoglobinuria. The haemolysis results from the crushing action on red cells in surface capillaries caused by repeatedly striking a hard surface. March haemoglobinuria has also been described in long-distance runners, in bongo drum players and in karate practitioners.

Severe and extensive burns are frequently accompanied by intravascular haemolysis induced by thermal injury to the red cells. Subjecting red cells to temperatures above 49°C, even for relatively short periods, causes irreversible denaturation of spectrin and membrane disruption. In most cases, the haemolysis is acute and self-limiting, resolving within 48 hours of the initial injury. The intravascular haemolysis is made worse by the sequestration of minimally heat-damaged red cells in the spleen.

7.3 PATHOPHYSIOLOGY OF HAEMOLYTIC DISORDERS

The signs and symptoms produced by the various haemolytic disorders are very similar. A haemolytic state is defined by the presence of a shortened red cell lifespan and a compensatory increase in the rate of erythropoiesis. These two features are responsible for the characteristic physiological changes that permit the recognition of haemolytic disorders on clinical grounds:

- **anaemia** is frequently absent because of the compensatory increase in the rate of erythropoiesis. Severe, decompensated haemolysis can lead to severe anaemia, particularly where folate deficiency is also present.
- **jaundice** due to increased breakdown of haem liberated from lysed red cells. The primary breakdown product of haem, bilirubin, is a bright yellow pigment and is responsible for the characteristic yellow discoloration of jaundice (see also *Box 7.12*).
- **reticulocytosis** as a sign of an appropriate erythropoietic response. Reticulocytosis may be suppressed in the presence of folate deficiency.
- **pigment gallstones** are composed of precipitated bilirubin crystals and are found in relatively young people with chronic congenital haemolysis.
- **splenomegaly** is a common feature of haemolysis but is typically slight. Marked splenomegaly may indicate the presence of an underlying condition such as lymphoma as the cause of the haemolysis.
- **haemoglobinuria**. The passage of dark red or even black urine is strongly indicative of intravascular haemolysis.
- **intractable leg ulcers** are relatively common in chronic haemolytic states such as HS and sickle cell disease.
- **aplastic crisis**. Acute arrest of erythropoiesis accompanied by a dramatic fall in circulating red cell count following parvovirus infection is associated with chronic haemolytic disorders such as HS.

Box 7.12 Bilirubin conjugation

The form of bilirubin that predominates in haemolytic jaundice is unconjugated and circulates tightly bound to albumin. Because unconjugated bilirubin is not excreted into the urine, an increase in this form of bilirubin leads to jaundice, but no increase in bilirubin excretion in urine, i.e. *acholuric jaundice*.

- **growth retardation and delayed puberty** are seen in association with severe congenital disorders such as homozygous β-thalassaemia that have a haemolytic component.
- **hypertrophic skeletal changes** due to expansion of erythropoietic marrow are only seen in severe congenital haemolytic disorders.

Once a haemolytic disorder is suspected on clinical grounds, further enquiry may provide useful indicators of the mechanism or cause of the haemolysis:

- **family history**. If the disorder is present in other family members, especially if several generations are involved, a hereditary condition may be suspected. Construction of a pedigree chart can sometimes provide information about the possible mode of inheritance of the disorder.
- **ethnic origin**. Some inherited haemolytic disorders are associated with particular ethnic groups. For example, G-6-PD deficiency is most common in Mediterranean and Chinese populations. However, such associations cannot be used to *exclude* any possible cause of haemolysis.
- **patient history**. Neonatal jaundice may be indicative of congenital conditions such as HS or G-6-PD deficiency whereas a late age of onset suggests an acquired condition. This information must be interpreted with caution because diagnosis of a mild congenital disorder may be missed until adulthood.

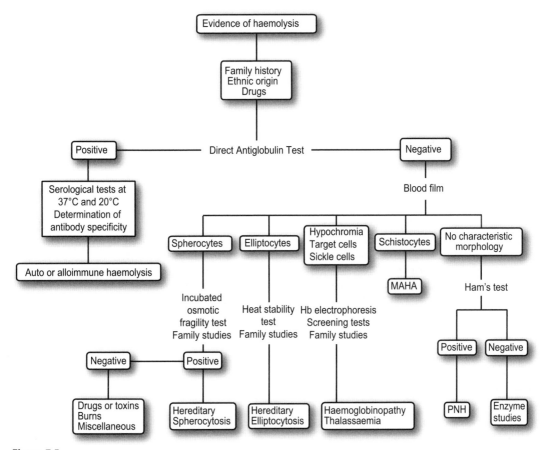

Figure 7.5
Simplified schema for investigation of the haemolytic disorders.

■   **triggering events**. A history of drug ingestion, infection, exposure to cold, surgery or other event, which appears to be associated with the onset of haemolysis, may provide evidence of the cause of an acquired condition.

Clinical findings are seldom sufficient to enable a definitive diagnosis of a particular haemolytic condition to be made; laboratory investigation plays a central role in the accurate diagnosis of haemolysis. The various laboratory features of the different haemolytic disorders can all be grouped under two headings: signs of increased haemolysis and signs of an increased rate of erythropoiesis. A detailed consideration of the laboratory investigation of haemolysis is beyond the scope of this book, but a simplified schema is shown in *Figure 7.5*.

SUGGESTED FURTHER READING

An, X. & Mohandas, N. (2008) Disorders of red cell membrane. *Br. J. Haem.* **141:** 367–375.

Dhaliwal, G., *et al.* (2004) Hemolytic anemia. *Am. Fam. Physician,* **69:** 2599–2606.

Gehrs, B.C. & Friedberg, R.C. (2002) Autoimmune hemolytic anemia. *Am. J. Hematol.* **69:** 258–271.

Mohandas, N. & Gallagher, P.G. (2008) Red cell membrane: past, present, and future. *Blood,* **112:** 3939–3948.

Petz, L.D. (2008) Cold antibody autoimmune hemolytic anemias. *Blood Rev.* **22:** 1–15.

SELF-ASSESSMENT QUESTIONS

1.   Differentiate between the terms haemolytic disorder and haemolytic anaemia.
2.   Name the four most abundant phospholipids in the red cell membrane.
3.   Which of the following are integral proteins?
      a.   AE1
      b.   ankyrin
      c.   glycophorin C
      d.   spectrin
      e.   glucose transport protein
4.   What is the trivial name for band 5?
5.   Which of the two forms of spectrin (α and β) is synthesized more rapidly?
6.   Why is splenectomy an effective measure in hereditary spherocytosis?
7.   Name the five major forms of hereditary elliptocytosis.
8.   What is the reason for progressive red cell water depletion in hereditary xerocytosis?
9.   Outline the mechanism of haemolysis in paroxysmal cold haemoglobinuria.
10.   Why is IgG anti-D routinely administered to all Rh-negative women during pregnancy?
11.   Outline the four mechanisms involved in drug-induced immune-mediated haemolysis.

Disorders of red cell metabolism

Learning objectives
After studying this chapter you should confidently be able to:

■ **Describe the requirements for energy and reducing power in mature red cells**
The mature red cells require a supply of energy to maintain the intracellular cation balance, to maintain the biconcave discoid shape and to drive the early steps of glycolysis. Reducing power is required to combat membrane lipid oxidation, to maintain haemoglobin in the Fe^{2+} state and to detoxify environmental oxidants.

■ **Differentiate between the primary functions of the Embden–Meyerhof pathway, hexose monophosphate pathway and glutathione cycle**
The Embden–Meyerhof pathway is the primary supplier of the energy needs of the mature red cell, while its reducing power is provided by interaction of the hexose monophosphate pathway and glutathione cycle.

■ **Describe the physiological importance of the Rappaport–Luebering shunt**
The Rappaport–Luebering shunt helps to modulate the oxygen affinity of adult haemoglobin by producing 2,3-DPG, which binds to β-globin chains, thereby stabilizing the haemoglobin molecule in the low oxygen affinity configuration.

■ **Explain the importance of the Rappaport–Luebering shunt in determining the clinical severity of defects of the Embden–Meyerhof pathway**
Defects of enzymes located above the Rappaport–Luebering shunt tend to be clinically severe because the shortage of 2,3-DPG that ensues leads to increased oxygen affinity, exacerbating the effects of anaemia. Conversely, enzyme defects below the Rappaport–Luebering shunt tend to be ameliorated by the accumulation of 2,3-DPG that results.

■ **Explain the phenomenon of episodic haemolysis in G-6-PD deficiency**
In the great majority of cases of G-6-PD deficiency, there is sufficient residual reducing power present to deal with day-to-day oxidant stress. When there is an acute increase in oxidant stress, G-6-PD-deficient cells have no reserve reducing capacity and acute haemolysis results. The reticulocytes that are produced in response to this haemolytic crisis are relatively richer in G-6-PD, so the haemolysis tends to be self-limited.

As red cells mature they lose their nucleus, mitochondria and ribosomes. Absence of the nucleus and ribosomes makes the mature red cell incapable of protein synthesis and the lack of mitochondria deprives the cell of the most efficient means of energy production, oxidative phosphorylation. The cell is thus entirely dependent upon the relatively inefficient mechanism of anaerobic glycolysis via the Embden–Meyerhof pathway (*Figure 8.1*; see also *Box 8.1*) to provide its energy requirement. Protection of the red cell against oxidative stresses is provided mainly via the hexose monophosphate pathway (*Figure 8.1*). Because of the dependence of the red cell upon the proper functioning of these two pathways, defects in the enzymes that catalyse them can be catastrophic.

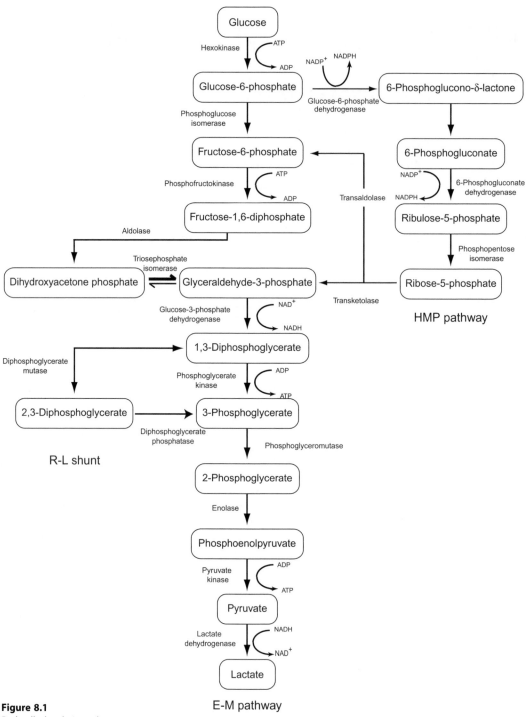

Figure 8.1
Red cell glycolytic pathways.

Box 8.1 Red cells and hypoxia

The ability of cells to extract energy anaerobically from glucose in the form of ATP represents an extremely important survival mechanism. Anaerobic glycolysis can provide a short-term energy reserve for vital organs when oxygen supply is cut off and aerobic glycolysis ceases. For example, at birth, changes in the fetal blood circulation temporarily starve all of the major organs except the brain of oxygenated blood. During this period, the energy demands of the fetal organs are met via anaerobic glycolysis. In other words, if anaerobic glycolysis did not exist, nor could we!

The glucose that is used by the red cell in the two glycolytic pathways is derived from plasma via a specific transport protein in the red cell membrane. Normally, about 95% of red cell glucose is metabolized via the Embden–Meyerhof pathway while the remainder enters the hexose monophosphate pathway.

8.1   THE EMBDEN–MEYERHOF PATHWAY

The primary role of the Embden–Meyerhof pathway in the economy of the mature red cell is the generation of ATP. Large quantities of energy are released from ATP during its conversion to ADP, and ATP should be thought of as an energy store for use by the cell. The Embden–Meyerhof pathway is also a source of nicotinamide adenine dinucleotide (NADH), which acts as a cofactor for the enzyme methaemoglobin reductase in the conversion of methaemoglobin to functional haemoglobin. 2,3-diphosphoglycerate (2,3-DPG) is formed via a diversion from the main pathway known as **the Rappaport–Luebering shunt** (*Figure 8.1*). This molecule functions to modulate oxygen delivery to the tissues by altering the oxygen affinity of haemoglobin as described in *Chapter 6*.

There are three main requirements for energy within normal red cells, as follows.

- **Maintenance of intracellular cation balance.** The intracellular concentrations of Na^+ and K^+ differ markedly from those of the surrounding plasma. This difference is maintained by an active process, which pumps Na^+ from the cell into the plasma and K^+ into the cell from the plasma. The energy required to drive this process is provided via the conversion of ATP to ADP by a membrane-bound ATPase. Failure of the cation pump results in rapid loss of K^+ and water, and leads to the premature death of the red cell.
- **Maintenance of cell shape.** Maintenance of the cytoskeleton determines the characteristic biconcave shape and deformability of the red cell and is an energy-consuming process. Failure of energy production results in loss of deformability and shape changes, which shorten the lifespan of the cell.
- **Phosphorylation of glucose and fructose-6-phosphate.** The early stages of the Embden–Meyerhof pathway involve the phosphorylation of glucose to glucose-6-phosphate and fructose-6-phosphate to fructose-1,6-diphosphate. Failure of these steps results in failure of the pathway and a consequent reduction in ATP synthesis. Low levels of ATP lead to failure of these early phosphorylation steps, thus establishing a vicious circle, which culminates in the death of the cell.

The reaction steps of the Embden–Meyerhof pathway

The first reaction of the Embden–Meyerhof pathway involves the phosphorylation of glucose to form glucose-6-phosphate (G-6-P). This reaction consumes a mole of ATP for every mole of glucose phosphorylated and is catalysed by the enzyme hexokinase in the presence of divalent metal ions such as Mg^{2+}. The catalytic action of hexokinase is inhibited by the product of the reaction, G-6-P, thus providing an important control mechanism on the rate of glycolysis. An important effect of this reaction is to 'lock' the intermediates of glycolysis within the red cell: the red cell membrane is impermeable to phosphorylated sugars.

G-6-P is subsequently converted to its isomer, fructose-6-phosphate (F-6-P) in an isomerization reaction catalysed by the enzyme phosphoglucose isomerase (see also *Box 8.2*).

F-6-P is further phosphorylated, again at the expense of ATP, to form fructose-1,6-diphosphate (F-1,6-DP), a reaction catalysed by the enzyme phosphofructokinase (see also *Box 8.3*). High levels of ATP inhibit the catalytic function of phosphofructokinase. Thus, in the presence of adequate levels of ATP, glycolysis is inhibited and, conversely, when the supply of energy falls glycolysis is stimulated. This mechanism provides the most important regulator of the rate of glycolysis.

The cleavage of F-1,6-DP into dihydroxyacetone phosphate and glyceraldehyde-3-phosphate (Ga-3-P) is catalysed by the enzyme aldolase. These two products are isomers and are interconvertible under the influence of the enzyme triose phosphate isomerase. Because Ga-3-P is constantly consumed in the next step of the pathway, the dynamic equilibrium that exists between dihydroxyacetone phosphate and Ga-3-P is shifted to the right. Thus, in effect, one mole of F-1,6-DP is cleaved to form two moles of Ga-3-P.

The next reaction involves the conversion of Ga-3-P to 1,3-diphosphoglycerate (1,3-DPG). This reaction is catalysed by the enzyme glyceraldehyde-3-phosphate dehydrogenase and results in the formation of NADH, for which a supply of nicotinamide adenine dinucleotide (NAD) is needed.

At this stage of the Embden–Meyerhof pathway, two moles of ATP have been consumed and none generated. However, everything is now in place to commence production of ATP. 1,3-DPG has a high potential to donate one of its phosphoryl groups to ADP thus forming 3-phosphoglycerate (3-PG) and ATP. This reaction is catalysed by the enzyme phosphoglycerate kinase. However, remember that one mole of glucose has been converted into two moles of 1,3-DPG. Thus, for each mole of glucose that enters the Embden–Meyerhof pathway, two moles of ATP are generated by this reaction. This balances the energy equation of the pathway: two moles of ATP have been expended and two moles have been generated.

The final stages of the Embden–Meyerhof pathway are designed to generate two further moles of ATP in the conversion of 3-PG to lactate. This outcome requires the synthesis of a molecule that, like 1,3-DPG, has a high phosphoryl group transfer potential. The first step

---

Box 8.2 Elucidating the pathway

Otto Meyerhof worked at the University of Heidelberg and was awarded a Nobel Prize in 1922 for his work on anaerobic muscle metabolism. Gustav Embden was Director of the Physiological Institute at Frankfurt Sachsenhausen and shared Meyerhof's interest in muscle metabolism, although the two men did not collaborate. The full Embden–Meyerhof pathway was not elucidated until 1949, 16 years after Embden's premature death. Rappaport and Luebering described the mode of 2,3-DPG formation the following year.

Box 8.3 BPG or DPG?

Strictly, phosphorylated intermediates such as fructose-1,6-diphosphate (F-1,6-DP) and 2,3-diphosphoglycerate (2,3-DPG) should be called fructose-1,6-bisphosphate (F-1,6-BP) and 2,3-bisphosphoglycerate (2,3-BPG) because the two phosphate groups are located on separate carbon atoms. However, the abbreviations F-1,6-DP and 2,3-DPG have been used so extensively that to replace them with the correct forms would be confusing. The diphosphate nomenclature has therefore been retained in this book.

towards achieving this goal occurs under the influence of the enzyme phosphoglyceromutase and involves the rearrangement of 3-PG to form 2-phosphoglycerate (2-PG). 2-PG is converted into phosphoenolpyruvate (PEP) in the presence of the enzyme enolase. Enol phosphates such as PEP have a high phosphoryl group transfer potential. In the presence of the enzyme pyruvate kinase, PEP donates its phosphoryl group to ADP, resulting in the formation of two moles of ATP and two moles of pyruvate per mole of glucose metabolized. Thus, although two moles of ATP have been consumed by the early reactions of the Embden–Meyerhof pathway, four moles of ATP are generated by subsequent reactions resulting in a net gain of two moles of ATP per mole of glucose metabolized. Pyruvate is subsequently converted into lactate under the influence of the enzyme lactate dehydrogenase. This reaction generates the NAD needed for the conversion of Ga-3-P to 1,3-DPG.

The Rappaport–Luebering shunt

1,3-DPG, in addition to its direct conversion to 3-PG, can be converted in the presence of the enzyme diphosphoglycerate mutase into 2,3-diphosphoglycerate (2,3-DPG). This diversion from the main Embden–Meyerhof pathway is called the Rappaport–Luebering shunt and is of prime physiological importance because of the role that 2,3-DPG plays in modulating the oxygen affinity of haemoglobin A (see *Chapter 6*). The unique role of 2,3-DPG in red cells is underlined by its high concentration within these cells. Most other cells of the body contain only traces of the substance.

2,3-DPG can be converted to 3-PG under the influence of the enzyme 2,3-diphosphoglycerate phosphatase, thus completing the shunt. However, the co-product of this reaction is free phosphate rather than ATP.

8.2 THE HEXOSE MONOPHOSPHATE PATHWAY

The hexose monophosphate pathway generates reducing potential for the red cell in the form of nicotinamide adenine dinucleotide phosphate (NADPH), which is an essential component of the glutathione cycle as shown in *Figure 8.2* (see also *Box 8.3*). Reduced glutathione (GSH) is the most important antioxidant within red cells. Under normal circumstances, hexose monophosphate pathway activity consumes about 5% of the G-6-P formed as the first step of glycolysis. However, the rate of activity can be increased when required to deal with an increased level of oxidants.

Reducing power is required by the red cell for three main reasons.

- **Combating membrane lipid oxidation**. Oxidation and peroxidation of membrane lipids would cause an increase in membrane rigidity and permeability and so render the red cell liable to destruction in the spleen.
- **Reduction of methaemoglobin**. Oxidation of the ferrous (Fe^{2+}) iron in haem to the ferric (Fe^{3+}) form results in the formation of methaemoglobin, which is incapable of oxygen transport. Small quantities of methaemoglobin are constantly formed within the red cell. It is essential that accumulation of methaemoglobin is prevented by its rapid reduction to functional haemoglobin.
- **Detoxification of oxidants**. In the process of methaemoglobin formation, highly reactive oxygen radicals such as superoxide and hydroxyl radical are formed, which lead to the generation of the powerful oxidant hydrogen peroxide. Ingestion of oxidant drugs such as primaquine and the sulphonamides also results in the formation of hydrogen peroxide. Detoxification of these substances via the glutathione cycle is essential if severe oxidant damage to the cell is to be avoided.

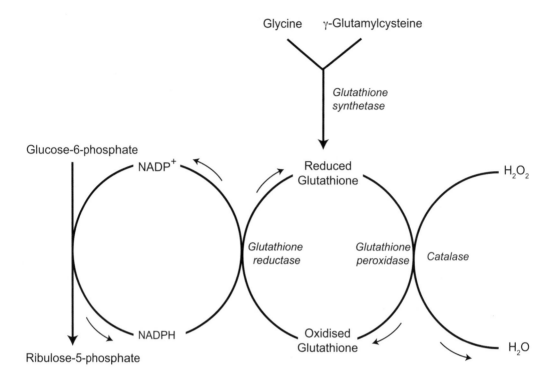

Figure 8.2
The glutathione cycle.

The reaction steps of the hexose monophosphate pathway

The first reaction of the hexose monophosphate pathway involves the dehydrogenation of G-6-P to form 6-PG via an intermediate called 6-phosphoglucono-δ-lactone (see also *Box 8.4*). The conversion of G-6-P into 6-phosphoglucono-δ-lactone is the rate-determining step of the hexose monophosphate pathway and is catalysed by the enzyme G-6-PD. This reaction is accompanied by the generation of NADPH.

6-PG is then decarboxylated in the presence of the enzyme 6-phosphogluconate dehydrogenase to form ribulose-5-phosphate (Ru-5-P) and, in the process, another mole of NADPH is formed. Thus, for each mole of glucose that enters the hexose monophosphate pathway, two moles of NADPH are generated. NADPH formation is the physiologically relevant role of this pathway in red cells.

Ru-5-P is subsequently converted into ribose-5-phosphate (R-5-P) under the influence of the enzyme phosphopentose isomerase. R-5-P is used by other cells in the synthesis of nucleotides and nucleic acids. In red cells, however, R-5-P is converted into F-6-P and Ga-3-P in the presence of the enzymes transaldolase and transketolase respectively. These substances are then metabolized via the Embden–Meyerhof pathway.

The conversion of G-6-P to R-5-P constantly consumes NADP⁺ and generates NADPH. The NADPH thus formed acts as a reducing agent in the reduction of oxidized glutathione (GSSG)

Box 8.4 Enzyme classification

Enzymes are classified into six major classes, each with several subclasses:

Class 1 – oxidoreductases catalyse redox reactions and include dehydrogenases, oxidases and peroxidases.

Class 2 – transferases catalyse the transfer of functional groups such as amino groups (aminotransferases) and phosphoryl groups (kinases).

Class 3 – hydrolases catalyse the transfer of functional groups to water and include peptidases, esterases and deaminases.

Class 4 – lyases catalyse the addition or removal of the elements of water, ammonia or carbon dioxide and include the decarboxylases and the dehydratases.

Class 5 – isomerases catalyse isomerization reactions and include the epimerases, the racemases and the mutases.

Class 6 – ligases catalyse synthetic reactions where two molecules are joined together and include the synthetases and carboxylases.

---

in the presence of the enzyme glutathione reductase. In this process, $NADP^+$ is formed which is then utilized in the generation of more R-5-P. Reduced glutathione (GSH) is required for the detoxification of oxidants as described above. In this process, GSH is cycled back to GSSG.

8.3   THE PURINE SALVAGE PATHWAY

Red cells are incapable of *de novo* synthesis of purines because the enzyme 5′ phosphoribosyl-1-pyrophosphate (PRPP) amidotransferase is absent. However, an active purine salvage pathway exists which can generate ATP from preformed bases. Adenine can penetrate red cells where, in the presence of PRPP and the enzyme adenine phosphoribosyl transferase, it is converted to adenosine monophosphate (AMP). AMP can then be phosphorylated to form first ADP and then ATP in the presence of the enzyme adenylate kinase.

The existence of the purine salvage pathway in red cells is exploited in the storage of blood for transfusion. The addition of adenine to the storage medium provides a supplementary source of fuel for ATP synthesis and so prolongs the useful life of the stored red cells. However, purine salvage is of doubtful physiological significance.

8.4   DISORDERS OF RED CELL METABOLISM

The mature red cell has lost its nucleus and mitochondria in the process of maturation. This has two important metabolic effects.

■ Loss of the mitochondria means that the cell depends completely upon glycolysis via the Embden–Meyerhof pathway for the fulfilment of its energy requirement, and on the hexose monophosphate pathway for its reducing power. Thus, a defect or a deficiency in any of the enzymes that catalyse these pathways can have serious deleterious effects on the overall economy of the cell and may lead to a shortening of red cell lifespan.

■ Loss of the nucleus means that the cell has no means of synthesizing more protein to compensate for enzyme deficiency.

By common agreement, the definition of an enzyme deficiency relates to suboptimal activity of the enzyme under physiological conditions: both quantitative and qualitative enzyme disorders are encompassed by this term (see also *Box 8.5*).

Box 8.5 Understanding terminology

Red cell disorders that are characterized by an enzyme deficiency are known as the *red cell enzymopathies*. This name is derived from the Greek word for disease – *pathos*. Thus, enzymopathies are disorders of enzymes. Similarly, the disorders that are characterized by abnormal haemoglobin synthesis are known as the *haemoglobinopathies*. Learning the meaning of word fragments like this is a useful way of working out what haematological terms mean.

Disorders of the Embden–Meyerhof pathway

Failure of the Embden–Meyerhof pathway is associated with deficiency of ATP within the red cell and a consequent collapse of energy-dependent processes. The result, in most cases, is a shortening of red cell lifespan. Defects of the Embden–Meyerhof pathway are manifest as a congenital non-spherocytic haemolytic anaemia (CNSHA) of highly variable severity (see also *Box 8.6*). This clinical heterogeneity arises partly because of the great variety of mutations that are encountered, but is also related to the position of the affected enzyme relative to the Rappaport–Luebering shunt.

Abnormalities of all of the enzymes of the Embden–Meyerhof pathway have been described, although most are extremely rare. The most common defect, pyruvate kinase deficiency, accounts for more than 90% of cases of glycolytic enzyme deficiency that are associated with haemolysis.

Box 8.6 Congenital or inherited?

Congenital means present at birth. Congenital conditions are not necessarily inherited and inherited conditions are not necessarily congenital. For example, spina bifida is present at birth but is not inherited, and Huntington's chorea is an autosomal dominant inherited disorder that usually does not appear until middle age.

Pyruvate kinase deficiency

Pyruvate kinase (PK) catalyses the conversion of phosphoenol pyruvate (PEP) to pyruvate and exists in several isoenzyme forms in different tissues of the body. The PK isoenzymes are encoded by two genes: *PKM2*, which is located at chromosome 15q22, and *PKLR* which is located at chromosome 1q21. Each of these genes encodes two distinct PK isozymes as shown in *Table 8.1*.

Because of this tissue specificity, a deficiency of red cell PK is not reflected in white cells and platelets (see also *Box 8.7*). PK deficiency is inherited as an autosomal recessive trait, being expressed only in homozygotes and compound heterozygotes. More than 100 mutations of the PK genes have been described, including mis-sense mutations, splicing mutations, insertions and deletions. Most individuals who express disease are compound heterozygotes for two different variant enzymes. It is this genetic heterogeneity that is the major determinant of the clinical variability of this disorder.

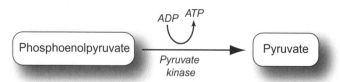

Figure 8.3
The role of pyruvate kinase in red cell metabolism.

Table 8.1 Pyruvate kinase genes and isozymes

Gene	Isozymes	Tissue
PK-M2	PK-M1	Mature muscle and brain
	PKM2	All fetal tissues
		Red cell precursors
		Mature white cells, platelets, lung, kidney, spleen, adipose tissue
PKLR	PK-L	Hepatocytes
	PK-R	Mature red cells

Box 8.7 Recognition of pyruvate kinase

Pyruvate kinase deficiency was first recognized in 1960 by William Valentine and colleagues at the University of California in Los Angeles. Detailed investigation of several families with congenital non-spherocytic haemolytic anaemia, pointed to a deficiency of this enzyme as the most likely cause of their condition. Amazingly, the original paper describing this important discovery was submitted for publication in *Science* but was rejected as being of limited interest!

Pathophysiology. The clinical severity of pyruvate kinase deficiency is highly variable, ranging from a severe CNSHA to a clinically silent, compensated form. In most cases, there is a moderate reduction in haemoglobin concentration to 6–10 g/dl. The haemoglobin concentration is usually stable but can fall suddenly during an infection. Some degree of jaundice and splenomegaly is usually present. Neonatal jaundice is relatively common and, occasionally, may be severe enough to require an exchange transfusion. The continuous presence of excess bilirubin in the plasma can result in the formation of pigment gallstones at a relatively young age. In common with other chronic haemolytic conditions, there is an increased incidence of folate deficiency in affected individuals.

Although most individuals with PK deficiency are moderately anaemic, clinical symptoms of anaemia may be minimal or absent. This anomaly is explained by the position of PK in the Embden–Meyerhof pathway. Deficiency of PK causes an accumulation of PEP and other intermediates from higher up the Embden–Meyerhof pathway. Most importantly, the concentration of red cell 2,3-DPG may treble. As explained in *Chapter 6*, 2,3-DPG binds to β-globin chains, thereby stabilizing the haemoglobin molecule in the low oxygen affinity configuration. Thus, although the haemoglobin concentration is reduced in PK deficiency, the capacity for oxygen delivery to the tissues is increased and the effects of the anaemia are minimized. There have been a number of reports of PK-deficient individuals with reduced haemoglobin concentrations who regularly indulge in middle-distance running!

There are no characteristic features of red cell morphology associated with PK deficiency. Moderate reticulocytosis is usually present and irregularly contracted red cells (pyknocytes) may be seen, but these are not diagnostic. The severity of the anaemia is diminished by splenectomy (see also *Box 8.8*).

Box 8.8 Understanding terminology

Splenomegaly means an enlarged spleen and is a relatively common finding in haematological disease. Similarly, hepatomegaly means enlargement of the liver, and hepatosplenomegaly means enlargement of both.

Hexokinase deficiency

Hexokinase catalyses the phosphorylation of glucose to form glucose-6-phosphate (G-6-P) in the presence of divalent metal ions such as Mg^{2+}. The inhibition of hexokinase activity by the product of this reaction provides an important mechanism for the control of the rate of glycolysis.

Four hexokinase isozymes have been identified (Hk-1-4), each encoded by a distinct gene. The HK1 gene encodes the hexokinase found in red cells, platelets and lymphocytes and is located on chromosome 10. Hk-1 deficiency has no clinically significant effect on platelet or white cell function because of the presence of Hk-3 in these cells.

Hexokinase activity diminishes rapidly with increasing red cell age. This phenomenon leads to a reduction in glycolytic activity and a relative lack of ATP within senescent red cells and contributes to their demise.

Hexokinase deficiency is extremely rare but most reported cases have shown an autosomal recessive mode of inheritance (*see also Box 8.9*). Occasional examples of autosomal dominant inheritance have also been reported.

The sequelae of hexokinase deficiency are similar to those for PK deficiency in most respects. However, because hexokinase acts above the Rappaport–Luebering shunt, deficiency leads to an increased haemoglobin oxygen affinity due to lack of 2,3-DPG. This is manifest as severe symptoms of anaemia in the presence of a moderately reduced haemoglobin concentration.

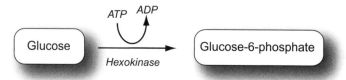

Figure 8.4
The role of hexokinase in red cell metabolism.

Box 8.9 Acquired hexokinase deficiency

Acquired hexokinase deficiency can sometimes occur in Wilson's disease, a rare inherited disorder in which excessive amounts of copper accumulate in the body. The build-up of copper leads to damage in the kidneys, brain, and eyes, and can inhibit hexokinase leading to intermittent haemolysis.

Disorders of the hexose monophosphate pathway

Defects of the hexose monophosphate pathway result in an increased susceptibility of the red cell to oxidant stress. All defects are rare except deficiency of G-6-PD, which is by far the most common red cell enzymopathy, affecting almost 1% of the world's population.

Box 8.10 G-6-PD and antimalarials

The widespread use of antimalarial prophylactic drugs in US soldiers in the Korean War led to the observation that pamaquine triggered an acute and severe, but self-limited haemolytic anaemia in about one in ten black soldiers. US military-funded studies of a group of 'volunteers' from the Stateville Penitentiary, Illinois, showed that this phenomenon was caused by an intracellular red cell defect. However, it was not until 1956 that Paul Carson and colleagues traced this form of drug-induced haemolysis to a deficiency of G-6-PD.

Glucose-6-phosphate dehydrogenase deficiency

G-6-PD catalyses the dehydrogenation of G-6-P to form 6-phosphoglucono-δ-lactone with the simultaneous reduction of NADP to form NADPH. Deficiency of G-6-PD has been reported in most populations of the world, but is most commonly seen in western and central Africa, the Mediterranean region, the Middle East and SE Asia. For example, in some parts of Saudi Arabia, almost one-third of the population carry an abnormal G-6-PD gene. In common with thalassaemia and sickle cell disease, G-6-PD deficiency is associated with malarial areas because female carriers have increased resistance to malarial infection. These are all examples of a balanced polymorphism in which two alleles are maintained in a stable equilibrium, because of selection pressure caused by the heterozygote state conferring an advantage (e.g. malarial resistance) over either of the homozygous states.

The gene that encodes G-6-PD is located on the tip of the q arm of the X chromosome, close to the factor VIII gene. The normal form of G-6-PD is designated G-6-PDB or Gd^B and the normal gene is denoted *Gd^B*. This form of G-6-PD is present in 99% of Caucasians and in about 70% of people of African descent. A functionally normal variant G-6-PD isoenzyme, Gd^A is found in about 20% of people of African descent (see also *Box 8.10*).

G-6-PD deficiency results from the synthesis of structurally abnormal enzyme variants that have impaired stability or catalytic activity (see also *Box 8.11*). More than 350 different G-6-PD variants have been described but only a few are associated with clinically severe disease. The most common variant of G-6-PD is found in about 10% of black people and is designated Gd^{A-}. All other abnormal G-6-PD variants are designated by their area of greatest incidence, e.g. Gd^{MED} is most prevalent in the Mediterranean region, India and SE Asia, while Gd^{CANTON} is most prevalent in Chinese populations.

G-6-PD deficiency is inherited in a sex-linked recessive manner, i.e. it is transmitted by symptomless female heterozygotes to affected male hemizygotes. Because of the relatively high incidence of aberrant genes in some populations, female homozygotes are not uncommon.

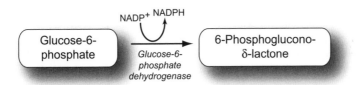

Figure 8.5
The role of G-6-PD in red cell metabolism.

Box 8.11 Enzyme classification

The World Health Organization (WHO) classification of G-6-PD variants takes account of the severity of the enzyme deficiency and the severity of haemolysis:

Class I variants have very severe enzyme deficiency (<10–20% of normal) and have chronic haemolytic anaemia.
Class II variants also have severe enzyme deficiency (<10% of normal), but usually only intermittent haemolysis.
Class III variants have moderate enzyme deficiency (10–60% of normal) with intermittent haemolysis usually associated with infection or drugs.
Class IV variants have no enzyme deficiency or haemolysis.
Class V variants have increased enzyme activity.

Pathophysiology

The red cell is protected from oxidative damage by the constant regeneration of GSH via the glutathione cycle. The hexose monophosphate pathway provides the continuous supply of NADPH required to drive the glutathione cycle. Thus, red cells that are deficient in G-6-PD develop a secondary deficiency of GSH and are highly susceptible to oxidative damage. This can lead to a reduction in red cell lifespan in three ways:

- cross-linking and aggregation of membrane cytoskeletal proteins causes a decrease in red cell deformability thereby promoting sequestration in the liver and spleen;
- peroxidation of membrane lipids also causes a loss of deformability and intravascular haemolysis;
- oxidation of thiol and other groups in globin chains leads to the aggregation and precipitation of denatured globin within the cell, forming Heinz bodies. These inclusion bodies bind to the inner aspect of the red cell membrane via disulphide bonds between globin and the cytoskeleton, and are 'pitted' from the cell during its passage through the spleen, resulting in the formation of 'bite' cells and premature haemolysis.

Despite the large number of G-6-PD variants, individuals with G-6-PD deficiency typically exhibit one of two patterns of haemolysis: CNSHA or episodic haemolysis (see also *Box 8.12*).

Chronic non-spherocytic haemolytic anaemia. CNSHA is associated with extremely unstable or severely dysfunctional G-6-PD variants (see also *Box 8.11*). A large number of such variants exist but all are rare; many have only been described in a single family. This form of G-6-PD deficiency presents as life-long haemolytic anaemia of variable severity, which does not respond to splenectomy. The condition may be complicated by sporadic haemolytic or aplastic crises, which may be triggered by infection or ingestion of oxidant drugs.

Episodic haemolysis. The most common G-6-PD variants are characterized by episodes of acute haemolysis induced by increased oxidant stress. In the vast majority of cases of G-6-PD deficiency, red cell enzyme activity is sufficient to combat the oxidative stresses imposed by everyday life and red cell survival is almost normal. However, exposure to increased oxidant stress exposes the inability of the red cell to respond by increasing hexose monophosphate pathway activity and leads to acute intravascular haemolysis. Broadly, three sets of triggers of acute haemolysis in G-6-PD-deficient individuals have been identified.

- **Ingestion of oxidant drugs** can trigger acute intravascular haemolysis in G-6-PD-deficient individuals. A wide range of drugs has been implicated as shown in *Table 8.2*. Most of the offending drugs are taken up by the red cell where they mediate the transfer of electrons from intracellular reducing agents such as NADPH and GSH to molecular oxygen, thereby forming superoxide, hydrogen peroxide and hydroxyl radicals within the red cell. The inability of G-6-PD-deficient red cells to detoxify these powerful oxidants leads to acute intravascular haemolysis. This oxidation also occurs in non-deficient people, but an intact hexose monophosphate pathway is usually capable of neutralizing this effect.
- **Ingestion of the common broad (or fava) bean**, *Vicia faba*, may trigger acute intravascular haemolysis in individuals with some types of G-6-PD deficiency. This form

---

Box 8.12 G-6-PD and reticulocytes

The self-limited nature of the haemolysis is explained by the higher concentration of G-6-PD present in reticulocytes. The marked reticulocyte response that follows the primary haemolytic episode effectively raises the circulating G-6-PD level, and thereby reduces the sensitivity of the circulating red cells to oxidant stress.

Table 8.2 Drugs commonly implicated as triggers of acute haemolysis in G-6-PD deficiency

Drug family	Drug examples	Uses
Antimalarials	Chloroquine	Malaria prophylaxis and treatment
	Mefloquine	Malaria prophylaxis
	Amodiaquine	Malaria treatment
	Primaquine	Malaria prophylaxis and treatment
Sulphonamides and sulphones*	Sulphamethoxazole	Antibacterial (bladder and some GI infections)
	Sulphasalazine	Ulcerative colitis, Crohn's disease
	Cotrimoxazole	Antibacterial (urinary, respiratory, otitis media)
	Dapsone	Leprosy, dermatitis herpetiformis
Cardiovascular	Procainamide	Anti-arrhythmic
	Quinidine	Anti-arrhythmic
Cytotoxic/antibacterial	Chloramphenicol	Eye infections
	Nalidixic acid	Antibacterial (urinary tract)
	Nitrofurantoin	Antibacterial (urinary tract)
Miscellaneous	Aspirin	Non-narcotic analgesic and anti-inflammatory
	Probenicid	Gout
	α-methyldopa	Antihypertensive
	Dimercaprol	Treatment of heavy metal poisoning
	Hydralazine	Antihypertensive
	Mestranol	Oral contraceptive
	Phenylhydrazine	Polycythaemia (no longer used)
	Vitamin K	Haemorrhagic disease of the newborn

*Most members of this group of antibacterials have been implicated as triggers of acute haemolysis in G-6-PD-deficient individuals but, other than those listed, they have been superseded and are little used nowadays.

of haemolysis is known as favism and is associated particularly with the Gd^{MED} variant of G-6-PD. The Gd^{A-} variant is not associated with favism. The substances present in broad beans that elicit the haemolysis are thought to be vicine and convicine. These compounds are metabolized to the oxidants divicine and isouramil in the intestine, leading to a decrease in GSH and production of hydrogen peroxide and free radicals within red cells, creating a severe oxidant stress. G-6-PD-deficient red cells are unable to cope with this acute oxidant stress and acute haemolysis results. Haemolysis is most common following ingestion of fresh, raw broad beans but has been reported following ingestion of cooked, dried and frozen beans and even inhalation of broad bean pollen. At least one report exists of haemolysis in a breast-fed infant following maternal ingestion of broad beans.

■ **Infection** is a relatively common trigger of acute intravascular haemolysis in G-6-PD-deficient individuals. Haemolysis is seen most commonly following pneumococcal infection or viral hepatitis. The exact mechanisms that trigger haemolysis remain obscure but release of oxidants from activated neutrophils, ingestion of antimicrobial drugs, hyperthermia and acidosis probably all contribute.

In the absence of acute haemolysis, the blood of a G-6-PD-deficient individual appears essentially normal. During a haemolytic crisis, however, moderate anisocytosis, bite cells and

---

Box 8.13 Heinz bodies

Heinz bodies appear on Romanowsky-stained blood films as small purple irregular bodies in the cytoplasm of red cells. They are seen in cases of G-6-PD deficiency, particularly after the administration of oxidant drugs such as primaquine, in the presence of unstable haemoglobin variants such as Hb Hammersmith, and after removal of the spleen (splenectomy).

Heinz bodies are named after R Heinz, who was director of the Institute of Pharmacology at Erlanger, where he described the appearance of these inclusion bodies in guinea pig blood following the administration of acetylphenylhydrazine. Heinz bodies are removed during passage of the red cell through the spleen. This process damages the red cell and leads to the formation of red cells that appear on the blood film to have been nibbled by mice! These are known as 'bite' cells. *Anisocytosis* means variation in red cell size. *Poikilocytosis* means variation in red cell shape. If both phenomena are present together, the result is described as *anisopoikilocytosis*.

---

occasional spherocytes are typically present. Heinz bodies may be present in acute drug-induced haemolysis or favism, but are seldom seen otherwise (see also *Box 8.13*). Methaemoglobinaemia may be present but is seldom severe.

G-6-PD deficiency is the most common cause of neonatal jaundice worldwide. Normal neonatal red cells typically have suboptimal activity of the glutathione cycle and so, when a deficiency of G-6-PD is superimposed upon this, are highly susceptible to oxidant-induced haemolysis. However, the degree of jaundice observed is frequently more severe than expected, due to the relative inability of the neonatal liver to conjugate bilirubin and, possibly, to a deficiency of hepatic G-6-PD. In some cases, the cause of acute haemolysis in a G-6-PD-deficient neonate can be traced to an oxidant drug used by the mother during labour, or to the use of sulphonamides to combat neonatal infection. In most cases, however, no trigger can be identified.

8.5   LABORATORY INVESTIGATION OF A SUSPECTED ENZYMOPATHY

Because the red cell enzymopathies are mostly rare conditions, it is essential first to eliminate the more common causes of haemolysis. A clinical and family history may provide useful clues to guide the investigation. For example, evidence of a family history of haemolysis, unexplained neonatal jaundice or a pattern of episodic haemolysis with identifiable triggers such as drug or fava bean ingestion increase the index of suspicion.

A blood film examination can help to guide the investigation. Although red cell enzymopathies are typically not associated with marked or specific abnormalities in red cell morphology, certain findings are associated with particular abnormalities. For example, prominent basophilic stippling is a characteristic finding in pyrimidine-5'-nucleotidase deficiency homozygotes; Heinz bodies may be present after acute oxidant haemolysis in G-6-PD or glutathione deficiency; echinocytes may be seen in pyruvate kinase, hexokinase or other glycolytic enzyme deficiencies that lead to a shortage of ATP. A raised reticulocyte count confirms increased marrow activity, although a normal count does not exclude chronic haemolysis because of the potential masking effect of folate deficiency.

Where other causes of haemolysis have been excluded and clinical or family history suggests enzymopathy, specific enzyme assays should be undertaken (see also *Box 8.14*). It is sensible to test sequentially for the most common enzymopathies before moving to the rarer types.

Because of the huge variety of mutations that cause abnormalities of red cell enzymes, genetic screening is not routinely useful. However, there are certain circumstances where molecular approaches may be helpful:

Box 8.14 G-6-PD and reticulocytes

Misleading results can be obtained for G-6-PD assay results during or immediately following acute haemolytic episodes. The concentration of G-6-PD in a red cell decreases with the age of the cell. Thus, if the reticulocyte count is raised significantly, such as during acute haemolytic episodes, the normal distribution of circulating red cell ages is skewed and the overall G-6PD level may be artificially high, masking a deficiency. Wherever possible, assay of G-6-PD (or other age-dependent enzymes) should be performed during periods of normal erythropoietic activity.

- if the specific mutation within a family is identified, specific testing for that abnormality in other family members or as antenatal diagnosis is possible;
- certain mutations are known to be more prevalent in particular ethnic groups, for example, a restricted number of mutations of pyruvate kinase are prevalent in the Pennsylvania Amish people and so can usefully be screened for.

SUGGESTED FURTHER READING

Alberto, Z., *et al.* (2007) Pyruvate kinase deficiency: the genotype–phenotype association. *Blood Reviews,* **21:** 217–231.

Cappellini, M.D. & Fiorelli, G. (2008) Glucose-6-phosphate dehydrogenase deficiency. *The Lancet,* **371:** 64–74.

Glader, B. (2009) Hereditary hemolytic anemias due to red blood cell enzyme disorders. In: *Wintobe's Clinical Hematology* (Greer, J.P., Foerster, J., Rodgers, G.M., *et al.*, eds), Vol. 1, pp. 933–955. Lippincott Williams and Wilkins, Philadelphia.

Gordon-Smith, E.C. (2005) Disorders of red cell metabolism. In: *Postgraduate Haematology* (Hoffbrand, A.V., Catovsky, D. & Tuddenham, E.G.D., eds), pp. 133–150. Blackwell Science, Oxford.

Voet, D. & Voet, J.G. (2004) Glycolysis. In: *Biochemistry*, 3rd edition pp. 581–625. John Wiley and Sons, New York.

An Introduction to G6PD Deficiency – http://rialto.com/g6pd/
G6PD Deficiency Favism Association – http://www.g6pd.org/favism/english/index.mvc

SELF-ASSESSMENT QUESTIONS

1. Why are mature red cells particularly vulnerable to disorders of their glycolytic enzymes?
2. Why are red cells unable to derive energy via oxidative phosphorylation?
3. What chemical reaction is responsible for the liberation of energy in red cells?
4. Why do red cells require energy?
5. Why is 2,3-DPG physiologically important?
6. Why do red cells require reducing power?
7. Name the most common enzyme defects of the Embden–Meyerhof and hexose monophosphate pathways.
8. Why is hexokinase deficiency clinically more severe than pyruvate kinase deficiency?
9. Name the two normal variants of G-6-PD and the populations with which they are associated.
10. List three common triggers of acute haemolysis in G-6-PD deficiency.
11. What is favism?

CHAPTER 9

Non-malignant leucocyte disorders

Learning objectives
After studying this chapter you should confidently be able to:

■ Review the non-malignant quantitative disorders of neutrophils
Quantitative neutrophil disorders are extremely common and frequently indicate an underlying disease process. Neutrophilia is the body's normal response to bacterial infection. It is often accompanied by a 'left shift' and toxic granulation. Other causes of neutrophilia include inflammatory conditions, tissue destruction, haemorrhage and haemolysis, metabolic abnormalities and some drugs (e.g. steroids). Neutropenia is common during infections, as an idiosyncratic response to a drug or other chemical, as a consequence of antineoplastic therapies, in deficiency of vitamin B_{12}, folate or copper, during inflammation and, rarely, as an autoimmune condition.

■ Review the non-malignant qualitative disorders of neutrophils
The inherited qualitative neutrophil disorders are rare and include leucocyte adhesion deficiency and chronic granulomatous disease.

■ Review the non-malignant morphological abnormalities of neutrophils
Apart from Pelger–Hüet anomaly, all of the conditions characterized by morphological abnormalities of neutrophils are rare. Such abnormalities include May–Hegglin anomaly, Alder–Reilly anomaly, Chédiak–Higashi syndrome, Jordan's anomaly, specific granule deficiency and Undritz anomaly.

■ Outline the main causes of eosinophilia and basophilia
Reactive eosinophilia occurs in response to a defined event such as an allergic reaction. Transient reactive eosinophilia is most commonly associated with acute reactive processes such as non-specific inflammation, allergic reactions, drug reactions, or during the recovery phase of a viral or bacterial infection. Chronic reactive eosinophilia is associated with persistent infections, parasitic infestation, autoimmune disease, atopic disease, certain endocrinopathies, and some malignant diseases. A wide range of disorders in which eosinophilia is present also exist, but the reason for the eosinophilia is often obscure. Conditions associated with an increase in basophils are far less common than those associated with eosinophilia, but such increases have been reported in myxoedema, in hypersensitivity reactions and in various myeloproliferative states.

■ Outline the non-malignant quantitative disorders of monocytes
Monocytopenia is rare, and usually only occurs as part of a generalized leucopenia as in, for example, autoimmune diseases, although it can occur during corticosteroid administration and in some rare malignancies (e.g. hairy cell leukaemia). Monocytosis is much more common and frequently occurs in inflammatory conditions, particularly chronic infections.

Overall, non-malignant disorders of neutrophils are far more frequently encountered than the malignant diseases such as the leukaemias. The most common abnormalities are the acquired quantitative disorders such as neutrophilia and neutropenia. Inherited non-malignant leucocyte disorders are, for the most part, rare conditions.

9.1 DISORDERS OF NEUTROPHILS

Quantitative neutrophil disorders

The quantitative neutrophil disorders are manifest as an increased number of circulating neutrophils (neutrophilias) and those where the neutrophil count is lower than normal (neutropenias).

Physiological 'pseudoneutrophilia'

Neutrophilia is by far the most commonly encountered neutrophil abnormality; however, the classification is contextual, in that neutrophil numbers vary considerably for physiological as well as for pathological reasons. The astute haematologist needs to be aware of these physiological fluctuations to avoid misdiagnosis. For example, normal physiological variations in circulating neutrophil counts with age need to be taken into account when assessing the normality or otherwise of a given blood sample. In the newborn infant, the circulating neutrophil count is often raised relative to that of one-week-old infants. This is almost certainly a normal physiological response to the rigours of birth (see *Table 9.1*). The neutrophil count usually subsides rapidly over a couple of days until the neutrophil count appears to be reduced relative to that of a 6–9 year old child. From that time until around the age of 7–9 years, lymphocytes will dominate over neutrophils, with the normal adult proportions appearing by puberty. From then on, an approximate ratio of 60:40 neutrophils to lymphocytes persists until the end of life. This means that different reference ranges for neutrophil counts are required for different age groups and that determination of normality, neutropenia and neutrophilia must be made by comparison to the appropriate age range (see *Table 9.1*).

Many other normal variations in neutrophil count exist:

- it is normal for the neutrophil count to rise during pregnancy, with the highest levels seen as term approaches. Immediate post-delivery neutrophil counts are frequently significantly raised. This, as with other 'pseudoneutrophilias', presents a potential difficulty of interpretation as to when a raised neutrophil count in a pregnant woman indicates a pathological rather than a physiological change.
- people of African descent have been shown to have slightly lower neutrophil and monocyte counts and higher eosinophil counts. These differences appear to be most marked for indigenous Africans.
- there is a normal diurnal variation in neutrophil count, with highest levels in the afternoon. However, it is unusual for diurnal changes in the neutrophil count to fall outside the reference range.
- strenuous exercise is associated with a significant leucocytosis and neutrophilia. This is caused by release of neutrophils from the marginated pool to the circulating pool. In this

Table 9.1 Reference ranges for neutrophil count at different ages

Age	Total WBC ($\times 10^9$/l)	Neutrophil count	
		%	$\times 10^9$/l
Birth	9.0–30.0	65–90	6.0–26.0
1 week	5.0–21.0	30–50	1.5–10.0
1–4 years	5.0–14.5	30–60	1.5–8.5
5–10 years	4.5–13.5	45–60	2.1–8.0
Adult	4.5–11.0	46–70	2.1–7.7

case, the neutrophil count generally returns to normal levels within a few hours. Similar, transient rises are seen following convulsive seizures.

Neutrophilia

Neutrophilia is the body's normal response to bacterial infection. It is often accompanied by a 'left shift' of the cells, meaning that the circulating cells have fewer lobes to their nuclei, an indication of immaturity and of premature release. In extreme cases this numerical increase and appearance of immaturity may mimic leukaemia, the so-called 'leukaemoid reaction', in which very early forms are released from marrow. The neutrophil series cells are, however, non-clonal, as is seen in the leukaemias and other haematological malignancies. Another phenomenon that may be exhibited in acute severe responses is 'toxic granulation', which is the presence of intensely staining granules within the cytoplasm. Occasionally, toxic neutrophils may exhibit ribosomal aggregates that stain pale blue with Romanowsky stains due to the acidic nature of their RNA. These are known as Döhle bodies and are insignificant if they are accompanied by other toxic changes explicable by the clinical state of the patient. Rarely, the presence of Döhle bodies may provide clues to a diagnosis of May–Hegglin anomaly, a rare genetic disorder discussed in *Chapter 19*.

Other causes of neutrophilia besides bacterial infections include inflammatory conditions (Crohn's disease, collagen disease, rheumatoid arthritis, etc.), tissue destruction (trauma and surgery, tissue necrosis and infarction, neoplasia), haemorrhage and haemolysis, metabolic abnormalities (e.g. metabolic ketosis, uraemia, gout, etc.) and certain drugs (e.g. steroids).

Neutropenia

Neutropenia is defined as a reduction in the absolute number of neutrophils in the peripheral circulation below that which is normal for age, gender, ethnicity and taking account of various physiological conditions, including pregnancy and recent exercise. Neutropenia may be classified into mild (absolute neutrophil count (ANC) $1.0–1.5 \times 10^9/l$), moderate (ANC $0.5–1.0 \times 10^9/l$) and severe (ANC $< 0.5 \times 10^9/l$). These categories correspond well to the clinical risk of severe bacterial and fungal infection.

Acquired neutropenias

There are many causes of acquired neutropenia, including:

- **infection.** Many types of infection are associated with neutropenia, including viral infections (e.g. human immunodeficiency virus (HIV), Epstein–Barr virus (EBV), cytomegalovirus (CMV), hepatitis viruses, mumps, measles, etc.), severe or deep-seated bacterial infections (e.g. brucellosis, tuberculosis, septicaemia, etc.), fungal (e.g. histoplasmosis), parasitic (e.g. malaria, leishmaniasis) and rickettsial (e.g. typhus). The mechanisms vary from direct attack on the haemopoietic mechanisms (e.g. HIV, EBV) to increased utilization and destruction (e.g. septicaemia).
- **idiosyncratic drug or chemical reactions.** The list of drugs that have been associated with neutropenia is extremely long and includes antimicrobial drugs, analgesics, antipsychotics, anticonvulsants, antihistamines, allopurinol and colchicine, among many others. The highest risk classes of drugs include thionamide antithyroid drugs, macrolide antibiotics (e.g. erythromycin) and the anti-arrhythmic procainamide. Severe drug-related neutropenia is rare (1–10 cases per 10^6 population per year) and has been associated most frequently with the antipsychotic clozapine, antithyroid drugs and sulfasalazine. Drug-induced neutropenia is more common in patients over the age of 60 years, and women are more commonly affected than men. In many cases, definitive proof that the drug is responsible for the induction of neutropenia is lacking. There are three recognized mechanisms for drug-induced neutropenia:

□ **antibody-mediated destruction** occurs when a drug binds to neutrophils, acts as a hapten and stimulates the formation of antibodies that then mediate the destruction of circulating neutrophils either directly or by complement-mediated lysis. The drugs most commonly associated with hapten formation are aminopyrine, propylthiouracil, penicillin, and gold compounds. Withdrawal of the offending drug typically corrects the problem.

□ **acceleration of neutrophil apoptosis** occurs when metabolites of certain drugs (e.g. the antipsychotic clozapine) bind to neutrophils, causing depletion of intracellular glutathione, toxicity and cell death.

□ **inhibition of granulopoiesis.** β-lactam antibiotics (e.g. cephalosporins) and some anticonvulsant drugs (e.g. carbamazepine and valproic acid) have been shown to directly inhibit marrow CFU–GM in a dose-dependent manner, leading to neutropenia.

■ **iatrogenic causes.** Neutropenia is an inevitable consequence of cytotoxic chemotherapy for malignant disease. Radiotherapy can have similar effects.

■ **micronutrient deficiencies** such as vitamin B_{12} and folic acid or copper are frequently associated with neutropenia.

■ **immune mechanisms.** Primary autoimmune neutropenia (AIN) is caused by the development of antibodies directed against neutrophil surface antigens, resulting in splenic sequestration and destruction. In infancy, the condition causes severe neutropenia but life-threatening infection is rare. Most cases occur in infants aged 6–12 months and frequently remit spontaneously. In adults, AIN usually occurs in patients with other autoimmune conditions such as rheumatoid arthritis, systemic lupus erythematosus (SLE) or Sjögren's syndrome. Alloimmune neutropenia can occur in neonates (NAIN) and is caused by IgG maternal antibodies directed against fetal neutrophil antigens in a similar manner to haemolytic disease of the newborn. NAIN can cause severe neutropenia, but consequent serious infection is rare. The condition remits in the first months of life and seldom requires clinical intervention.

■ **inflammatory conditions** such as rheumatoid arthritis and SLE are sometimes associated with neutropenia. Various contributory factors have been demonstrated including circulating immune complexes, autoimmune neutropenia, increased margination and suppression of marrow neutrophil precursors by large granular T lymphocytes. In Felty's syndrome, a condition characterized by rheumatoid arthritis, splenomegaly, and neutropenia, the neutropenia results from splenic sequestration and destruction of neutrophils. Immune neutropenias have also been reported as a complication of bone marrow transplantation, and of the transfusion of blood and blood products.

■ **haematological malignancy** and solid tumours that have metastasized to the bone marrow can be associated with neutropenia due to occupation of the marrow space by malignant cells. This causes physical constraint of normal haemopoiesis and suppression of haemopoiesis either directly or indirectly by cytokines released from tumour cells or by immune mechanisms.

■ **splenomegaly** of whatever cause is often accompanied by a degree of neutropenia due to splenic sequestration.

Inherited neutropenias
The inherited neutropenias are covered in *Chapter 17*.

Qualitative defects of neutrophils

Leucocyte adhesion defects
The neutrophil membrane contains numerous adhesion molecules, including integrins and selectins. Integrins are cell surface receptors that mediate cell:cell adhesion and adhesion to

components of the extracellular matrix such as fibronectin, vitronectin, collagen and laminin. Integrins also function as signal transduction molecules, playing a significant role in cell migration, survival, proliferation and differentiation.

Three forms of neutrophil integrin exist. All are heterodimers formed by association of CD18 with one of three variant forms of CD11:

- **CD18:CD11a** is present on neutrophils, macrophages, T cells and B cells and functions primarily as a receptor for intercellular adhesion molecule-1 (ICAM-1, CD54), which is present on vascular endothelium, monocyte/macrophages and lymphocytes. This complex also binds to ICAM-2 and ICAM-3 and is important in recruitment of neutrophils and other immune cells to sites of infection. CD18:CD11a is also known as leucocyte function-associated antigen 1 (LFA-1).
- **CD18:CD11b** is only found on leucocytes, specifically neutrophils and monocyte/macrophages. It functions as a receptor for the complement component iC3b and also for fibrinogen, coagulation factor X and bacterial lipopolysaccharide. Binding of this integrin to cell-associated iC3b triggers phagocytosis of the target cell. This integrin is also known as macrophage-1 antigen (MAC-1).
- **CD18:CD11c** (also known as p150,95) functions as a receptor for the complement component iC3b and also for fibrinogen.

Three forms of leucocyte adhesion deficiency (LAD) have been defined:

- LAD-1 is the most common form of leucocyte adhesion deficiency by some way and is associated with recurrent bacterial and fungal infections; impaired recruitment of neutrophils and monocyte/macrophages to sites of infection with a lack of pus formation and poor wound healing. LAD-1 is an autosomal recessive disorder and is caused by mutations of the *CD18* gene at 21q22.3, with a consequent deficiency of all three integrins on the neutrophil surface. The circulating neutrophil count is usually raised, even between infections. The clinical severity of LAD-1 correlates with the degree of CD18 deficiency.
- LAD-2 is associated with the Bombay (hh) blood group phenotype, severe mental retardation, growth retardation and distinctive facial abnormalities in addition to the expected recurrent bacterial infections, lack of pus accumulation and a raised circulating white cell count. LAD-2 is an autosomal recessive disorder and is caused by mutation of the *SLC35C1* gene at 11p11.2, which encodes a GDP-fucose transporter. The neutrophils in LAD-2 express integrins normally and have no defect of integrin function. The impairment of neutrophil recruitment to sites of infection is caused by reduced fucosylation of P-selectin glycoprotein ligand 1 (PSGL-1) on the neutrophil surface, with a consequent impairment of tethering and rolling of leucocytes on activated endothelial cells.
- LAD-3 (also known as LAD-1 variant or LAD-1v) is caused by mutations in the *FERMT3* gene at 11q13, which encodes kindlin 3, an intracellular protein that interacts with the cytoplasmic tail of CD18 and acts as a regulator of integrin activation. This form of LAD differs from the others in that, in addition to the recurrent infections, platelet integrin function is also affected, leading to a bleeding tendency similar to Glanzmann's disease.

Chronic granulomatous disease

Chronic granulomatous disease (CGD) is a rare inherited disorder of neutrophils and other phagocytic leucocytes and is characterized by recurrent bacterial and fungal infections, granulomatous infiltration of major organs and, in the absence of treatment, early death. The increased susceptibility to bacterial and fungal infection in CGD results from failure of the post-phagocytic respiratory burst, and hence impaired destruction of ingested microbes. Adhesion, chemotaxis and phagocytosis are all normal. Failure to rapidly clear foci of infection from the tissues prompts the localized formation of granulomatous lesions. Over time, the accumulation of extensive granulomas can lead to a variety of clinical complications such as severe tissue necrosis, fibrosis, obstruction of the gastrointestinal and genito-urinary tracts and secondary organ failure.

During activation, neutrophils undergo a several hundred-fold increase in oxygen consumption, almost all of which is directed towards the synthesis of microbicidal oxygen derivatives such as superoxide (O_2^-), hydrogen peroxide (H_2O_2), hydroxyl radical (OH•), hypochlorous acid (HOCl) and chloramines. These antimicrobial products of the respiratory burst together constitute the oxygen-dependent microbicidal mechanisms of the neutrophil. The failure of the respiratory burst in CGD results from a deficiency or defect of one of the components of NADPH oxidase, the enzyme that catalyses the generation of superoxide.

NADPH oxidase is a membrane-bound complex that consists of a FAD moiety and a cytochrome, and functions as a catalyst for the one-electron reduction of molecular oxygen to superoxide. The cytochrome is a *b*-type cytochrome and has been found to be located in the plasma membrane and specific granules of neutrophils, but more recently has been found in the plasma membrane of several other cell types, including fibroblasts and mesangial cells. The cytochrome has a very low mid-point potential ($E_{m7.0}$ = –245 mV), which facilitates the reduction of molecular oxygen to superoxide and so is designated cytochrome b_{245}. An alternative designation, cytochrome b_{558}, relates to the absorbance of the α-band of the cytochrome on visible light spectroscopy, which occurs at 558 nm.

Cytochrome b_{245} is unusual in being a heterodimer, consisting of a small α-subunit of approximately 22 kDa (designated p22-*phox*) and a larger β-subunit of approximately 76–92 kDa (designated gp91-*phox*).

Besides the membrane-bound cytochrome b_{245}, the NADPH oxidase also requires the presence of several cytosolic proteins, including p47-*phox*, p67-*phox* and p40-*phox*.

The most common form of chronic granulomatous disease is inherited as an X-linked recessive disorder and is due to mutation of the *CYBB* gene at Xp21.1, which encodes the gp91-*phox* cytochrome *b* subunit. Both subunits of the cytochrome are deficient in this form of the disease, as both are needed for stable incorporation of the cytochrome into the plasma membrane.

Defects in the p47-*phox* constitute the next largest group of CGD patients. The *NCF1* gene that encodes p47-*phox* is located at 7q11. This form of CGD has an autosomal mode of inheritance.

Approximately 5% of CGD patients have a defect in the *CYTA* gene at 16p24 that encodes the p22-*phox*. Another 5% of patients have a defect in the *NCF2* gene at 1q25 that encodes the p67-*phox* gene.

Pseudo-chronic granulomatous disease

Profound deficiency of G-6-PD produces a clinical phenotype that is clinically similar to CGD apart from a co-existent congenital non-spherocytic haemolytic anaemia. In these cases, failure of the respiratory burst is caused by the failure of NADPH production via the hexose monophosphate pathway. This manifestation of G-6-PD deficiency is associated with the hyper-unstable variants of G-6-PD and so is extremely rare.

Morphological abnormalities of neutrophils

Pelger–Huët anomaly

The Pelger–Huët anomaly is a relatively common (prevalence about 1 in 1000–10 000) benign abnormality of granulocytes, characterized by nuclear hyposegmentation. The defect is seen most obviously in neutrophils, because the neutrophil nucleus most commonly has three to four segments. In Pelger–Huët anomaly, a substantial number of neutrophils have only two nuclear segments, creating the characteristic 'dumb-bell' or 'pince-nez' nuclear configuration.

In homozygotes, the neutrophil nucleus may not be segmented at all. Pelger–Huët anomaly is caused by mutations in the laminin B-receptor gene at 1q42.1. It is important to differentiate this condition from the 'left-shift' that frequently accompanies infection. There appear to be no clinical sequelae of being heterozygous for Pelger–Huët anomaly, but some of the very rare homozygotes described have had significant abnormalities such as mental retardation, macrocephalus, ventricular septal defect, and shortening of the metacarpals.

May–Hegglin anomaly

May–Hegglin anomaly (MHA) is a rare autosomal dominant disorder caused by mutation of the non-muscle myosin heavy chain-9 gene (*MYH9*) at 22q11.2, leading to macrothrombocytopenia secondary to defective megakaryocyte maturation and fragmentation (see *Box 19.3* in *Chapter 19*). MHA is characterized by variable thrombocytopenia with giant platelets containing few granules and the presence of large basophilic, cytoplasmic inclusion bodies (resembling Döhle bodies), consisting of precipitated myosin heavy chains in the neutrophils, eosinophils, basophils and monocytes. The condition is often asymptomatic but may be associated with purpura, easy bruising and mucous membrane bleeding, although this is seldom severe. Both neutrophil and platelet function are normal in MHA.

Alder–Reilly anomaly

The Alder–Reilly anomaly is characterized by the presence of abnormally large azurophilic and basophilic granules in neutrophils, which can be mistaken for 'toxic' granulation due to other causes. Differentiation from toxic granulation can be achieved by excluding causes of toxic granulation such as infection and also by finding similar inclusions that stain dark red or purple with Romanowsky stains in lymphocytes and monocytes.

The Alder–Reilly anomaly is associated with a family of genetic disorders known as the mucopolysaccharidoses (MPS). These disorders are characterized by an impaired ability to degrade the protein–carbohydrate complexes known as mucopolysaccharides. Each form of MPS involves deficiency of a different enzyme required for mucopolysaccharide degradation. The abnormal inclusions of the Alder–Reilly anomaly are seen most commonly in MPS type I (Hurler syndrome), MPS type II (Hunter syndrome), MPS type III (Sanfilippo syndrome) and MPS type VI (Maroteaux–Lamy syndrome). These disorders are further considered in the section on disorders of mononuclear leucocytes later in this chapter.

Chédiak–Higashi syndrome

Chédiak–Higashi syndrome (CHS) is an autosomal recessive disorder with moderate-to-severe neutropenia, recurrent infections, learning difficulties, a bleeding tendency, partial ocular and cutaneous albinism and numerous other phenotypic abnormalities. Most cases of CHS die in infancy or early childhood. The granulocytes in blood and bone marrow contain abnormally large primary granules. The microbicidal function of neutrophils in CHS is impaired due to delayed release of primary granule contents into the phagolysosome.

CHS is an autosomal recessive condition and is caused by mutation of the lysosomal trafficking regulator gene *LYST* at 1q42.1–42.2. There is a generalized disorder of lysosomal function throughout the body, which explains the wide spectrum of clinical manifestations of CHS.

Jordan's anomaly

Jordan's anomaly is characterized by marked 'vacuolization' of granulocytes, monocytes, and occasionally lymphocytes and plasma cells. These 'vacuoles' have been shown to be deposits of lipid that do not stain with Romanowsky stain, which explains their erroneous appearance as vacuoles. Jordan's anomaly has been noted in the rare inherited conditions neutral lipid storage disease with icthyosis (Dorfman–Chanarin syndrome), which is due to mutations in the *ABHD5* gene at 3p21 and neutral lipid storage without icthyosis but with mild myopathy, which is caused by mutations in the *PNPLA2* gene at 11p15.5.

Specific granule deficiency

Specific granule deficiency is an autosomal recessive disorder characterized by recurrent skin and sinus infections, impaired neutrophil chemotaxis, impaired bacterial killing, and absence of neutrophil secondary granules. In some cases, additional neutrophil morphological abnormalities are present. It is likely that there is more than one cause of this condition, but at least some cases are caused by mutations in the myeloid transcription factor *CEBPE* gene at 14q11.2.

Undritz anomaly

Undritz anomaly is a benign autosomal dominant condition that is characterized by hypersegmentation of neutrophil nuclei. There appears to be no clinically significant functional impairment in this condition. It is important to recognize, mainly to differentiate it from the much more common acquired nuclear hypersegmentation of neutrophils seen in vitamin B_{12} or folate deficiency.

9.2 DISORDERS OF EOSINOPHILS AND BASOPHILS

Eosinophilia

Eosinophilia is defined as an increase in the absolute eosinophil count above $0.5 \times 10^9/l$. In general, non-malignant causes of eosinophilia can be divided into idiopathic eosinophilia, reactive eosinophilia and eosinophilic syndromes.

Reactive eosinophilia occurs in response to a defined event such as an allergic reaction (*Table 9.2*), and can be short-lived (transient reactive eosinophilia) or more persistent (chronic reactive eosinophilia). Transient reactive eosinophilia is most commonly associated with acute reactive processes such as non-specific inflammation, allergic reactions, drug reactions, or during the recovery phase of a viral or bacterial infection. Chronic reactive eosinophilia is associated with persistent infections, parasitic infestation, autoimmune disease, atopic disease, certain endocrinopathies and some malignant diseases.

The most commonly encountered cause of chronic reactive eosinophilia worldwide is persistent worm (helminth) infection, including roundworms (nematodes), tapeworms (cestodes) and flukes (trematodes). In these cases, eosinophilia is thought to result from stem cell stimulation by eosinopoietic growth factors such as IL-4, IL-5 and IL-13 secreted by activated T cells, mast cells and tissue stromal cells, rather than a simple chemotactic response to factors emanating from the parasite, as was previously thought. In the developed world, parasitic infections are much less common and eosinophilia is seen most commonly in allergic and autoimmune disorders. The incidence of such disorders has increased significantly in recent decades. One possible explanation for this observation is that the lack of acute and chronic stimulation of the Th2 immune response during childhood by helminth infection leads to an exaggerated response to allergens.

The precise role played by eosinophils in helminth infections, as well as in allergic diseases (including asthma) is complex and incompletely understood. It is clear that eosinophils exert a range of toxic effects against helminths, involving the release of cationic proteins such as major basic protein (MBP), eosinophilic cationic protein (ECP), eosinophil peroxides (EPs), eosinophil-derived neurotoxin (EDN), platelet-activating factor (PAF), reactive oxygen species, and lysosomal hydrolases. Some of these substances are responsible for localized activation of mast cells, basophils and neutrophils, which contributes to the host response.

Table 9.2 Main causes of eosinophilia

Disorder
Idiopathic eosinophilia

Reactive eosinophilia
  Transient
    Infections
    Allergic reactions
    Drug reactions
    Chronic helminth infections
    Other chronic infections
    Autoimmune diseases
  Chronic
    cGvHD
    Atopic diseases
    Endocrinopathies
    Malignant disease

Eosinophilic syndromes
  Organ-restricted forms
    Eosinophil oesophagitis
    Eosinophil gastritis
    Eosinophilic panniculitis
    Eosinophilic cellulitis (Wells' syndrome)
    Acute eosinophilic pneumonia
    Chronic eosinophilic pneumonia
    Löffler's endocarditis
  Non-organ-restricted forms
    Hyper IgE syndrome
    Polymyalgia syndrome + eosinophilia
    Kimura disease
    Shulman's syndrome
    Churg–Strauss syndrome (CSS)
    Necrotizing vasculitis + eosinophilia
    Eosinophil-myalgia syndrome
    DRESS syndrome (drug rash with eosinophilia and systemic symptoms)
    Severe combined immunodeficiency + eosinophilia (Omenn syndrome)

However, the eosinophil response and the substances released as part of that response can also cause localized damage to surrounding tissue. In allergic diseases such as asthma, eosinophil-mediated bronchial inflammation and damage to the respiratory epithelium is a major pathogenetic mechanism. Until recently, the role of eosinophils in asthma and other allergic disorders was unquestioningly taken to be protective and responsive, the ingress of eosinophils serving to reduce the inflammatory activity. In particular, the histamine from eosinophils was thought to actively down-regulate the mast cell response in inflammation. This view is now being challenged as a result of *in vitro* experiments involving IL5 knockout mice and also using anti-IL-5 antibodies, which suggest in each case that the eosin response is reduced. The relevance, if any, of these findings to human pathology is still uncertain.

Basophilia

Conditions associated with an increase in basophils are far less common than those associated with eosinophilia, but such increases have been reported in myxoedema, in hypersensitivity reactions and in various myeloproliferative states. In particular, the development of severe basophilia in the course of chronic myeloid leukaemia is frequently an ominous sign, indicating the development of blast crisis.

9.3   DISORDERS OF MONONUCLEAR PHAGOCYTES

Quantitative monocyte disorders

Monocytopenia is rare, and usually only occurs as part of a generalized leucopenia as in, for example, autoimmune diseases, although it can occur during corticosteroid administration and in some rare malignancies (e.g. hairy cell leukaemia).

Monocytosis is much more common and frequently occurs in inflammatory conditions, particularly chronic infections and especially where the neutrophil response is compromised or ineffective, for example, infection with encapsulated micro-organisms. Common causative inflammatory diseases include infections (e.g. tuberculosis, syphilis and brucellosis), and also non-infectious inflammatory states, including systemic lupus erythematosus (SLE), rheumatoid arthritis and sarcoidosis among others.

Langerhans cell histiocytosis

Peripheral blood monocytes are essentially immature cells in transit between their site of formation in the bone marrow and their site of function as macrophages in the tissues. Macrophages are present in a wide variety of tissues, where they perform a variety of tissue-specific functions. Some tissue macrophages are more commonly known by an alternative name, e.g. bone macrophages are known as osteoclasts because of their function as bone-resorbing cells, and liver macrophages are known as Kupffer cells.

Most dendritic cells are derived from the same haemopoietic precursor cells as monocytes. Dendritic cells are found in almost all tissues, but especially those that are interface tissues with the external environment, where they perform a vital role in the processing and presentation of antigen. A proportion of dendritic cells are derived from lymphoid precursor cells. Within the tissues, cells of the mononuclear phagocyte system were formerly termed 'histiocytes'.

The most common disorder of myeloid-derived dendritic cells is Langerhans cell histiocytosis (LCH). Langerhans cells are dendritic cells found in the skin and mucosa, locations where they are particularly well placed to encounter and process antigenic material for presentation to lymphocytes. There is an ongoing debate about whether LCH is a malignant or a reactive process. The presence of a monoclonal proliferation of abnormal dendritic cells that may evolve into a more aggressive form suggests a malignant disease. However, the absence of identified cytogenetic abnormalities, the frequency of spontaneous remissions and the ongoing cytokine storm that accompanies LCH supports a reactive mechanism for the disease.

The presentation and clinical course of LCH is highly variable with relatively indolent forms that may present as solitary lesions, through to an acute, fulminant form of disseminated disease that used to be known as Letterer–Siwe disease (see *Box 9.1*).

Table 9.3 Lysosomal storage diseases

Degradative defect	Disorder	Enzyme defect	Gene	Locus	Inheritance
Defective glycosaminoglycan metabolism (mucopolysaccharidoses)	Hurler disease (MPS type IH); Hurler–Scheie syndrome (MPS type IH/S); Scheie syndrome (MPS type IS)	α-L-iduronidase	IDUA	4p16.3	AR
	Hunter syndrome (MPS type II)	Iduronate-2-sulphatase	IDS	Xq28	XR
	Sanfilippo (MPS type IIIA–D)	Heparan N sulphatase	SGSH	17q25.3	AR
		α-N-acetylglucosaminidase;	NAGLU	17q21	AR
		acetyl-coA: α glucosaminide acetyltransferase;	HGSNAT	8p11.1	AR
		N-acetylglucosamine 6-sulphatase	GNS	12q14	AR
	Morquio (MPS IVA, B)	Galactosamine 6-sulphate sulphatase	GALNS	16q24.3	AR
		β-galactosidase	GLB1	3p21.33	AR
	Maroteaux–Lamy syndrome (MPS type VI)	Arylsulphatase B	ARSB	5q11–13	AR
	Sly syndrome (MPS type VII)	β-glucuronidase	GUSB	7q21.1	AR
Defective glycan degradation	Aspartylglycosaminuria	Aspartylglucosaminidase	AGA	4q32–33	AR
	Fucosidosis – type I, II	α-fucosidase	FUCA-1	1p34	AR
	α-mannosidosis	α-mannosidosae	MAN2B1	19cen–q12	AR
	β-mannosidosis	β-mannosidase	MANBA	4q22–25	AR
	Sialidosis – type I, II	α-N-acetylneuraminidase	NEU1	6p21.3	AR
Defective degradation of glycogen	Pompe disease	Acid α-glucosidase	GAA	17q25.2–25.3	AR
Defective degradation of sphingolipid components	Niemann–Pick disease type A, B	Sphingomyelin phosphodiesterase-1 gene	SMPD1	11p15.4–15.1	AR
	Niemann–Pick disease type C1		NPC1	18q11–12	AR
	Niemann–Pick disease type C2		NPC2	14q24.3	AR
	Fabry disease	α-galactosidase	GLA	Xq22	XR
	Farber disease	Acid ceramidase	AC	8p22–21.3	AR
	Gaucher disease – type I–III	Glucocerebrosidase	GBA	1q21	AR
	GM1 Gangliosidosis – type I–III	β-galactosidase 1	GLBA-1	3p21.33	AR
	Tay-Sachs disease – type I–III	β-hexosaminidase (α chain)	HEXA	15q23–24	AR
	Sandhoff disease – type I	β-hexosaminidase (β chain)	HEXB	5q13	AR
	Krabbe disease	Galactosylceramidase	GALC	14q31	AR
	Metachromatic leukodystrophy – type I–III	Arylsulphatase A	ARSA	22q13.31–qter	AR

Table 9.3 Lysosomal storage diseases – *continued*

Degradative defect	Disorder	Enzyme defect	Gene	Locus	Inheritance
Defective degradation of polypeptides	Pycnodysostosis	Cathepsin K	CTSK	1q21	AR
Defective degradation or transport of cholesterol, cholesterol esters or other complex lipids	Neuronal ceroid lipofuscinosis – type 1	Palmitoyl-protein thioesterase	PPT1	1p32	AR
	Neuronal ceroid lipofuscinosis – type 2	Acid protease tri-peptidyl-peptidase-1	TPP1	11p15.5	AR
	Neuronal ceroid lipofuscinosis – type 3	CLN3 lysosomal membrane protein	CLN3	16p12.1	AR
	Neuronal ceroid lipofuscinosis – type 4	Unknown	CLN4	Unknown	AR/AD
	Neuronal ceroid lipofuscinosis – type 5	Unknown	CLN5	13q21.1–32	AR
	Neuronal ceroid lipofuscinosis – type 6	Unknown	CLN6	15q21–23	AR
	Neuronal ceroid lipofuscinosis – type 7	Lysosomal transporter	MFSD8	4q28.1–28.2	AR
	Neuronal ceroid lipofuscinosis – type 8	Unknown	CLN8	8p23	AR
	Neuronal ceroid lipofuscinosis – type 9	Regulator of dihydroceramide synthetase	CLN9	Unknown	AR
Multiple deficiencies of lysosomal enzymes	Galactosialidosis	Cathepsin A	CTSA	20q13.1	AR
	Mucolipidosis II (MLII I-Cell Disease; ML III Pseudo-Hurler polydystrophy)	UDP-N-acetylglucosamine-l-phosphotransferase	GNPTAB	12q23.3	AR
Transport and trafficking defects	Cystinosis	Cystinosin	CTNS	17p13	AR
	Mucolipidosis IV	Mucolipin-1	MCOLN1	19p13.3–13.2	AR
	Infantile sialic acid storage disease/Salla disease	Vesicular excitatory amino acid transporter	SLC17A5	6q14–15	AR

AR – autosomal recessive; AD – autosomal dominant; XR – X-linked recessive

> **Box 9.1 Histiocytosis X**
>
> A group of histiocytic disorders previously considered to be separate conditions (Hand–Schüller–Christian syndrome, Letterer–Siwe disease, eosinophilic granuloma, Hashimoto–Pritzker syndrome, self-healing histiocytosis and pure cutaneous histiocytosis) were grouped under the name of histiocytosis X in 1953. The X was intended to signify the lack of knowledge about the aetiology of the disease and the mystery surrounding the clinical and pathological links between the conditions included in this condition. In 1985 histiocytosis X was renamed as Langerhans cell histiocytosis (LCH) and this is now the preferred term.

LCH affects patients at all ages, although it is more common in children. The aetiology of this condition is unknown.

Lysosomal storage diseases

Lysosomes are cellular organelles that contain acid hydrolases and are responsible for the digestion of macromolecules, ingested material and waste disposal within the cell. Many inherited disorders of lysosomal function exist. All can be traced to a deficiency or defect of a specific lysosomal enzyme, activator protein or transport protein. The impact of the deficiency is the accumulation within the lysosome of the relevant enzyme substrate, hence the name given to this family of disorders, the lysosomal storage diseases.

In *Table 9.3*, the lysosomal storage diseases are categorized according to the defect of lysosomal degradation.

The lysosomal storage diseases are not really monocyte/macrophage disorders. They are generalized disorders that may be manifest in any cells that contain lysosomes. However, because monocyte/macrophages are particularly rich in lysosomes, these disorders are frequently identifiable on blood films using specialized staining techniques or by recognition of characteristic morphological changes in monocytes. Definitive diagnosis requires detailed genetic testing and specific enzyme assays.

The clinical picture of lysosomal storage diseases varies widely and depends on the nature of the accumulated substrate and the nature of the enzyme defect. Symptoms can vary from a relatively indolent course with mild symptoms through to severe and rapidly progressive neurological disease and early death. Most of these conditions present in childhood and are progressive disorders. Some of the conditions are not clinically manifest until later in life. There is no universally accepted effective treatment for these disorders, although some success has been achieved with stem cell transplantation.

9.4   DISORDERS OF LYMPHOCYTES

Functional disorders of lymphocytes, including immunodeficiency and hyperimmune states are the realm of immunology, and so are outside the scope of this book.

Lymphocytosis and lymphopenia

Circulating blood lymphocytes represent probably only around 2% of total body lymphocytes, and those that are in the blood at any one time are only there briefly, being cells in transit between different lymphoid tissues. There is an equilibrium between the lymphocytes in the blood and those in lymphoid tissue and, since such a low proportion are in the blood, it only takes a small change in that equilibrium to have a marked effect on blood lymphocyte numbers;

thus both lymphocytoses and lymphopenias can represent merely a transient redistribution. This is probably the reason for the diurnal variation that can occur in lymphocyte numbers, and for the decrease in lymphocytes that can be observed in response to corticosteroids, either therapeutic or endogenous, since there is a diurnal variation in steroid production. Lymphocyte numbers are higher at night than in the morning and, as with several other blood measurements, this should be borne in mind when sequential counts are performed.

Lymphopenia can occur in infections, particularly influenza and certain other viral infections, but it can also occur in miliary TB, pneumonia, malaria and HIV. It can also occur in a variety of other conditions including lymphoma and some other malignancies, in connective tissue disease, severe bone marrow failure, as a consequence of immunosuppressive, cytotoxic or radiotherapy, and in severe vitamin B_{12} and folate deficiency.

Lymphocytosis can also occur in a variety of conditions, but is usually a sign of an active immune response. A severe viral infection, especially Epstein–Barr virus and cytomegalovirus (CMV), but many other viruses, including rubella, frequently trigger such a response. Hepatitis, varicella, mumps, HIV and chickenpox can occasionally elicit such a response. Protozoal infections, particularly toxoplasmosis but also malaria, can trigger a lymphocytosis, as can a variety of bacterial and similar infections, including healing TB, syphilis, typhoid fever, brucellosis and diphtheria. One of the most marked examples of lymphocytosis can be seen in pertussis (whooping cough), where the count can rise to very high levels in young children. Finally, a variety of diverse non-infectious causes can cause a lymphocytosis, including serum sickness, drug reactions, metastatic melanoma and hyperthyroidism.

Morphologically abnormal, so-called 'atypical lymphocytes' are found in infectious mononucleosis (glandular fever) due to Epstein–Barr virus, which produces atypical reactive T-lymphocytes. CMV, other viruses and toxoplasmosis may produce a similar picture. The atypical lymphocytes frequently display cytoplasmic and nuclear abnormalities. The cytoplasmic margin often appears ragged, and gives the appearance of giving way to surrounding cells. The cytoplasm often shows an abnormal basophilia but with a perinuclear halo. The nucleus itself often appears open and active. The abnormal blood cell picture can persist for some time, but eventually returns to normal as recovery occurs.

SUGGESTED FURTHER READING

Bain, B.J. (2006) *Blood Cells: a practical guide.* Blackwell Publishing, Oxford.

Potasman, I. & Prokocimer, M. (2008) The added value of peripheral blood cell morphology in the diagnosis and management of infectious diseases — part 2: illustrative cases. *Postgrad. Med. J.* **84:** 586–589.

Prokocimer, M. & Potasman, I. (2008) The added value of peripheral blood cell morphology in the diagnosis and management of infectious diseases — part 1: basic concepts. *Postgrad. Med. J.* **84:** 579–585.

SELF-ASSESSMENT QUESTIONS

1. Differentiate between autoimmune neutropenia and neonatal alloimmune neutropenia.
2. Identify the genes involved in the three forms of LAD.
3. Which of the following best describes the defect of classical CGD?
   a. Mutation of the *CYBB* gene at Xp21.1, resulting in deficiency of both gp91-*phox* and p22-*phox*.

b. Mutation of the *CYBB* gene at Xp21.1, resulting in an isolated deficiency of gp91-*phox*.

c. Mutation of the *CYBB* gene at Xp21.1, resulting in an isolated deficiency of p22-*phox*.

d. Mutation of the *NCF1* gene at 7q11, resulting in deficiency of p47-*phox*.

e. Mutation of the *CYTA* gene at 16p24, resulting in deficiency of p22-*phox*.

4. Which of the following statements about Pelger–Huët anomaly are true?

a. Pelger–Huët anomaly is a rare abnormality of granulocytes.

b. Pelger–Huët anomaly is characterized by nuclear hyposegmentation.

c. Pelger–Huët anomaly is caused by mutations in the laminin B-receptor gene at 1q42.1.

d. Pelger–Huët anomaly is associated with a right shift.

e. Most cases of Pelger–Huët anomaly are homozygous for the genetic abnormality.

5. Which inherited neutrophil abnormality is characterized by hypersegmentation of neutrophil nuclei?

a. Jordan's anomaly

b. Chédiak–Higashi syndrome

c. Undritz anomaly

d. Alder–Reilly anomaly

e. May–Hegglin anomaly

6. Name the genes affected in the following conditions:

a. Jordan's anomaly

b. Chédiak–Higashi syndrome

c. Pelger–Huët anomaly

d. May–Hegglin anomaly

7. Is development of severe basophilia in a patient with CML a good or poor prognostic indicator?

Haematological malignancies

Learning objectives
After studying this chapter you should confidently be able to:

■ **Outline the WHO classification of the haematological malignances**
The WHO classification of haematological malignancies employs a combination of morphological, immunophenotypic, genetic and clinical features to define distinct disease entities and is the current standard in this regard.

■ **Review the aetiology of haematological malignancies**
Much has been learned about the aetiology of the haematological malignancies. Starting at the level of epidemiological associations and then tying these in with the discovery of non-random cytogenetic abnormalities provided a rationale for the search for underlying molecular abnormalities. Several examples of how cytogenetic and molecular abnormalities can lead to specific haematological malignancies are reviewed.

■ **Review the biology of malignancy**
We now know that all malignancy results from the stepwise accumulation of genetic mutations that lead to dysregulation of cell growth and survival. Broadly, there are three types of genes that are closely involved in the development of malignancy: (proto-)oncogenes, tumour suppressor genes and DNA repair genes. The ways in which abnormalities of each of these gene types can contribute to the development of malignancy are reviewed.

■ **Outline the principles of treatment for haematological malignancy**
The most widely employed modes of treatment in haematological malignancy are cytotoxic chemotherapy, haemopoietic stem cell transplantation, radiotherapy and supportive care.

Haematological malignancies are characterized by an uncontrolled clonal proliferation of haemopoietic cells. Numerous classification schemes exist for this complex group of disorders. In this book, the WHO classification (2008) is used, except where explicitly stated. The WHO classification system is summarized in *Tables 10.1* and *10.2*. The specific characteristics of each group are considered in detail in *Chapters 11–17*. This chapter concentrates on topics that are important across the spectrum of haematological malignancy.

10.1 CLASSIFICATION OF THE HAEMATOLOGICAL MALIGNANCIES

The most recent classification system for the haematological malignancies is the 2008 WHO classification of tumours of the haemopoietic and lymphoid tissues. This system employs a combination of morphological, immunophenotypic, genetic and clinical features to define distinct disease entities. The first step in the WHO system is to classify neoplasms according to their haemopoietic lineage as:

Table 10.1 The WHO classification of the myeloid neoplasms

Myeloid neoplasms*

   Acute myeloid leukaemia (AML)

      Acute myeloid leukaemia with recurrent genetic abnormalities

      Acute myeloid leukaemia with myelodysplasia-related changes

      Therapy-related myeloid neoplasms

      Acute myeloid leukaemia, not otherwise specified

      Myeloid proliferations related to Down syndrome

      Blastic plasmacytoid dendritic cell neoplasm

   Myeloproliferative neoplasms (MPN)

      Chronic myeloid leukaemia (CML)

      Chronic neutrophilic leukaemia (CNL)

      Chronic eosinophilic leukaemia (CEL)

      Polycythaemia vera

      Primary myelofibrosis

      Essential thrombocythaemia

      Myeloproliferative neoplasms, unclassifiable

   Myelodysplastic syndromes (MDS)

      Refractory cytopenia with unilineage dysplasia (RCUD)

         Refractory anaemia (RA)

         Refractory neutropenia (RN)

         Refractory thrombocytopenia (RT)

      Refractory anaemia with ring sideroblasts (RARS)

      Refractory cytopenia with multilineage dysplasia (RCMD)

      Refractory anaemia with excess blasts-1 (RAEB-1)

      Refractory anaemia with excess blasts-2 (RAEB-2)

      MDS with isolated del(5q)

      MDS, unclassifiable

      Childhood myelodysplastic syndrome

   Myelodysplastic/myeloproliferative neoplasms (MPN)

      Chronic myelomonocytic leukaemia (CMML)

      Atypical chronic myeloid leukaemia (aCML)

      Juvenile myelomonocytic leukaemia (JMML)

      Myelodysplastic/myeloproliferative neoplasm, unclassifiable

Neoplasms with myeloid and lymphoid lineage

   Myeloid/lymphoid neoplasms with eosinophilia and abnormalities of *PDGFRA, PDGFRB* or *FGFR1*

---

* For clarity, some rare or provisional entities have been omitted

Table 10.2 The WHO classification of the lymphoid neoplasms

Lymphoid neoplasms*

   Precursor lymphoid neoplasms

   B-lymphoblastic leukaemia/lymphoma NOS (B-ALL)

   B-lymphoblastic leukaemia/lymphoma with recurrent genetic abnormalities (B-ALL)

   T-lymphoblastic leukaemia/lymphoma (T-ALL)

   Mature B-cell neoplasms

   Chronic lymphocytic leukaemia/small lymphocytic lymphoma (CLL/SLL)

   B-cell prolymphocytic leukaemia (B-PLL)

   Lymphoplasmacytic lymphoma

   Waldenström macroglobulinaemia (WM)

   Splenic marginal zone lymphoma

   Hairy cell leukaemia (HCL)

   Extranodal MALT lymphoma

   Nodal marginal zone lymphoma

   Follicular lymphoma (FL)

   Primary cutaneous follicle centre lymphoma

   Mantle cell lymphoma (MCL)

   Diffuse large B-cell lymphoma (DLBCL)

   Primary mediastinal large B cell lymphoma

   Primary effusion lymphoma

   Plasma cell myeloma (MM)

   Solitary plasmacytoma of bone

   Extraosseous plasmacytoma

   ALK ± large B-cell lymphoma

   Plasmablastic lymphoma

   Burkitt lymphoma (BL)

   Heavy chain disease (HCD)

   Mature T-cell and NK-cell neoplasms

   T-cell prolymphocytic leukaemia (T-PLL)

   T-cell large granular lymphocytic leukaemia

   Aggressive NK cell leukaemia

   Adult T-cell leukaemia/lymphoma (ATLL)

   Extranodal NK/T-cell lymphoma, nasal type

   Enteropathy-associated T-cell lymphoma

   Hepatosplenic T-cell lymphoma

   Subcutaneous panniculitis-like T-cell lymphoma

   Mycosis fungoides

   Sézary syndrome

   Anaplastic large cell lymphoma, ALK+

   Peripheral T-cell lymphoma

   Angioimmunoblastic T-cell lymphoma

   Primary cutaneous T-cell lymphoma

   Hodgkin lymphoma

   Nodular lymphocyte-predominant Hodgkin lymphoma

   Classical Hodgkin lymphoma

      Nodular sclerosis classical Hodgkin lymphoma

      Lymphocyte-rich classical Hodgkin lymphoma

      Mixed cellularity classical Hodgkin lymphoma

      Lymphocyte-depleted classical Hodgkin lymphoma

   Post-transplantation lymphoproliferative disorders (PTLD)

* For clarity, some rare or provisional entities have been omitted

- myeloid neoplasms
- lymphoid neoplasms
- histiocytic/dendritic neoplasms
- neoplasms with myeloid and lymphoid lineage.

Myeloid neoplasms

The myeloid neoplasms are derived from bone marrow progenitor cells that are restricted to developing into red cells, granulocytes, monocytes, or megakaryocytes. One important exception to this is chronic myeloid leukaemia (CML), where the cell of origin is a pluripotent haemopoietic stem cell. The myeloid neoplasms can be further subdivided into three broad classes:

- acute myeloid leukaemias (AML; see *Chapter 11* and *Box 10.1*)
- myelodysplastic syndromes (MDS; see *Chapter 13*)
- myeloproliferative neoplasms (MPN; see *Chapter 14*)

Box 10.1 Acute and chronic leukaemias

The division of the leukaemias into acute and chronic types describes the natural history of the diseases in the absence of treatment. In these circumstances, acute leukaemia is typically fatal within weeks or months of diagnosis. In contrast, survival in chronic leukaemia is measured in years. Modern treatment methods have made the distinction in survival time between acute and chronic leukaemias much less clear, however.

Lymphoid neoplasms

The lymphoid neoplasms are derived from cells that normally develop into the different forms of T and B cells, and are further subdivided into neoplasms derived from T and B lymphoid precursors and those derived from mature T and B cells and plasma cells. Previous classification systems divided lymphoid neoplasms into the leukaemias (those that presented primarily with blood and bone marrow manifestations) and the lymphomas (those that presented with disease mainly manifest in lymph nodes and tissues). This distinction is not present in the WHO classification system, because it groups neoplasms according to their cell of origin. This means that several disorders previously considered to be separate diseases are now classified as single entities. For example, chronic lymphocytic leukaemia (CLL) and small lymphocytic lymphoma (SLL) are considered to be different manifestations of the same disease. However, the separation of diseases into acute and chronic leukaemias and Hodgkin and non-Hodgkin lymphoma remains clinically meaningful. In this book, the acute leukaemias are reviewed in *Chapter 11*, the chronic lymphoid leukaemias in *Chapter 12*, the lymphomas in *Chapter 15* and myeloma and related plasma cell disorders in *Chapter 16*.

Neoplasms with myeloid and lymphoid lineage

Some neoplasms express markers of both myeloid and lymphoid lineages. An important group here are classified as myeloid/lymphoid neoplasms with eosinophilia and abnormalities of *PDGFRA*, *PDGFRB* or *FGFR1* (see *Chapter 14*).

10.2   AETIOLOGY OF THE HAEMATOLOGICAL MALIGNANCIES

The question 'what causes haematological malignancy?' can be tackled in many ways. Much of our current understanding of the aetiology of haematological malignancy has been derived from epidemiological studies. Such studies are notoriously difficult to perform, bedevilled as they are by the rarity of some of the conditions under study, by lack of reliable historical data, by variations in diagnostic and recording practices and by the confounding influences of socio-economic factors such as access to health care. The results of such studies must always be interpreted with caution. An alternative approach is to study the differences between malignant cells and their normal counterparts. At first, this approach revealed cytogenetic abnormalities that were associated with particular haematological malignancies such as the Philadelphia chromosome and CML. As knowledge of molecular genetics improved, it gradually became clear that malignant cells have acquired multiple genetic and epigenetic abnormalities that are responsible for malignant transformation and progression. This section adopts a similar, chronological approach to unravelling the aetiology of haematological malignancies. Finally, in *Section 10.3*, knowledge of the underlying aetiology of haematological malignancies is used to illuminate discussion of their biology.

Aetiological associations

Although exposure to certain environmental conditions, drugs and chemicals has been shown to be associated with the development of haematological malignancy, proof of a cause / effect relationship is often lacking (see *Box 10.2*). In addition, only a relatively small proportion of individuals exposed to these carcinogenic factors actually develop a malignant condition, suggesting that other factors, such as genetic constitution, may be operating.

The following factors are widely regarded as being involved, or having the potential to be involved, in the aetiology of haemopoietic (and other) malignancy:

- ionizing radiation
- therapeutic drugs
- chemicals
- viruses
- familial and genetic factors.

Box 10.2 Cause and effect or association

It is important not to confuse association with cause and effect. For example, several epidemiological studies have shown that women treated with hormone replacement therapy (HRT) also had a reduced incidence of coronary heart disease (CHD). Some authorities suggested that these studies implied that HRT had a protective effect against CHD. In fact, prospective randomized controlled trials have shown that HRT causes a small, but significant increase in CHD risk. Careful review of the earlier epidemiological data showed that the women taking HRT in these studies were more likely to be from higher socio-economic groups with lifestyles that are known to decrease CHD risk. In this case, leaping to the 'obvious' conclusion was misleading. Proof of association is not the same as proof of causality.

Ionizing radiation

The atomic bombs that were dropped on Hiroshima and Nagasaki provided incontrovertible evidence that exposure to a dose of ionizing radiation in excess of 1 Gray is leukaemogenic. An increased incidence of CML, acute lymphoblastic leukaemia (ALL), AML and MDS, non-Hodgkin lymphoma (NHL) and multiple myeloma (MM) in survivors of these horrific events was identified in the late 1940s.

Interesting differences in the rates of different haematological malignancy provided some potential clues to the role of ionizing radiation in their induction. For example, an increased risk of developing CML was observed in people with lower radiation doses than those in whom AML or ALL developed. The excess risk of developing AML (about $\times 20$ overall) increased in line with age at the time of exposure, with a peak incidence after about 7–8 years. An increased risk of NHL and MM was seen in the survivors of Hiroshima, but not Nagasaki, which may have been attributable to differences in the spectrum of radiation emitted at these sites. Survivors had an excess risk of developing ALL of about 9 times, and the risk was highest in children. The excess risk of NHL and MM was highest in those aged under 25 years at the time of exposure.

Chronic exposure to therapeutic X irradiation has also been associated with an increased incidence of leukaemia, aplastic anaemia and solid tumours in heavily exposed tissue. Retrospective studies of cause of death in medical staff showed an excess of fatal leukaemia in radiologists prior to 1940. This excess disappeared following the introduction of adequate shielding and dosage monitoring in such staff.

The therapeutic use of ionizing radiation for malignant conditions, both for solid tumours and for haematological malignancies, has been associated with an increased risk of developing a secondary malignancy. Whilst the very mechanism used therapeutically, that of disrupting the DNA in target cells, is vital for the efficacy of radiotherapy, the same mechanism is also known to be mutagenic, and there are clear links between the use of radiotherapy and the subsequent development of haematological disorders such as CML. There is clear evidence that ionizing radiation induces strand breaks in double-stranded DNA that can result in cell death, optimal repair or mutations caused by suboptimal repair (see *Box 10.3*).

Box 10.3 Radiation dosage

The biological damage inflicted by ionizing radiation is largely determined by the dosage, which is defined in terms of the amount of energy transferred to the irradiated tissue. Dosage is expressed in Gray where 1 Gray is equivalent to the absorption of 1 joule of energy per kilogram of irradiated tissue. The older unit of dosage was the rad. 1 Gray = 100 rad.

Therapeutic drugs

The treatment of established malignancy frequently involves administration of cytotoxic drugs. The use of certain forms of cytotoxic drugs is associated strongly with an increased incidence of secondary (therapy-induced) MDS and AML. For example, treatment with alkylating agents increases the risk of secondary AML for up to 12 years, with a peak at around 5 years. About 10–20% of MDS cases and up to 30% of AML cases are secondary to previous cancer chemotherapy. Therapy-induced AML differs from *de novo* AML in a number of important respects:

■ at least 90% of therapy-induced AML cases have cytogenetic abnormalities, most commonly monosomy 5, 5q-, monosomy 7 and 7q-.
■ a preleukaemic phase (antecedent haematological disorder (AHD)) occurs in more than 65% of cases of therapy-induced AML but less than 25% of de novo cases.
■ therapy-induced AML is often refractory to treatment: the mean survival time from diagnosis is 4 months compared to 20 months for *de novo* cases.

Secondary MDS/AML is also associated with previous treatment with topoisomerase I inhibitors (e.g. irinotecan; see *Box 10.4*) and topoisomerase II inhibitors (e.g. etoposide).

Box 10.4 Topoisomerases

Topoisomerases are enzymes that are responsible for unwinding and then rewinding DNA so that genes can be expressed and DNA can be replicated. They act by binding to DNA and severing the phosphate backbone of the molecule. Inhibition of these enzymes is potentially genotoxic and mutagenic. Etoposide-related secondary AML frequently shows rearrangement of the MLL gene at 11q23. Interestingly, some studies have shown that a maternal diet rich in the bioflavonoids genistein or quercetin is associated with childhood AML or ALL with the same rearrangement.

The most likely explanation for the induction of MDS/AML by alkylating agents lies with their known mutagenic properties. Alkylating agents are capable of alkylating the nitrogen and oxygen molecules of all four DNA bases, phosphodiester bonds and the 2′ oxygen atom of ribose, resulting in inappropriate base pairing, strand breaks, complex rearrangements and the deletion of part or all of a chromosome. Mutations that alter the expression of normal cellular oncogenes can result in malignant change.

Chemicals

A large number of different chemicals have been suggested as possible inducers or promoters of haematological malignancy but, in most cases, the evidence is unconvincing. The exception is benzene: chronic exposure to benzene and its derivatives is associated with an increased incidence of hypoplastic anaemia and AML. Most cases have resulted from prolonged occupational exposure to relatively high concentrations of benzene. However, recent reports of an excess of AML in male cigarette smokers and in the children of women who continued to smoke heavily during pregnancy, have raised the possibility that chronic exposure to the low levels of aromatic compounds found in tobacco smoke may be leukaemogenic.

Antenatal exposure to alcohol has been associated with an increased risk of AML, as has prophylactic administration of vitamin K to neonates.

Epidemiological studies of rates of haematological malignancy in different occupations have revealed a slight excess incidence of myeloma, NHL, AML and CML in agricultural workers, possibly related to increased exposure to insecticides and herbicides. Similar studies have shown an excess of CLL and NHL in rubber industry workers, ALL in the children of nuclear industry workers, CML in welders and NHL in anaesthetists and those exposed to halomethane compounds. None of these associations are universally accepted as proven cases of cause and effect.

Viruses

There is a wealth of evidence for viral induction of leukaemia and solid tumours in animals, including higher primates. An estimated 15% of all human tumours worldwide are caused by viruses (see also *Box 10.5*). These oncogenic viruses can be divided into two types, the DNA

Box 10.5 Leukaemia transmission

The earliest demonstration that leukaemia could be transmitted between animals was made in 1908 at the Royal Veterinary School in Copenhagen by V. Ellermann and O. Bang. They showed that injecting leukaemic cells from chickens with avian myeloblastosis into healthy birds caused the development of the condition in the healthy birds. Further experiments showed that the same effect could be obtained by injecting carefully filtered, cell-free extracts. Three years later, P. Rous showed that solid tumours could be induced in chickens by the injection of cell-free extracts from similarly afflicted birds. These observations were not extended to mammals until 1936 when J.J. Bittner demonstrated the transmission of murine mammary carcinoma through maternal milk. The earliest clear demonstration of leukaemia induction by the injection of cell-free extracts was made in 1951 by L. Gross in New York who used new-born mice. Attempts to induce leukaemia in adult mice were unsuccessful.

viruses (papillomaviruses, adenoviruses and herpesviruses) and the RNA viruses, including retroviruses. Examples of the involvement of DNA viruses in the induction of human tumours include human papillomavirus (HPV) in cervical neoplasia, Epstein–Barr virus (EBV) in Burkitt lymphoma, Hodgkin disease and nasopharyngeal carcinoma, and hepatitis B virus (HBV) and C virus in primary hepatoma. The only convincing evidence for retroviral induction of neoplasia in humans comes from studies of the retrovirus human T lymphotropic virus I (HTLV-I). The accumulated evidence for the role of this virus in the aetiology of an unusual form of acute T cell leukaemia / lymphoma in southern Japan and the Caribbean is compelling.

Viruses can induce malignant transformation of host cells in three ways.

■ Retroviruses that contain an oncogene within their genome can induce malignant transformation in host cells by insertion of the viral oncogene into the host cell genome. This mechanism, known as direct mutagenesis, typically leads to an acute and rapidly progressive tumour.

■ Insertion of viral DNA at a specific point in the host DNA, enabling the viral regulatory sequences to influence the expression of host cellular proliferation genes (proto-oncogenes). This mechanism, known as insertional mutagenesis, is associated with a relatively long latency period and only a minority of infected animals develop neoplasia, since such changes merely establish an appropriate environment for subsequent oncogenesis.

■ HTLV-I differs in that the point of insertion of viral DNA into host DNA varies widely. HTLV-I is thought to be capable of transforming host T lymphocytes by a process known as transactivation. A viral protein designated TAX has been shown to transactivate the genes that encode the IL-2 receptor, IL-3, IL-4, GM–CSF and the oncogene *FOS*.

Numerous epidemiological studies have suggested a possible role for infectious agents in human haematological malignancy. The observation of an increased incidence of myeloma, NHL, AML and CML in agricultural workers raises the possibility that contact with oncogenic animal viruses may be involved. However, exhaustive studies of pet owners, slaughterhouse workers and children bitten by animals have failed to provide consistent confirmation of this observation.

Burkitt lymphoma is a form of NHL endemic to tropical Africa and Papua New Guinea and manifests as tumours of the jaw and abdomen with extensive extranodal involvement. Virtually all cases of African Burkitt lymphoma have definitive evidence of EBV infection and one of three chromosomal translocations: (t(8;14); t(8;22) or t(2;8)). EBV is a very common virus worldwide but infection in developed countries causes the self-limiting condition infectious mononucleosis. This relatively mild illness is associated with EBV infection during adolescence, which is common in developed countries. In Africa, primary infection with EBV usually occurs in the first year of life. It is suggested that EBV is implicated in the development of African Burkitt lymphoma via a multi-step route as follows.

■ Primary EBV infection occurs and 'immortalizes' infected B lymphocytes. This occurs in all infected individuals.

■ An immortalized B lymphocyte is stimulated to proliferate by some immunological challenge such as malaria infection, resulting in the formation of an immortalized B cell clone. The variety and frequency of immunological challenges in tropical Africa makes this step more likely.

■ In the process of cell proliferation, a single cell in the immortalized clone develops one of the three chromosomal translocations that induce malignant transformation. The result is Burkitt lymphoma.

Hodgkin disease (HD) is a heterogeneous condition that has been suspected of having an infectious aetiology since it was first described in 1832. Recent evidence has suggested that EBV is implicated in the pathogenesis of HD in a proportion of cases in children and adults over the age of 50 years. A multi-step aetiology similar to that for African BL is also proposed for HD.

Host factors and familial malignancy

Numerous case reports exist of families with a greater than expected number of cases of haematological malignancy, including leukaemia, lymphoma and myeloma. In some cases, it has been possible to discern an underlying inherited predisposition to the development of malignancy, whereas in others no clearly-defined link exists (see the subsection on familial malignancy later in this chapter).

The significantly increased risk of ALL in an identical twin of a confirmed case is well established. The risk of coincident development of ALL is highest in infancy. The most likely explanation for this phenomenon is the transmission of cells with increased malignant potential from one twin, in whom the cells arose, to the other via the shared placental circulation *in utero*.

Cytogenetics and haematological malignancy

The results of epidemiological studies suggested that the common property of factors that were strongly associated with an increased risk of haematological malignancy was that they were associated with damage to DNA. For example, ionizing radiation and alkylating agents are known to induce strand breaks in DNA, and benzene is a known mutagen. As this evidence was accumulating, a second strand of evidence was developing – that an increasing number of haematological malignancies were associated with cytogenetic abnormalities. The best example of this was the universal finding of an abnormality known as the Philadelphia chromosome in CML. The association between this abnormal chromosome and the disease was so strong that it became an essential component of the diagnosis for CML. For many years, no other abnormality was found that was so closely associated. Most chromosomal abnormalities could be found in more than one type of haematological malignancy and most forms of haematological malignancy could exist without specific cytogenetic abnormalities. However, it became increasingly clear that the incidence and distribution of cytogenetic abnormalities were non-random.

A large number of cytogenetic abnormalities associated with haematological malignancy have been identified. Many of these abnormalities are discussed in detail in the following chapters. To illustrate how identification of some of these abnormalities contributed to a growing understanding of the nature of malignant disease, three examples are reviewed here. Many other examples of specific rearrangements that are associated with particular haematological malignancies are reviewed in detail in the following chapters.

t(8;14)(q24;q32) and Burkitt lymphoma

Burkitt lymphoma is a form of NHL that is most closely associated with equatorial Africa and presents as tumours affecting the jaw and facial bones, particularly in children. The disease is also found sporadically in other parts of the world, where the disease frequently involves abdominal organs such as the ileum, caecum, ovaries or kidney and also in the setting of HIV–AIDS.

It was found that more than two-thirds of cases of Burkitt lymphoma carried the cytogenetic abnormality t(8;14)(q24;q32), which is a reciprocal translocation that involves breakage of chromosome 8 at 8q24, chromosome 14 at 14q32 and swapping of chromosomal material. The specificity of these breakpoints prompted investigation of the genes located there, and it was discovered that the translocation moved a gene called *MYC* located at 8q24 to the immunoglobulin heavy chain locus at 14q32. The immunoglobulin genes are among the most actively transcribed in the genome. Conversely, the *MYC* gene encodes a nuclear transcription factor that ordinarily is transiently transcribed. Relocation of *MYC* leads to its overexpression. This discovery led to the hypothesis that overexpression of a gene (*MYC*) that is involved in regulation of the activity of other genes is likely to be implicated in the malignant process of Burkitt lymphoma.

Subsequent identification of the variant translocations t(2;8)(p12;q24) and t(8;22)(q24;q11) in cases of Burkitt lymphoma, in which *MYC* is translocated to the immunoglobulin light chain κ gene locus at 2p12 or the immunoglobulin light chain λ gene locus at 22q11, lent considerable weight to the hypothesis.

t(15;17)(q22;q21) and acute promyelocytic leukaemia

Acute promyelocytic leukaemia (APL) is a subtype of AML that was originally described as a hyperacute fatal disease, associated with fulminant disseminated intravascular coagulation (DIC). Three strands of research came together to explain the pathophysiology of this disorder.

- In the mid-1970s, fundamental research on myeloid differentiation pointed towards the role of retinoic acid in the differentiation of granulocytic cells.
- In the mid-1980s, thawing of relations with China led to sharing of Chinese medical knowledge with the West, including their experience of treating APL with all-trans retinoic acid (ATRA), a derivative of vitamin A.
- In the early 1990s, the specific translocation t(15;17)(q22;q21) was identified in most cases of APL. This translocation was shown to involve the *PML* gene on chromosome 15q22 and the retinoic acid receptor gene (*RARα*) on chromosome 17q21, and to result in the formation of two novel fusion genes, both of which are transcribed. This discovery seemed to provide a rationale for the then puzzling efficacy of ATRA in this condition.

The *RARα* gene is mainly expressed in haemopoietic cells and regulates gene expression and cellular differentiation. In the absence of retinoic acid, the RARα protein binds to the transcriptional co-regulatory protein nuclear corepressor factor, resulting in suppression of gene transcription and promyelocytic differentiation. Conversely, in the presence of retinoic acid, transcriptional suppression is removed, promoting terminal differentiation of promyelocytes. The PML–RARα fusion protein binds more tightly to the nuclear corepressor factor, with the result that physiological concentrations of retinoic acid no longer relieve the transcriptional suppression, resulting in the promyelocytic differentiation block characteristic of APL.

The effect of ATRA in APL is to induce terminal differentiation of the leukaemic cells. It is not cytotoxic. However, when combined with conventional cytotoxic chemotherapy, ATRA has helped to transform APL from a near-universally fatal disease to an eminently curable one.

t(9;22)(q34;q11) and chronic myeloid leukaemia

The discovery of a minute chromosome 22 that characterized CML was the first example of a specific cytogenetic abnormality that could be used for diagnostic purposes. The Philadelphia chromosome, as it became known, is formed by the reciprocal translocation t(9;22)(q34;q11). Molecular analysis subsequently showed that the translocation involves the *ABL* gene at 9q34 and the *BCR* gene at 22q11 and results in the creation of two novel fusion genes. The normal ABL protein (p145^{abl}) is a cytoplasmic and nuclear protein tyrosine kinase that is involved in the processes of cell division, differentiation, adhesion and stress response, while the normal BCR protein (p160^{bcr}) is involved in the activation of GTP-binding proteins within cells. The *BCR–ABL* fusion gene product (BCR–ABL) functions as a tyrosine kinase and is constitutively active, i.e. it does not require activation by other cellular messaging proteins. BCR–ABL has been shown to activate cell cycle regulators and to inhibit DNA repair, resulting in dysregulated cell growth and increased genomic instability.

The creation of a hybrid *BCR–ABL* gene is required, but is not sufficient, for the development of CML. There is strong evidence that the acquisition of this abnormality is a relatively late step in CML leukaemogenesis.

10.3   BIOLOGY OF MALIGNANCY

Accumulating knowledge of the nature of the non-random cytogenetic and molecular abnormalities in malignant disease led to the now confirmed understanding that all malignancy results from the stepwise accumulation of genetic mutations that lead to dysregulation of cell growth and survival, the defining feature of malignancy (see *Figure 10.1*). This section focuses on the biology of malignant disease as a whole, although the underlying principles apply equally to haematological malignancies. More specific details of the molecular abnormalities that underlie specific haematological malignancies are reviewed in the following chapters.

Broadly, there are three types of genes that are closely involved in the development of malignancy: (proto-)oncogenes, tumour suppressor genes and DNA repair genes.

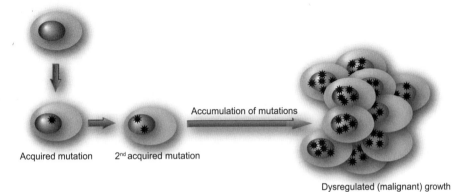

Accumulation of mutations

Acquired mutation   2nd acquired mutation

Dysregulated (malignant) growth

Figure 10.1
The accumulation of gene mutations leading to development of malignancy.

Oncogenes and malignancy

Oncogenes were first defined as viral genes that were associated directly with malignant transformation of infected cells. It was not long before it was recognized that, in humans, oncogenes were mutated forms of normal genes that encode growth factors, growth factor receptors, intracellular signalling molecules, nuclear transcription factors, cell cycle regulators and apoptotic proteins. These normal genes are essential for cellular growth, differentiation and survival and are known as proto-oncogenes (see *Figure 10.2*). Mutation of a proto-oncogene can cause overexpression of its protein product, or expression of an abnormal protein that is more active in promoting cell growth or survival and so may contribute to a progressive loss of control over cell growth and death, the hallmark of malignancy.

A useful working definition of oncogenes in humans is 'abnormal genes whose *presence* can stimulate the development of malignancy'. *Table 10.3* lists some proto-oncogenes, the function of their protein products, and examples of the abnormalities that can turn them into oncogenes.

Tumour suppressor genes and malignancy

Tumour suppressor genes are another family of genes closely involved in the regulation of cell growth and survival. In general, the protein products of normal tumour suppressor genes inhibit cell growth mechanisms and promote cell death mechanisms (see *Figure 10.3*). Tumour

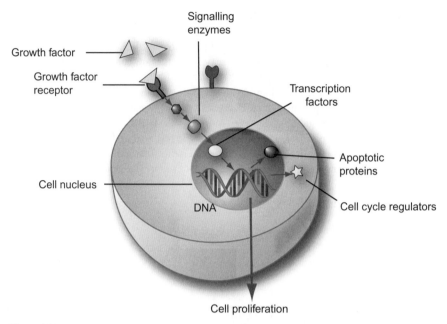

Figure 10.2
Normal mechanisms of regulation of cell growth and death encoded by proto-oncogenes.

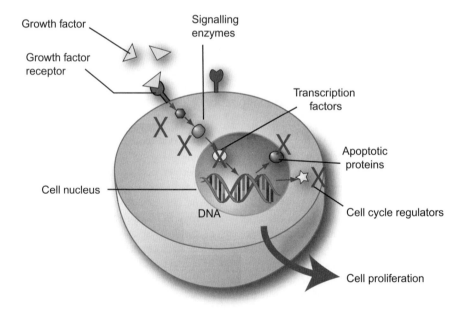

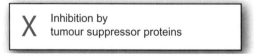

Figure 10.3
The function of the protein products of tumour suppressor genes.

Table 10.3 Proto-oncogenes and related oncogene activation

Proto-oncogene	Protein function	Altered oncogene product function
RAS	GTPase enzyme in mitotic signalling pathway	Mutation that blocks enzyme activity
MYC	Transcription factor	Gene overexpression
FOS, JUN	Combine to form transcription factor	
RAF	Protein kinase enzyme in mitotic signalling pathway	Mutations that permanently activate the enzyme
EGFR	Growth factor receptor	Gene overexpression or mutation that permanently activates the receptor
PDGF	Growth factor	Gene overexpression
BCL-2	Inhibitor of apoptosis	
ABL	Protein kinase enzyme with multiple functions	Mutations that permanently activate the enzyme or gene overexpression
SRC	Protein kinase enzyme with multiple functions	
PIK3CA	Subunit of signalling complex	
AKT	Protein kinase enzyme with multiple functions	

suppressor genes, therefore, can be usefully defined as 'normal genes whose *absence* can stimulate the development of malignancy'.

Loss of tumour suppressor gene function due to mutations can make cells susceptible to unregulated growth and malignant transformation (see *Figure 10.4*). For example, the *P53* and *RB* genes are tumour suppressor genes that directly inhibit cell cycle progression. Loss of the normal function of these genes through mutations can cause inappropriate progression through the cell cycle.

Mutations in tumour suppressor genes are recessive, i.e. both genes must be mutated for the suppressive effect to be lost and malignancy development to be stimulated. For example, there are two forms of an eye tumour known as retinoblastoma. About 40% of cases are diagnosed in young children and it is common for tumours to be present in both eyes. This form of the disease is caused by inheriting an abnormal form of the *RB* gene from both parents. In other words, these patients have no normally functional *RB* gene and so a reduced tumour suppressive effect and bilateral tumours develop early in life. There may be a family history of retinoblastoma.

In the other, sporadic, form tumours tend to develop later in life and usually only in one eye. Typically, a family history of retinoblastoma is absent. These cases are caused by inheriting one normal and one abnormal *RB* gene. The presence of the normal *RB* gene means that tumour suppression is present and there is no intrinsically increased tendency to develop retinoblastoma. However, if a random event damages the functional *RB* gene, then the tumour suppressive effect is lost and retinoblastoma will develop.

Some known tumour suppressor genes whose functional loss is associated with the development of malignancy are listed in *Table 10.4*.

DNA repair genes and malignancy

Another class of genes implicated in the development of cancer are the DNA repair genes. These encode proteins that correct errors in DNA introduced during replication or by external factors such as exposure to ionizing radiation or alkylating agents. Mutation in DNA repair genes can

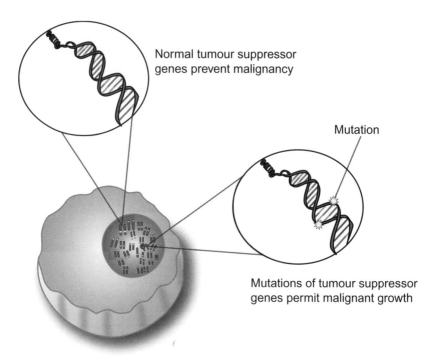

Normal tumour suppressor genes prevent malignancy

Mutation

Mutations of tumour suppressor genes permit malignant growth

Figure 10.4
Tumour suppressor gene mutation and the development of malignancy.

Table 10.4 Tumour suppressor genes and associated malignancies

Gene	Function of protein	Associated malignancy
APC	Inhibitor of mitotic signalling	Familial adenomatous polyposis coli, colorectal cancer
RB	Cell cycle inhibitor	Retinoblastoma
P53	DNA damage response, stress response	Li–Fraumeni syndrome, lymphoma, leukaemia, ovarian, colorectal, lung, pancreatic, prostate and skin cancers
WT1	Transcription factor. Binds to p53 protein	Wilm's tumour (childhood renal cancer)
P16^{INK4A}	Cyclin-dependent kinase inhibitor	Melanoma
BRCA-1, BRCA-2	DNA damage response	Breast and ovarian cancers
VHL	Regulation of gene expression by oxygen	Von Hippel–Lindau syndrome, renal cancer
NF1, NF2	GTPase enzyme in mitotic signalling pathway	Neurofibromatosis, brain cancers

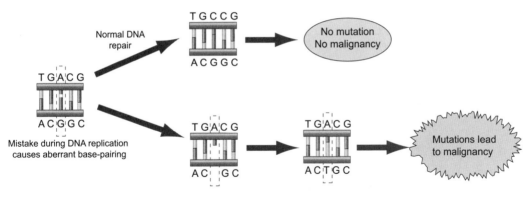

Figure 10.5
DNA repair and the development of malignancy.

allow errors in DNA to accumulate and can contribute to the development of malignancy (see *Figure 10.5*).

For example, in the inherited condition xeroderma pigmentosum, mutation of the *XPA* gene means that those affected cannot effectively repair the DNA damage caused by exposure to ultraviolet radiation. These people commonly develop basaliomas and other skin cancers at a young age and so must avoid sunlight. Mutations in DNA repair genes are also implicated in the development of an unusual form of colorectal cancer called hereditary non-polyposis colorectal cancer (HNPCC). Other disorders associated with defective DNA repair and an excess cancer risk include ataxia-telangiectasia, Fanconi anaemia and Bloom syndrome.

Other genes implicated in malignancy
Although the most important classes of genes involved in the development of malignancy are the oncogenes, tumour suppressor genes, and DNA repair genes, a variety of other genes may contribute. Examples include genes that encode proteins responsible for activation or deactivation of carcinogens, cell cycle regulators, cell senescence proteins and cell differentiation factors. Other mutations, for example in adhesion molecule genes, may facilitate tumour invasion or metastasis.

Familial malignancy
Malignancy is caused by mutations in genes that lead to dysregulated cell growth and survival. This does not mean that malignancies are inherited conditions: the majority of malignancies are caused by acquired mutations that are not heritable, i.e. they are somatic mutations. About 90% of malignancies develop in people with no previous family history of that particular form of malignancy.

Sporadic reports of families that seem to share an increased tendency to develop malignancy have existed for decades. Some of these early cases may have been explicable by shared exposures to environmental carcinogens. However, in many cases, it has been possible to define a shared inheritance of a germline mutation of a proto-oncogene, tumour suppressor gene or DNA repair gene. Some of these inherited conditions and the malignancies they are associated with are summarized in *Table 10.5*.

However, there is not always such a neat explanation for cases of apparent familial haematological malignancy. Some of these cases demonstrate a phenomenon known as

Table 10.5 Inherited conditions that predispose to haematological (and sometimes other) malignancies

Inherited condition	Mode of inheritance	Defect	Associated haematological malignancies
Genomic instability			
Diamond–Blackfan	AR, AD	Heterogeneous	AML
Familial platelet disorder (FPD)	AD	*RUNX1* mutation	AML, MDS
Kostmann syndrome	AD, AR	Heterogeneous	AML
Amegakaryocytic thombocytopenia		*MPL* gene at 1p34	AML
Shwachman–Diamond	AR	*SBDS* gene at 7q11	ALL, AML, JMML
Tumour suppressor defects			
Down syndrome	Somatic, +21	*TEL-AML1* fusion gene in some cases	AML, ALL
Li–Fraumeni syndrome	AD	*P53* gene at 17p13	NHL, ALL, CML, JMML, AML
Dyskeratosis congenita	X, AD, AR	*DKC1* gene at Xq28, heterogeneous	Uncertain
DNA repair defects			
Ataxia telangiectasia	AR	*ATM* gene at 11q22–23	AML, TALL, T-PLL, T NHL, B NHL
Bloom syndrome	AR	*BLM* gene at 15q26	AML, ALL, NHL
Fanconi syndrome	AR, X	*FANCA-FANCJ* genes	AML
Immunodeficiency			
Wiskott–Aldrich syndrome	X	*WASP* gene at Xp11.23–11.22	ALL, HD, NHL
Severe combined immunodeficiency disease (SCID)	AR, X	Heterogeneous	B NHL
Common variable immunodeficiency	AR, AD	Heterogeneous	B NHL

'anticipation', which means that the age of onset of a familial condition decreases with each successive generation. This phenomenon has been associated with the accumulation of unstable trinucleotide repeat sequences within one or more genes in the inherited degenerative neurological condition Huntington disease, suggesting that there may be an as yet uncharacterized genetic basis in affected families.

Some other families have been reported to show various immune abnormalities or HLA (human leucocyte antigen) associations in those that develop haematological malignancy; however, a definitive explanation is lacking.

Several inherited conditions exist that similarly result in an increased risk of developing specific solid tumours. The best-known examples of these are:

■ familial adenomatous polyposis, which is caused by mutations in the *APC* gene at 5q21–q22 or the *MUTYH* gene at 1p34.3–p32.1. In either case, the result is a markedly increased (approaching 100%) tendency to develop colon cancer

■ Li–Fraumeni syndrome which, in addition to an increased risk of developing haematological malignancies, also results in increased rates of premenopausal breast cancer, childhood soft tissue sarcomas, osteosarcoma, brain tumours and adrenal cortical carcinomas

■ germline mutation of either the *BRCA-1* or *BRCA-2* genes, which leads to a significantly increased risk of both breast and ovarian cancer.

The cell cycle

As a cell grows, differentiates and divides, it progresses through four distinct phases referred to as the cell cycle (see *Figure 10.6*). The phases of the cell cycle are known as G_1, S, G_2 and M. Growth and differentiation take place in the G_1, S and G_2 phases, collectively known as interphase, because it was once regarded as a resting stage. It is now known to be a period of intense cellular metabolic activity. Mitosis, the process of cell division, takes place during the M phase.

During the G_1 phase, the immature cell grows and differentiates to carry out specialized functions. The cell is also engaged in RNA and protein synthesis during this phase. Following the G_1 phase, the cell enters the S (synthesis) phase, in which it replicates its DNA in preparation for mitosis. Next the cell enters G_2, a second growth phase in which the replicated DNA condenses into chromosomes. The cell is then ready to begin dividing.

In M phase, the cell undergoes mitosis, during which the cell divides into two identical daughter cells, each of which receives a full complement of genetic material. Following mitosis, actively proliferating cells directly enter the G_1 phase to prepare for further replication. Non-proliferating cells enter a quiescent state referred to as G_0. Cells in phases G_1, S, G_2 or M are said to be cycling, while those in G_0 are dormant, or non-cycling. The cell cycle is tightly regulated in normal cells. Dysregulation of the cell cycle is a major factor in the development of haematological malignancy.

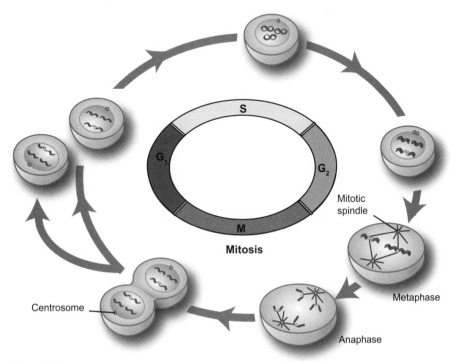

Figure 10.6
The phases of the cell cycle.

Regulation of the cell cycle

The passage of a cell through the cell cycle is regulated by cytoplasmic proteins such as:

- cyclins
  - ☐ G_1 cyclin (cyclins D1–3)
  - ☐ S-phase cyclins (cyclins E and A)
  - ☐ mitotic cyclins (cyclins B and A)
- cyclin-dependent kinases (CDKs)
  - ☐ G_1 CDK (CDK4)
  - ☐ S-phase CDK (CDK2)
  - ☐ M-phase CDK (CDK1)

The levels of the various cyclins in the cytoplasm rise and fall with the different stages of the cell cycle. In contrast, the cytoplasmic levels of the CDKs remain relatively constant. CDKs must bind to their designated cyclin to be activated. Once active, CDKs phosphorylate (add phosphate groups to) various cytoplasmic proteins that regulate cell cycle processes.

When a cell is stimulated to grow, entry into the G_1 phase of the cell cycle is accompanied by increased expression of cyclin D1, which is bound by CDK4 and CDK6. This leads to phosphorylation of the retinoblastoma protein (RB), reversing its inhibitory effect on the transcription factor E2F. Activation of E2F triggers expression of cyclin E, which binds to CDK2. This complex phosphorylates the cyclin D inhibitory protein P27^{Kip1}, tagging it for degradation. The result is that expression of cyclin A increases, allowing progression to S phase. Cyclin D1 is also involved in preparing the chromosomes for replication by modifying local chromatin structure and transcription of genes involved in cellular proliferation and differentiation. Overexpression of cyclin D1 is implicated in the development of several cancers including parathyroid adenoma, breast, prostate and colon cancers, lymphoma and melanoma. For example, the translocation t(11;14)(q13;q32) is found in about 15% of cases of myeloma and results in dysregulation of cyclin D1 expression.

During S phase, expression of cyclin A is induced and binds to CDK2. This complex, known as the S-phase promoting factor (SPF), enters the nucleus and prepares the cell for DNA duplication. As the cell passes into the G_2 phase of the cell cycle, cyclin E levels reduce and the levels of cyclins A and B begin to rise.

The level of cyclin B continues to rise until M phase, where it falls rapidly due to degradation. Cyclin B bound to CDK1 is known as mitosis promoting factor (MPF) and it triggers cellular changes that drive mitosis, including assembly of the mitotic spindle, dissolution of the nuclear envelope and chromosomal condensation. Degradation of cyclin B is regulated by a complex of several proteins known as anaphase-promoting complex (APC), which assembles in the early part of M phase, triggering destruction of the cohesins, thereby allowing separation of the duplicated chromosomes. The APC also promotes synthesis of cyclin D in preparation for entry into a new circuit of the cell cycle.

The changes in concentration of the cyclins during the cell cycle are depicted in *Figure 10.7*.

Cell cycle checkpoints

The cell has several systems for interrupting the cell cycle if something goes wrong. These are known as checkpoints and allow the cell to confirm that the course of the cycle up to that point has been conducted correctly and that no errors have been introduced. In effect, these checkpoints act as a decision point to:

- continue to the next phase of the cell cycle
- pause the cell cycle to repair or correct a problem
- abort the cell cycle and trigger apoptosis.

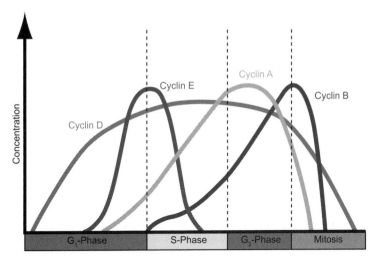

Figure 10.7
Changes in cyclin concentration during the cell cycle.

Several cell cycle checkpoints have been discovered (see *Figure 10.8*) including:

- the restriction checkpoint
- the G_2 checkpoint
- the anaphase checkpoint.

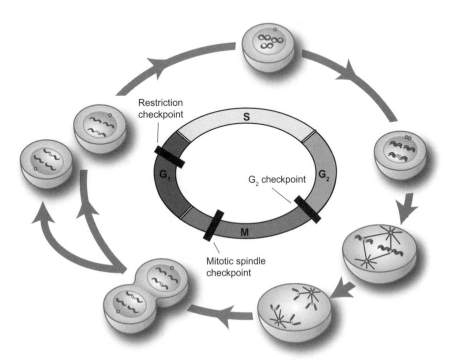

Figure 10.8
Major checkpoints of the cell cycle.

Restriction checkpoint. The restriction checkpoint is located at the end of G1 phase and functions as a decision point on whether to permit entry into S phase. This checkpoint is largely governed by the action of the cyclin-dependent kinase inhibitor protein p16^{INK4}. This protein inhibits CDK4 and CDK6, preventing binding to, and therefore activation of cyclin D. Any cell that passes into S phase must overcome the inhibitory effect of p16^{INK4}. This happens, for example, following growth factor-induced increases in cyclin D concentration.

Loss of expression of the *P15^{INK4A}* and *P16^{INK4A}* genes is very common in myeloma and has been shown to contribute to the dysregulated growth of myeloma cells. *P53* is the most commonly mutated gene in human malignancies. About 5% of newly-diagnosed MM patients carry a *P53* mutation, but the frequency increases with advancing disease. This gene normally causes cells to stop growing in the G$_1$ phase of the cell cycle or causes cell death if the DNA is damaged. Loss of *P53* function:

- can cause loss of restriction checkpoint control over cell cycle progression, resulting in cells with damaged DNA being allowed to continue growing
- is important in advanced MM and is associated with progression to an aggressive form of the disease
- is associated with poor prognosis in MM patients treated with standard dose chemotherapy.

P53 mutations are also common in other haematological malignancies such as AML. Mutation of other components of the *P53* pathway is also frequently seen. For example, mutations of the nucleophosmin (*NPM1*) gene are found in more than half of cases of AML that have a normal karyotype. Nucleophosmin is thought to play an important role in centrosome assembly, processing of pre-RNA molecules and has chaperone activity. The mutations seen in *NPM1* are diverse but all generate a nuclear export signal that relocalizes NPM1 protein to the cytoplasm, interfering with its function.

G$_2$ checkpoint. The G$_2$ checkpoint acts as the decision point at the interface between G$_2$ and M phase. The role of this checkpoint is to prevent damaged DNA from being passed on to the next generation. The major regulators of the G$_2$ checkpoint are the protein kinases Wee1 and Mt1 and the phosphatase Cdc25. These kinases maintain CDK1 in an inactive state by phosphorylation. Dephosphorylation of CDK1 by Cdc25 allows it to bind to cyclin B and to drive the cell into early M phase. However, if damaged DNA is detected at the G$_2$ checkpoint, two parallel cascades that inactivate the Cdc2–cyclin B complex are activated. The first cascade rapidly inhibits progression into mitosis by inactivating Cdc25 so that it no longer activates CDK1. The second cascade is slower and involves phosphorylation of the transcription factor and tumour suppressor p53, resulting in the CDK1–cyclin B complex being exported from the nucleus, dissociation of the CDK1–cyclin B complex within the nucleus, and inhibition of CDK1, preventing formation of the CDK1–cyclin B complex.

Mitotic spindle checkpoint. The purpose of the mitotic spindle checkpoint (also known as the anaphase checkpoint) is to ensure that, when cells divide, each daughter cell is correctly allocated one copy of each chromosome. This is extremely important because loss or gain of chromosomes generates aneuploidy, which may be lethal or may cause cancer development or progression. The spindle checkpoint acts to prevent this from happening by sensing whether the sister chromatids are correctly attached to opposite poles. Failure to achieve correct alignment triggers the release of Mad2 (this is normally bound to Mad1 in a Mad1/Mad2 complex). Mad2 binds to the anaphase-promoting complex (APC) to form an APC/Mad2 complex, thereby preventing entry into anaphase. In effect, Mad2 release acts as a 'wait signal' until all of the chromatids are properly attached to opposite spindle pole bodies. Once correct attachment is achieved, Mad2 is degraded and anaphase can proceed.

Growth factors

Intracellular cell cycle control proteins such as CDK, cyclin, and P53 are not solely responsible for regulating cell proliferation. Cells also receive extracellular signals from growth factors to divide. Growth factors are highly specific plasma proteins whose primary function is to stimulate cellular growth and proliferation. There are about 50 known growth factors. Other classes of molecules, such as steroid hormones, can also function as growth factors.

Growth factors can be divided into classes based on their specificity. Broad-specificity factors, such as platelet-derived growth factor (PDGF) and epidermal growth factor (EGF), affect many classes of cells. At the opposite extreme lie narrow-specificity factors, such as erythropoietin (EPO), which induces proliferation primarily of red blood cell precursors.

Growth factors exert their activity by interacting with specific receptor proteins expressed on the surfaces of cells. Cells only respond to growth factors for which they express the appropriate receptor protein. Although some growth factors circulate in the blood, most originate from cells in the neighbourhood of the affected cell and act as local mediators of growth.

When a growth factor binds to a receptor on the surface of a target cell, the activated receptor stimulates a series of intracellular processes that activate the genes involved in cell cycling. For example, growth factor signalling can activate the genes *FOS*, *MYC* and *JUN*, which encode transcription factors that act to increase expression of cyclins, thereby promoting progression through the cell cycle.

Programmed cell death and its regulation

In the normal course of events, cells are continually dying and being replaced. For example, following a traumatic injury such as a superficial burn, damaged cells die and are gradually replaced by new cells as the wound heals. This is an example of a type of cell death called necrosis. Sometimes, the body needs to control the timing of a cell's death; for example, during fetal development the separation of the fingers and toes is achieved by triggering the death of the cells that join them together. This is achieved by a process known as programmed cell death (PCD) or apoptosis, which can be likened to cell suicide.

Apoptosis can be triggered by many different events and circumstances, such as internal damage that cannot be repaired, viral infection, ionizing radiation, chemical toxins or by an immune response. Apoptosis functions as a protective mechanism by removing damaged cells or limiting the spread of viral infection.

Cells that undergo apoptosis experience a characteristic series of changes during their death throes:

- the cell shrinks and develops bubble-like blebs on its surface
- the nuclear chromatin begins to break down
- the mitochondria break down, with the release of cytochrome c
- the cell then breaks up into a series of fragments, each enclosed by a surface membrane
- during the breakup of the cell, a phospholipid called phosphatidylserine is exposed on the cell surface
- phagocytic cells, including macrophages and dendritic cells, recognize the phosphatidylserine and engulf the cell fragments
- an inflammatory response to the death of the cell is prevented by the secretion of the cytokines IL-10 and TGF-β by the phagocytes.

Regulation of cell survival, or cell death, is as important as regulation of cell proliferation to ensure normal tissue growth and function. In many tissues, cells are programmed to die if they do not receive specific signals for survival. The decision on whether or when a cell undergoes apoptosis depends on the balance between positive (or antiapoptotic) signals that tell the cell that it should continue to survive and negative (or proapoptotic) signals that tell it to die. Normally, for a cell to continue to survive, the strength of the positive signals should outweigh that of the negative signals. These signals are determined by the changing concentration of proapoptotic and antiapoptotic proteins within the cell. For example, the internal balance of the cell can be tipped in favour of apoptosis either by a reduction of antiapoptotic proteins, such as BCL-2 or an increase in proapoptotic proteins, such as BAD or BAX. There are three different mechanisms for apoptosis:

- the intrinsic or mitochondrial pathway of apoptosis
- the extrinsic or death receptor pathway of apoptosis
- caspase-independent apoptosis.

Mitochondrial apoptosis. Bcl-2 is an antiapoptotic protein that is normally present on the outer membranes of mitochondria. The presence of functional Bcl-2 prevents the cell from undergoing apoptosis. Damage to the cell sufficient to trigger apoptosis causes two related proapoptotic proteins, BAD and BAX, to be expressed on the mitochondrial surface. These bind to Bcl-2, blocking its protective effect. The result is that the mitochondria leak an enzyme called cytochrome c that triggers a cascade of protein activation that culminates in the death of the cell. Key components of this apoptotic cascade are a family of proteins called the caspases.

The death receptor pathway of apoptosis. Death receptors are cell surface receptor proteins that trigger apoptosis when they bind to their ligand. All of the death receptors belong to a family of proteins called the tumour necrosis factor (TNF) superfamily. The best-characterized death receptors are the Fas and TNF receptors. When Fas is bound to its ligand (FasL), an intracellular signalling cascade is triggered that results in activation of the caspase cascade, causing cell death by apoptosis. Cytotoxic T lymphocytes express FasL on their surface and kill target cells by binding to Fas on the target cell surface.

Caspase-independent apoptosis. Certain specialized cells such as neurons and retinal pigment epithelial cells show another mechanism of apoptosis that does not require caspase activation but shows all of the other hallmarks of apoptosis. This mechanism involves translocation of a mitochondrial protein called apoptosis-inducing factor (AIF) to the cell nucleus where it causes DNA fragmentation, leading to cell death.

Apoptosis and malignancy

Apoptosis plays an important role in preventing the development of malignancy. If a damaged cell is unable to undergo apoptosis, due to mutation or biochemical inhibition, it may be permitted to continue dividing and may progress to full malignancy. Malignant cells employ many different tricks to evade apoptosis.

- Human papillomavirus (HPV) infection is a known cause of cervical cancer. One of the mechanisms involved is that the virus produces a protein that inactivates P53, the protein responsible for triggering apoptosis in cells with damaged DNA.
- EBV, the cause of glandular fever, is also implicated in the development of Burkitt lymphoma and nasopharyngeal carcinoma. The virus expresses a protein that is similar to Bcl-2 and also induces the infected cell to up-regulate its own expression of Bcl-2. The result is resistance to apoptosis.
- Many B cell leukaemias and lymphomas express high levels of Bcl-2, and so block apoptotic signals.
- Lung and colon cancer cells often secrete elevated levels of a soluble 'decoy' molecule that binds to FasL, preventing it from binding Fas and so facilitating evasion of cytotoxic T lymphocyte-mediated destruction.

■   Many malignant cells express high levels of FasL, and so can kill cytotoxic T lymphocytes that try to kill them by binding to Fas on their cell surface.

Epigenetic control of gene transcription

A single human cell contains about two metres of DNA within a nucleus that is only about 5 μm in diameter. To achieve this, chromosomal DNA is highly organized and condensed, a process that has a profound impact on gene expression.

The ability to switch genes on and off either permanently or temporarily is vital to cellular and tissue growth and differentiation. For example, differentiation from precursor cells into specialized cells requires the silencing of certain genes and the regulated expression of others that confer the specialized functions of the mature cell. Once the cell line has matured, the new pattern of gene expression must be passed on to daughter cells during cellular division to preserve the specialized functions. Regulation of gene expression in this way, which does not involve any change to the DNA composition and can be passed on during cell division, is known as epigenetic control.

Within each cell, human DNA is combined with histone proteins that create a scaffolding to form chromatin. Histones carry a positive charge, which facilitates association with negatively charged DNA strands. Small spherical bodies called nucleosomes are formed, which consist of a core of histones around which are wrapped two turns of DNA.

The nucleosomes in the chromosome can be further condensed through the process of histone deacetylation, which increases the positive charge of histone proteins, creating a greater attraction between them and the negatively charged DNA wrapped around them. This causes a change in the shape of the chromatin that draws nucleosomes closer together into a compact group. The genes in this condensed chromatin (heterochromatin) are permanently silenced, and so are never expressed. Less tightly condensed chromatin, known as euchromatin, contains genes that may or may not be expressed, depending on the needs of the cell.

The expression of a gene within a segment of euchromatin requires that the segment has a more 'relaxed' structure. This is accomplished via histone acetylation, which neutralizes the positive charge and reduces histone–DNA attraction. Following transcription, deacetylation restores the compact structure. Chromatin acetylation and deacetylation are catalysed by histone acetyltransferase (HAT) and histone deacetylase (HDAC) enzymes, respectively.

An additional epigenetic control mechanism involves methylation of CpG dinucleotides. Areas of DNA where these dinucleotides are found in higher concentrations, known as 'CpG islands', are commonly found in or near the promoter regions of genes: about half of all genes have CpG islands associated with their promoters.

Methylation of CpG islands associated with gene promoters inhibits transcription and such genes are said to be 'silenced'. Gene silencing via methylation plays an important role in normal physiology, for example in altering gene expression patterns associated with cellular differentiation. The DNA methylation pattern of a cell is heritable and reversible. DNA methylation is catalysed by DNA methyltransferase enzymes.

Aberrant epigenetic changes have been shown to be involved in malignant transformation. The pattern of gene silencing by either or both methylation and histone modification is frequently altered in malignant cells. Normally, CpG islands associated with active genes are unmethylated, while scattered CpG dinucleotides are usually methylated. In some malignant cells, CpG islands associated with tumour suppressor genes are hypermethylated, resulting in aberrant gene silencing and promotion of malignant change. For example, the $P15^{INK4B}$ gene is methylated and therefore silenced in 38–50% of all patients with MDS, and in up to 83% of advanced disease. Other genes that are often methylated in MDS include the *CDH1*, *CDH13*, *CALC1*, *P73* and *RARβ* genes. *CDH1* and *CDH13* encode cadherin proteins, which promote cell adhesion, *CALC1* encodes the hormone calcitonin, which inhibits bone resorption, *P73* encodes a proapoptotic factor and inhibitor of cell proliferation, and *RARβ* is a tumour suppressor.

10.4 PRINCIPLES OF TREATMENT FOR HAEMATOLOGICAL MALIGNANCY

Theoretically ideal treatment for malignancy requires the selective and total removal or destruction of malignant cells in the absence of significant toxicity to normal cells, although this ideal is seldom attainable in practice. The widespread dissemination of malignant cells in most types of haematological malignancy, coupled with the extreme sensitivity of normal haemopoietic and other rapidly dividing tissue, make severe toxicity unavoidable. For example, a typical tumour load at diagnosis for AML is about $5 \times 10^{11} - 5 \times 10^{12}$ cells: this compares to a total normal haemopoietic stem cell load of less than 1×10^9. Any treatment that is sufficiently toxic to destroy the leukaemic cells would completely ablate the normal haemopoietic tissue with which it is associated. To overcome this problem, cytoreductive therapy needs to be 'pulsed', allowing recovery of normal tissue between treatments. Simplistically, normal tissue recovers more successfully between pulses of treatment than do malignant cells. Thus, with continued therapy, the malignant cell load progressively reduces, while normal cell counts are maintained within tolerable limits.

The most widely employed modes of treatment in haematological malignancy are cytotoxic chemotherapy, haemopoietic stem cell transplantation, (less commonly) radiotherapy and supportive care.

Cytotoxic chemotherapy

Cytotoxic chemotherapy involves the administration of highly toxic drugs in an attempt to poison the malignant cells. The main advantage of this approach over radiotherapy is that it is effective against disseminated tumours such as leukaemia. However, because the drugs are delivered via the bloodstream, poorly vascularized areas are not effectively treated. In particular, destruction of malignant cells in the cerebrospinal fluid requires additional intrathecal therapy. The main disadvantage of cytotoxic chemotherapy is that it is not selective for malignant cells: both normal and malignant cells are poisoned by cytotoxic drugs. This means that most cytotoxic agents are associated with severe side-effects that frequently limit the dose that can be used or the duration of treatment that can be tolerated. Since the rationale for cytotoxic chemotherapy is to maximize malignant cell kill, this limitation can significantly limit the effectiveness of monotherapy. As a result, it is far more common for cytotoxic drugs to be administered in repeated cycles of defined drug combinations, with the intention of inducing an additive or, ideally, a synergistic effect on the malignant cells. This approach has been shown to improve significantly the results obtained. Combinations of drugs are selected according to the following general principles:

- each drug chosen must demonstrate efficacy against the disease when used as a single agent
- drugs with different mechanisms of action should be used
- the major toxicity of each drug should differ from others in the combination
- there should be no synergistic toxicity associated with the combination
- each drug must be used as closely as possible to its optimum dose and treatment schedule, consistent with acceptable toxicity.

In practice, compromises are often required, but each combination should be as close to this ideal as possible.

The precise mode of action of many cytotoxic drugs remains obscure. Some drugs have been shown to exert particular toxic effects by *in vitro* experiments, and are classified according to this activity. It is likely, however, that their activities *in vivo* are more complex. In general, all cytotoxic drugs interfere with one or more essential cellular growth and survival processes, triggering apoptosis. Cytotoxic drugs can be classified in many different ways. In this book, they are grouped according to their mode of action or other similarities in their properties:

- alkylating agents
- antimetabolites
- epigenetic modifiers
- antineoplastic antibiotics
- plant alkaloids and terpenoids
- corticosteroids
- targeted therapies
- miscellaneous agents.

Alkylating agents

Alkylating agents are polyfunctional molecules with highly reactive alkyl groups that form crosslinks between the side chains of proteins and nucleic acids. These crosslinks interfere with the function of cellular enzymes and DNA/RNA replication, and attempts to repair the DNA damage make matters worse by inducing strand breaks and increasing the rate of mutation. Commonly prescribed alkylating agents include cyclophosphamide, ifosfamide, melphalan, chlorambucil, busulfan, procarbazine and nitrosourea.

The alkylating agents are cell cycle-nonspecific, i.e. they attack cells in any stage of the cell cycle, although some of the toxicities are more pronounced during S phase. Toxic side effects are therefore manifest most severely in rapidly dividing tissue, leading to pancytopenia, alopecia, gonadal atrophy and ulceration of mucous membranes. The alkylating agents are teratogenic and mutagenic, leading to an increased development of secondary malignancy. In addition, some toxicities are more common or more pronounced with certain alkylating agents. For example, alopecia and bladder toxicity are associated with cyclophosphamide due to hepatic microsomal enzyme metabolism to form acrolein, which is excreted via the urinary system, leading to side effects such as haemorrhagic cystitis and even bladder cancer.

Antimetabolites

Antimetabolites are analogues of compounds involved in essential biosynthetic pathways. Because of their biochemical nature, the antimetabolites act primarily on cells in S phase. For example, methotrexate is a close structural analogue of folic acid and therefore acts as a competitive inhibitor of the enzyme dihydrofolate reductase, leading to failure of thymidine and purine nucleotide synthesis. The most important toxicities of methotrexate are myelosuppression, mucositis and hepatic, pulmonary and CNS damage.

Other commonly prescribed antimetabolites include:

- cytosine arabinoside, which is an analogue of deoxycytidine formed by substitution of an arabinose moiety for deoxyribose. The antimetabolite activity of this drug is exerted in two ways:
    - via competitive inhibition of the enzyme DNA polymerase-α, which results in inhibition of DNA replication and synthesis
    - by competing with cytidine for incorporation into DNA during replication. The arabinose moiety is responsible for steric hindrance of molecular rotation within the DNA, resulting in inhibition of DNA replication.
- 6-mercaptopurine (6-MP), which is a purine (hypoxanthine) analogue and is activated within the cell by the enzyme hypoxanthine guanine phosphoribosyltransferase (HGPRT) to 6-MP ribose triphosphate. This substance is erroneously incorporated into DNA and

interferes with DNA replication. Other examples of purine analogues that act in a similar way are azathioprine and 6-thioguanine. 6-MP is generally well tolerated, but significant genetic variation in the thiopurine methyl transferase (*TPMT*) gene, which is involved in 6-MP detoxification, can result in markedly increased myelosuppression. Pre-treatment genotyping for *TPMT* may be advisable.

■   5-fluorouracil, which inhibits thymidylate synthase, preventing the methylation of deoxyuridylate to form deoxythymidylate and leading to the induction of both double-stranded and single-stranded DNA breaks.

■   6-azauridine, which is a synthetic analogue of uridine that inhibits de novo pyrimidine synthesis and so interferes with DNA and RNA synthesis and protein synthesis.

■   hydroxyurea, which inhibits the enzyme ribonucleotide reductase, leading to a reduction in deoxyribonucleotide availability; this inhibits DNA replication and repair.

Epigenetic modifiers

With the recognition that epigenetic mechanisms are commonly subverted in malignant disease, and that these changes are potentially reversible, a new class of antineoplastic agents was developed, the epigenetic modifiers. Two groups of epigenetic modifiers exist:

■   histone deacetylase inhibitors such as suberoylanilide hydroxamic acid (SAHA), which act by inhibition of the enzymes that deacetylate histones, resulting in reversal of gene silencing. SAHA has been used in the treatment of cutaneous T cell lymphoma and Sézary syndrome.

■   hypomethylating agents, such as decitabine and azacitidine, which act by inhibition of DNA methyltransferases, thereby reversing aberrant hypermethylation of CpG islands and consequent gene silencing. Decitabine and azacitidine are incorporated into DNA during replication. Their presence inhibits the action of DNA methyltransferase. Azacitidine is also incorporated into RNA during gene transcription. Both agents are used to treat MDS.

Although HDAC inhibitors and hypomethylating agents are thought to act primarily by reversal of aberrant epigenetic mechanisms, it is very likely that they have multiple, as yet uncharacterized effects *in vivo*.

Antineoplastic antibiotics

The most widely used antineoplastic antibiotics are anthracyclines, which include doxorubicin, daunorubicin, epirubicin and idarubicin. All of these agents act by inserting themselves between DNA base pairs, a process known as intercalation. In this position, they inhibit topoisomerase II, preventing religation of double-stranded DNA breaks and promoting apoptosis. There is also some evidence that anthracyclines inflict cellular damage by the generation of toxic oxygen radicals and other poorly characterized mechanisms.

Important side-effects of anthracycline therapy include cardiotoxicity, myelosuppression, mucositis and severe tissue necrosis following accidental extravasation. Dose-limiting cardiotoxicity prompted the development of liposomal forms of doxorubixcin.

Plant alkaloids and terpenoids

There are three major groups of plant alkaloid antineoplastic agents, the vinca alkaloids, the podophyllotoxins and the taxanes.

The vinca alkaloids are all derived from the Madagascan periwinkle and include vincristine, vinblastine, vinorelbine and vindesine. These agents are widely used in the treatment of haematological malignancies, including ALL, NHL and myeloma. They act by binding to tubulin and inhibiting its assembly into microtubules, thereby impairing formation of the mitotic spindle and leading to arrest of mitosis during metaphase. Side effects of vincristine therapy include neurotoxicity, alopecia and severe tissue necrosis following accidental extravasation.

The podophyllotoxins are derived from the American mayapple. The most common members of this group are etoposide and teniposide. Both of these agents act by inhibiting topoisomerase II. Side effects of etoposide therapy include vomiting, alopecia, peripheral neuropathy and myelosuppression.

The taxanes, including paclitaxel and docetaxel, are derivatives of the Pacific yew tree. They act by binding to and stabilizing GDP-bound tubulin, thereby leading to enhanced microtubule assembly and stabilization and mitotic arrest. The taxanes and vinca alkaloids are sometimes both grouped as mitotic spindle poisons, although their sites of tubulin binding and mechanism of action are different.

Corticosteroids

Prednisone and dexamethasone are widely used in the treatment of lymphoid malignancies, including ALL, myeloma and NHL. They induce apoptosis in lymphoid cells by binding to membrane glucocorticoid receptors. An important feature of the corticosteroids is their relative tolerability and lack of myelosuppressive activity. Side effects of glucocorticosteroid therapy include water and salt retention, hypokalaemia, osteoporosis, muscle wasting and neutrophilia.

Targeted therapies

The 'holy grail' of antineoplastic therapy has long been the so-called 'magic bullet' – the drug that specifically attacks malignant cells while leaving surrounding normal cells unscathed and the patient free of toxic side effects. Unfortunately, such a perfect antineoplastic agent does not exist now, and nor is it likely to in the future. However, there has been significant progress in this direction, with the development of drugs that preferentially target malignant cells. The two major classes of targeted chemotherapy widely used in haematological malignancy are:

- monoclonal antibodies
- signal transduction inhibitors.

The rationale for the use of monoclonal antibodies in haematological malignancy is that they can be used to specifically target malignant cells by binding to surface membrane proteins and either deliver some toxic insult or trigger apoptosis. The most successful such agent is rituximab, which is a chimeric mouse–human monoclonal antibody directed against the B cell antigen CD20. The precise mechanism of action of rituximab remains unclear, but it has been shown to bind to both malignant and normal B cells and to induce antibody-dependent cell-mediated cytotoxicity (ADCC) by natural killer cells, T cells, and macrophages, complement-mediated cytolysis and apoptosis due to CD20 crosslinking. Rituximab is widely used in the treatment of B cell NHL and CLL.

There are two clinically available anti-CD20 monoclonal antibodies that are conjugated with radioactive isotopes, allowing the targeted delivery of toxic radiation to B cells, ^{90}Y-Ibritumomab Tiuxetan and ^{131}I-Tositumomab.

Signal transduction inhibitors are designed to interfere with intracellular signalling pathways that are constitutively active in malignant cells and are involved in driving the malignant processes. The prototypical member of this group is the BCR–ABL inhibitor imatinib mesylate. This agent has transformed the treatment of CML and changed it from a near-universally fatal condition into one that can be effectively managed or cured in the majority of cases. Imatinib acts by binding to the ATP-binding site of the BCR–ABL fusion oncoprotein and inhibiting its tyrosine kinase activity. This effectively 'switches off' an important feature of the leukaemic process and induces disease responses in the great majority of cases of CML. Two second-generation BCR–ABL inhibitors (dasatinib and nilotinib) have been developed that can be used when imatinib resistance develops.

Several other tyrosine kinase inhibitors are available clinically that target other constitutively activated signal transduction molecules, including sunitinib, sorafenib and erlotinib, which target multiple pathways including platelet-derived growth factor receptor (PDGFR), epidermal growth factor receptor (EGFR), vascular endothelial growth factor receptor (VEGFR) and the stem cell factor receptor (KIT).

Miscellaneous agents

Immunomodulating agents. The immunomodulating drugs (IMiDs) include thalidomide and its derivatives, lenalidomide and pomalidomide.

Thalidomide was synthesized in 1953 and was initially marketed as an anti-convulsant for epilepsy treatment. Clinical experience subsequently suggested that it would be effective as a sedative or sleep aid and, in 1957, thalidomide was marketed for morning sickness and nausea in pregnancy. The drug went into general use the following year, and was widely prescribed in Europe, Australia, Asia, Africa and the Americas.

The earliest suspicions that thalidomide might cause fetal malformation were reported almost simultaneously by Hamburg paediatrician Dr Widukind Lenz and by the Australian gynaecologist Dr William McBride. The first 'thalidomide baby' was born in December 1956, and was followed by thousands of others in more than 46 countries.

Fetal malformations occurred early in pregnancy (28–42 days post-conception) and were thought to be due to inhibition of normal blood vessel formation. Malformations observed included deafness, blindness, cleft palate, malformed internal organs and phocomelia (a congenital defect in which the hands and feet are attached to abbreviated arms and legs). Thalidomide was withdrawn in 1961.

Since then, thalidomide has been used cautiously in the treatment of a range of conditions, but its teratogenic properties have limited its widespread use. More recently, thalidomide has been shown to be a highly effective agent in the treatment of MM, both alone and in combination with other agents and for front-line as well as relapsed/refractory disease.

The most significant problem associated with the use of thalidomide in MM is the adverse event profile of the drug, including somnolence, constipation, depression, thrombosis and peripheral neuropathy. Additionally, because of the teratogenicity of thalidomide, its clinical use is only permitted when coupled with a rigorous safety programme designed to minimize the risk of fetal exposure. Because of these shortcomings a rational investigation and development programme was launched to try to design analogues of thalidomide that retained its efficacy profile but reduced the toxicity of the drug. The initial focus of this effort was to produce molecules with enhanced inhibition of the cytokine tumour necrosis factor alpha (TNF-α), but with reduced side effects. Two distinct classes of thalidomide analogues were developed; the SelCIDs® (selective cytokine inhibitory drugs) and the second generation IMiDs.

The second generation IMiDs were developed by altering the structure of thalidomide. One type of alteration, the addition of an amino group to the fourth carbon of the phthaloyl ring of thalidomide, produced molecules with up to 50 000 times greater potency in inhibiting TNF-α than thalidomide *in vitro* and resulted in the derivative lenalidomide, which is also an effective treatment for MM, but with significantly reduced neurotoxicity.

The mechanism of action of the IMiDs is not fully characterized, but they are known to inhibit vascular endothelial growth factor (VEGF) and basic fibroblast growth factor (bFGF), thereby interfering with neoangiogenesis, to inhibit TNF-α and IL-6 synthesis, to stimulate IL-2 and IFN-α synthesis, and to modulate T cell function.

Proteasome inhibitors. Bortezomib is a modified dipeptidyl boronic acid that reversibly inhibits the chymotrypsin-like activity of the 26S proteasome, preventing the degradation of ubiquitinated proteins. The 26S proteasome is a large protein complex made up of over 30 protein subunits that plays an essential role in orchestrating the turnover of specific intracellular proteins, thereby maintaining cellular protein homeostasis. Many of the proteins regulated by proteasome degradation are critical for the control of cellular processes, including the orderly progression of the cell cycle, cell division, and cell survival. Inhibition of the 26S proteasome prevents targeted proteolysis and thereby affects multiple signalling cascades within the cell. Bortezomib inhibits 26S proteasome function by binding tightly and reversibly to a threonine residue in the chymotrypsin-like active site of the proteasome enzyme complex. This activity is sufficient to block all other proteasome catalytic activities.

In particular, bortezomib down-regulates NFκB. This transcription factor is involved in the activation of transcription of many genes that inhibit apoptosis and promote proliferation. Because malignant cells depend upon proteins regulated by the proteasome for proliferation, metastasis and survival, inhibiting protein degradation via proteasome inhibition can lead to cell death and inhibit growth.

Bortezomib is widely used in the treatment of MM and NHL and is particularly important for the treatment of patients with renal impairment and certain high-risk cytogenetic abnormalities.

Differentiating agents. As discussed previously in this chapter, in acute promyelocytic leukaemia, the specific translocation t(15;17)(q22;q21) creates a PML–RARα fusion protein, resulting in a promyelocytic differentiation block. ATRA acts as a differentiating agent in this condition and is capable of inducing remissions in the majority of cases when administered as monotherapy. Most of these remissions are temporary without the addition of conventional chemotherapy. This combination of treatment approaches has helped to transform APL from a near-universally fatal disease to an eminently curable one.

Arsenic trioxide is another effective agent in acute promyelocytic leukaemia that functions, at least partly, as a differentiating agent by degrading the PML–RARα fusion protein.

Enzymes. Normal blood cells meet their requirement for the amino acid asparagine by endogenous synthesis. In contrast to normal lymphoid tissue, however, the leukaemic blast cells in ALL have a relative deficiency of the enzyme L-asparagine synthetase, and so have a requirement for the uptake of asparagine from the extracellular fluid. Intravenous infusion of the bacterial enzyme L-asparaginase rapidly destroys the extracellular pool of asparagine, thereby selectively depriving the tumour cells and destroying their capacity to synthesize proteins that incorporate this amino acid.

Side effects of L-asparaginase therapy include sensitization to a bacterial product, disturbances of pancreatic and hepatic function and inhibition of protein synthesis leading to a deficiency of albumin, fibrinogen, antithrombin III, insulin and lipoproteins. In some cases, antithrombin III deficiency has been associated with thrombosis.

Haemopoietic stem cell transplantation

Haemopoietic stem cell transplantation (HSCT) is intended as a manoeuvre to allow intensification of cytotoxic chemotherapy and radiotherapy, without regard to collateral toxicity on normal haemopoietic tissue, with 'rescue' by infusion of normal haemopoietic stem cells to induce recovery. There are several forms of HSCT, and each has its own advantages and disadvantages that make it best suited for particular disease settings.

Autologous transplantation

Autologous transplantation is widely used in the treatment of MM, but is only available for patients under the age of 68–70 years. In this form of HSCT, the transplanted stem cells are derived from the patient after induction chemotherapy. Following collection of stem cells, high-dose chemotherapy is given to maximize the malignant cell kill. This also damages normal haemopoietic tissue and could prove lethal without the reinfusion of the stored stem cells. The advantages of this approach are that, because the transplanted material is of host origin, there is no need for TBI (total body irradiation), i.e. the conditioning regimen is less intense. This allows autologous HSCT to be offered to older patients. However, there are two major disadvantages of this approach:

■ there is a high probability that the transplanted material is contaminated with malignant cells, which may promote disease relapse
■ because the transplanted cells are of host origin, they do not mount a 'graft versus tumour' immune response. This has been shown to be an important determinant of the improved results seen with autologous transplantation.

Modern approaches attempt to mitigate the disadvantages of autologous HSCT by offering further treatment immediately after post-transplant recovery, either as consolidation/maintenance chemotherapy or as a second 'tandem' transplant. Despite this, few autologous HSCT patients are cured by this or subsequent treatment.

Allogeneic transplantation

Allogeneic HSCT is a significantly more rigorous procedure, and is seldom offered to patients older than 50–55 years. In this form of HSCT, the transplanted materials are obtained from an HLA-matched donor. In the case of the donated material being from an identical twin, the procedure is known as a syngeneic HSCT. Because the transplanted material is immunocompetent, allogeneic HSCT requires the complete ablation of the haemopoietic and immune system of the recipient and therefore requires very large doses of chemotherapy and radiotherapy as part of the conditioning regimen, which carry significant toxicity. Despite recent advances in supportive care, allogeneic HSCT carries a significant transplant-related morbidity and mortality that limit its use.

The major advantages of allogeneic HSCT are that there is no possibility of graft contamination with malignant cells, so there is a lower risk of relapse and also that the graft can mount an immune response against any residual malignant cells, which helps to eradicate them. There are, however, disadvantages:

■ the rigorous conditioning required induces prolonged and profound haemopoietic aplasia, with a marked infection and bleeding risk; this also limits availability to younger, fitter patients.
■ graft versus host disease (GvHD), in which the transplanted immune cells mount an immune response against recipient tissues, is common and can be difficult to control.
■ the need for a matched donor can be problematic. In the small minority of cases with an identical twin, the availability is limited only by willingness to donate. The next most likely source of a match is among siblings, but even here, the likelihood of a match is only about 25%. For the majority of patients, who have no suitable sibling match, an unrelated matched donor must be found and the search often proves fruitless.
■ the need for medium- to long-term immunosuppression post-transplant increases the risk of infection and secondary malignancy.

Allogeneic transplantation can effect a cure of the underlying malignancy in some cases. There has been substantial interest in developing a form of HSCT that takes the best features of autologous and allogeneic transplants, while reducing the risks of each. The so-called reduced intensity conditioning allogeneic HSCT (sometimes called a 'mini-allo' HSCT) employs a less rigorous conditioning regimen prior to allogeneic HSCT. The aim here is to establish a chimeric haemopoietic system that contains both donor and host cells. This maximizes the benefits of the graft versus tumour effect, while limiting the toxicity of the procedure. The inevitable GvHD is a disadvantage of this technique but treatments for this are improving. Reduced intensity conditioning allogeneic HSCT remains an experimental procedure but has shown promise, particularly when used in tandem transplant manoeuvres.

Radiotherapy

Ionizing radiation is a common component of treatment for many types of solid malignancy (radiotherapy), but its use in haematological malignancy is more restricted. It acts by inducing direct and indirect damage to the DNA of cells exposed to a concentrated source of radiation. Direct effects involve disruption of chemical bonds in DNA and cellular proteins, while indirect damage is caused by the free radicals generated by the ionization of water and dissolved oxygen. Direct radiation damage is greatest where heavy particles such as protons, neutrons or alpha particles are used. In some cases, the radiation-induced damage is sufficient to kill the malignant cells, but sub-lethal damage is passed on to daughter cells, increasing their susceptibility to subsequent therapies. In much the same way as cytotoxic chemotherapy is delivered in cycles, the antineoplastic effect of radiotherapy can be maximized relative to its toxic effects by fractionation of the total dose into several smaller doses with time for recovery of normal tissue between cycles.

In haematological malignancy, there are three main settings where radiotherapy may be useful:

- for localized tumours such as stage I HD or localized NHL, radiotherapy can be accurately targeted at the tumour and may be curative.
- although many haematological malignancies are highly radiosensitive, the disseminated nature of the disease limits the usefulness of radiotherapy, except in specialized circumstances such as eradication of disease from the CNS or for relief of localized symptoms, i.e. palliation.
- as part of the preparation for allogeneic haemopoietic stem cell transplantation, total body irradiation (TBI) can be used to destroy haemopoietic tissue. TBI is administered following induction chemotherapy and aims to completely ablate the haemopoietic tissue of the recipient to improve the chances of a successful graft, while minimizing the chances of GvHD.

Supportive care

Cytopenias

Although there have been major advances in the treatment of haematological malignancies over the past two decades, much of the credit for the improved progression-free and overall survival is attributable to improved supportive care. Both the diseases themselves as well as some of the treatments are associated with significant morbidity and mortality. Particularly common problems include cytopenias, recurrent or severe infection, pain, nausea and emesis and haemorrhage.

Cytopenias secondary to myelosuppression (anaemia, neutropenia and thrombocytopenia) can be treated by repeated transfusion of packed red cells for anaemia, platelet concentrates for thrombocytopenia or, less commonly, granulocyte concentrates for neutropenia associated with severe infection. Myelosuppression has been a major dose-limiting toxicity until recently, because of the risk of fatal infection or haemorrhage. The advent of recombinant growth factors has changed this picture dramatically.

Recombinant erythropoietin is an effective and established treatment for chemotherapy-induced anaemia. There has been some controversy recently about the possibility that erythropoietin therapy may be associated with encouragement of disease progression or reduced survival due to increased thrombotic risk. Current guidance continues to recommend recombinant erythropoietin for chronic, symptomatic anaemia secondary to chemotherapy for patients with moderate to severe anaemia (Hb < 10 g/dl). There is clear evidence of the superiority of this treatment over transfusion in this patient group. The evidence is much less clear for patients with mild anaemia. Most authorities warn against attempting to restore the haemoglobin concentration above 12 g/dl with erythropoietin because of the increased risk of thrombosis. In patients with MDS, responses to erythropoietin are improved by the concomitant administration of recombinant granulocyte colony-stimulating factor (G–CSF).

The mainstay of treatment for severe thrombocytopenia remains platelet transfusion, despite the associated risk of infection and sensitization. The transfusion of platelets may delay the onset of thrombocytopenia and prevent or reduce the severity of bleeding. Platelet support to prevent or combat haemorrhage during treatment and recovery may be required. Prophylactic platelet transfusions may be given in the absence of a bleeding episode if the platelet count falls below 10×10^9/l. Transfusion at higher levels may be necessary in patients with signs of haemorrhage, high fever, hyperleucocytosis, rapid fall of platelet count or coagulation abnormalities. Early recombinant thrombopoietic growth factors proved to be unsuitable for clinical use, and this set back the development of newer agents. Currently, the only clinically available recombinant growth factor suitable for the treatment and prevention of thrombocytopenia is interleukin-11 (IL-11), although several others are in development.

Neutropenia secondary to myelosuppression with associated infectious mortality is another major dose-limiting toxicity for chemotherapy. The development of recombinant G–CSF and granulocyte–macrophage colony-stimulating factor (GM–CSF) has made possible significant intensification of chemoradiotherapy regimens because of their ability to limit or to shorten the duration of neutropenia. Randomized clinical trials have shown a significant reduction in the duration of neutropenia, duration of antibiotic use and incidence of febrile neutropenia but no reduction in induction-related deaths or infection-related deaths associated with the use of these growth factors.

Granulocyte transfusion therapy can be used for patients with severe neutropenia with a bacterial or fungal infection that is unresponsive to treatment. This approach is used less frequently than platelet or red cell transfusion because of limited supply and safety issues associated with granulocyte transfusion.

Infectious complications

Patients with haematological malignancy are often highly susceptible to infection. The effects of chemotherapy, including myelosuppression and mucosal damage, may make patients even more vulnerable to serious infections. The prompt and effective treatment of established infection and attempts to prevent infection are vitally important components of treatment. The infections are usually bacterial but viral, fungal and protozoal infections also occur with increased frequency. Measures taken to reduce the risk of infection include nursing in isolation facilities, antibiotic therapy to reduce gut and other commensal flora, and vigorous microbiological surveillance.

The risk of infection is related to both the severity and the duration of the neutropenia. Careful instruction in personal hygiene, dental care and recognition of early signs of infection are required in all patients with neutropenia and if the neutrophil count falls below 0.1×10^9/l, prophylactic oral antibiotics and protective isolation may be required. Empiric broad-spectrum antimicrobial therapy is recommended for AML patients with a fever over 38°C (100.4°F). Central and peripheral blood cultures should be taken, as should urine and stool microbiological cultures.

In the last decade, there has been a shift in the organisms responsible for sepsis in neutropenic patients, with Gram-positive organisms, such as *Streptococcus viridans* and *Staphylococcus* species becoming more common causes of sepsis, replacing the Gram-negative organisms, such as *Klebsiella*, *Pseudomonas* and *Escherichia coli*, that were previously implicated. Although antibiotic prophylaxis has not been shown to have an effect on overall mortality, it has been reported to reduce both the incidence and the morbidity of Gram-negative infections. The choice of therapy should be guided by local microbiological advice on the most prevalent local bacterial strains.

Antifungal drugs can also be given empirically if antibacterial therapy is not effective within 48–72 hours of their initiation. It is standard practice to start antifungal agents after 4–7 days of fever in patients with severe neutropenia and inconclusive blood culture results.

Other supportive care needs

During treatment, nausea and vomiting are common so anti-emetic therapy is commonly used.

Acute tumour lysis syndrome (ATLS) is a specific condition caused by the rapid breakdown of malignant cells, resulting in electrolyte disturbances and acute renal failure, and is characterized by hyperuricaemia, hyperphosphataemia, hyperkalaemia, hypocalcaemia *and* oliguria. Physicians should monitor patients for this syndrome and may prescribe fluids, sodium bicarbonate and allopurinol (a drug used to reduce uric acid in the blood) to rid the body of unwanted chemicals and cell remains. Allopurinol may be used prophylactically during induction chemotherapy to avoid hyperuricaemia. Patients considered at higher risk of ATLS include those with elevated presentation and pre-chemotherapy white cell counts, elevated serum creatinine and raised uric acid levels at presentation, as well as those with the cytogenetic abnormality inv(16).

Extremely high leukaemic cell counts (hyperleucocytosis) can lead to circulatory problems such as leucostasis (blockage of blood flow) due to sludging in the microcirculation and raised blood viscosity leading to haemorrhage in the lungs and brain due to cell rigidity and stickiness. Hyperleucocytosis is primarily treated with chemotherapy, although leucopheresis may be required.

SUGGESTED FURTHER READING

Knowles, M. & Selby, P. (eds) (2005) *Introduction to the Cellular and Molecular Biology of Cancer.* Oxford University Press.

Pardee, A.B. & Stein, G.S. (eds) (2009) *The Biology and Treatment of Cancer: Understanding Cancer.* Wiley–Blackwell.

Pecorino, L. (2008) *Molecular Biology of Cancer: Mechanisms, Targets, and Therapeutics.* Oxford University Press.

Swerdlow, S.H., Campo, E., Harris, N.L., *et al.* (eds) (2008) *WHO Classification of Tumours of Haematopoietic and Lymphoid Tissues, Volume 2.* WHO Press.

SELF-ASSESSMENT QUESTIONS

1. Which of the following classes of cytotoxic drugs are strongly implicated in the development of secondary malignancy?
    a.   antimetabolites
    b.   alkylating agents
    c.   topoisomerase inhibitors
    d.   proteasome inhibitors
2. What virus is associated with Burkitt lymphoma?
3. Which two genes are involved in the specific translocation t(15;17)(q22;q21) identified in most cases of APL?

4. Which of the following genes function as proto-oncogenes and which as tumour suppressor genes?
   a. *RB*
   b. *P53*
   c. *ABL*
   d. *RAS*
   e. *VHL*

5. Name each of the cell cycle checkpoints being described:
   a. *This checkpoint functions as a decision point on whether to permit entry into S phase.*
   b. *The role of this checkpoint is to prevent damaged DNA from being passed on to the next generation.*
   c. *The purpose of this checkpoint (also known as the anaphase checkpoint) is to ensure that, when cells divide, each daughter cell is correctly allocated one copy of each chromosome.*

6. Name the family of antineoplastic drugs to which the following agents belong:
   a. cyclophosphamide
   b. decitabine
   c. melphalan
   d. 5-fluorouracil
   e. bortezomib
   f. cytosine arabinoside
   g. thalidomide

Acute leukaemias

Learning objectives
After studying this chapter you should confidently be able to:

■ Describe in detail the FAB and WHO classification systems for the acute leukaemias
Classification is critically important for the acute leukaemias because it helps to determine treatment and prognosis. The systems for classification are evolving. The current 'gold standard' system is the WHO system, which takes account of recent developments in immunophenotyping, cytogenetics and molecular diagnostics to identify clinically distinct subtypes.

■ Review the pathophysiology of the acute leukaemias
Despite the variety of acute leukaemias, most symptoms are traceable to infiltration of blood, bone marrow and other tissues by leukaemic cells with consequent bone marrow and organ failure and metabolic disturbances.

■ Review the cytogenetic and molecular basis of the acute leukaemias
Increasing knowledge of non-random cytogenetic abnormalities and the genes affected has begun to permit greater insight into the molecular and cellular processes that help to drive leukaemic transformation and progression. Several specific examples are discussed.

■ Identify characteristic features of the different forms of acute leukaemia
Some of the subtypes of acute leukaemia have specific clinical or laboratory characteristics that set them apart. For example, acute promyelocytic leukaemia is unique in that it can be successfully treated using all-trans-retinoic acid, a vitamin A derivative. Several other examples are discussed.

■ Outline the approaches to treatment of the acute leukaemias
The treatment of acute leukaemia is highly systematized, with specific phases of treatment that are near-universally observed. Improvements in treatment outcomes have resulted from an intensive programme of international clinical trials. A large proportion of patients with acute leukaemia are treated as part of this ongoing trial effort.

The acute leukaemias are a heterogeneous group of malignant disorders that are characterized by the uncontrolled clonal proliferation and accumulation of poorly differentiated blast cells in the bone marrow and other body tissues (see *Box 11.1* and *Box 11.2*). The acute leukaemias can be broadly divided into acute myeloid leukaemia (AML) and acute lymphoblastic leukaemia (ALL). Each of these can be further subdivided as described in this chapter.

11.1 CLASSIFICATION OF THE ACUTE LEUKAEMIAS

History of acute leukaemia classification

The classification of acute leukaemia was a fairly uncertain and subjective process until 1976, when the FAB classification was agreed upon by an expert group of haematologists from France,

Box 11.1 Rudolf Virchow (1821–1902)

The name leukaemia was coined by Virchow in 1847. He described the disease some two years earlier, the year before he lost his first university appointment in Berlin, apparently a victim of his 'uncompromisingly radical political attitudes'! His seminal observation was made at the autopsy table when he noted massive splenomegaly and a peculiar appearance of the blood in a recently deceased patient. The normal ratio of pigmented (red) cells and colourless (white) cells seemed to be reversed in the blood of the deceased. He described this condition as '*weisses Blut*', which translates as 'white blood' in English or 'leukaemia' in Greek.

Box 11.2 John Bennett (1812–1875)

It is generally believed that John Bennett in Edinburgh discovered leukaemia simultaneously with Virchow. Bennett was described as 'a man of brilliance but short temper, certain of his own virtues, pugnacious, and unable to suffer fools'! Bennett also made his original observation at the autopsy table in a patient with a very similar case history. Bennett felt the blood had pus in it because microscopic examination revealed the presence of a huge number of cells usually associated with the presence of pus. He described the condition as 'pyaemia'. A major disagreement between Virchow and Bennett was conducted in the journals for several years. During the decades that followed Virchow, now reinstated to his position but still maintaining his enlightened social and political views, made some seminal observations about leukaemia. These were all made without the ability to stain and count blood cells and it is remarkable how close his guesses were to the truth as it is known today.

the USA and Britain. This system represented an attempt to improve the reproducibility and comparability of the classification process by defining a fairly objective set of criteria for the classification of the acute leukaemias. As shown in *Table 11.1*, the FAB group recommended that the acute lymphoblastic leukaemias should be coded into three variants, which are designated L1–L3 according to the predominant morphology of the leukaemic lymphoblasts, and that the acute myeloid leukaemias should similarly be coded into eight subtypes, which are designated M0–M7. The classification was made only after the examination of both peripheral blood and bone marrow films, including the performance of a 500 cell differential count.

In cases of doubt, a number of different cytochemical stains could be used to supplement morphological examination, as shown in *Table 11.2*.

The FAB system was used worldwide, and is still used by many haematologists to describe the morphology of acute leukaemia (see *Box 11.3*). However, the system did not correlate well

Box 11.3 Progress in diagnostics

The study of haematological morphology parallels developments in microscopy and chemistry. The simple microscope of van Leeuwenhoek (c. 1700) revealed the red blood cells, whereas the colourless white blood cells were not reliably identified until about 1830 by Addison and Gulliver. The major breakthrough occurred with the work of Paul Ehrlich (1854–1915), who is regarded as one of the founding fathers of cytochemistry. It was his interest and enthusiasm, including the testing of thousands of new stains, which led to the reliable identification of the subtypes of white blood cells. The early stains developed detected lipids and carbohydrates and assessed the acidic or basic nature of the cell. Enzyme detection did not really progress until the 1940s with the development of the azo dyes, which can be used to detect intracellular enzymes such as esterases, phosphatases and dehydrogenases. By the mid-1970s cytochemistry was the best diagnostic tool available for acute leukaemia. The next advance came with the use of monoclonal antibodies and immunocytochemistry, which resulted in improvements in diagnosis, and reclassification of some types of leukaemia.

Table 11.1 Summary of the FAB classification scheme for the acute leukaemias

Acute lymphoblastic leukaemia		
Designation	Alternative	Bone marrow appearances
L1		Homogeneous population of small lymphoblasts with scanty cytoplasm and scanty nucleoli. Nucleus occasionally cleft
L2		Heterogeneous population of large lymphoblasts with moderately abundant cytoplasm and one or more nucleoli. Nucleus commonly indented or cleft
L3	Burkitt's type	Homogeneous population of large lymphoblasts with prominent nucleoli and deeply basophilic, vacuolated cytoplasm
Acute myeloid leukaemia		
M0		Identified by ultrastructural myeloperoxidase activity
M1	AML without maturation	Monomorphic with one or more distinct nucleoli, occasional Auer rod and at least 3% myeloperoxidase positivity
M2	AML with maturation	50% or more myeloblasts and promyelocytes with single Auer rods common. Dysplastic myeloid differentiation may also be present
M3	Acute promyelocytic leukaemia (APL)	Dominant cell type is promyelocyte with heavy azurophilic granulation. Bundles of Auer rods confirm diagnosis. Microgranular variant exists (M3v)
M4	Acute myelomonocytic leukaemia (AMMoL)	As M2 but > 20% promonocytes and monocytes
M5	Acute monoblastic leukaemia (AMoL)	> 80% monoblasts is poorly differentiated (M5a). > 80% monoblasts, promonocytes and monocytes is well differentiated
M6	Acute erythroleukaemia (AEL)	> 50% bizarre, dysplastic nucleated red cells with multinucleate forms and cytoplasmic bridging. Myeloblasts usually > 30%
M7	Acute megakaryoblastic leukaemia (AMegL)	Fibrosis, heterogeneous blast population with cytoplasmic blebs. Platelet peroxidase positive

with clinical outcome and, as knowledge of the pathogenesis of acute leukaemia grew, it became obvious that a new system was required that would take account of these developments.

The WHO classification of acute leukaemia

The FAB system is based purely on the appearance of the leukaemic cells; it takes no account of cytogenetic or other laboratory or clinical findings. The WHO classification system represents an attempt to improve upon and replace the FAB system and takes account of recent developments in clinical and laboratory knowledge of the acute leukaemias. The WHO classification system for acute leukaemias is summarized in *Tables 11.3–11.5*.

The WHO system categorizes cases of AML into clinical and biological groups as follows:

- **AML with recurrent genetic abnormalities**, which includes AML with the well-defined cytogenetic abnormalities t(8;21)(q22;q22); (*AML1/ETO*), inv(16)(p13q22) or t(16;16)

Table 11.2 The substances stained by, and applications of basic cytochemical stains

Method	Substances stained	Main uses
Sudan black	Neutral fats, phospholipids & lipoproteins	Identification of granulocyte precursors, including Auer rods
Peroxidase	Myeloperoxidase	Identification of neutrophil and eosinophil precursors, including Auer rods
Periodic acid Schiff (PAS)	Glycogen	Fine block positive in M6 erythroblasts; coarse block positive in ALL
Chloroacetate esterase	Esterase isoenzymes 1, 2, 7 & 8	Differentiation of granulocytic and monocytic maturation (M4 & M5)
Non-specific esterase	Esterase isoenzymes 3, 4, 5 & 6	
Acid phosphatase	Acid phosphatase	Useful in T ALL & HCL
TdT	Terminal deoxynucleotidyl transferase (TdT)	Differentiation of ALL and AML*

*rarely positive in AML

Table 11.3 WHO classification of myeloid neoplasms and acute myeloid leukaemias

AML with recurrent cytogenetic abnormalities
With t(8;21)(q22;q22), *(AML 1/ETO)*
With inv(16)(p13q22) or t(16;16)(p13;q22), *(CBFβ/MYH 11)*
Acute promyelocytic leukaemia t(15;17)(q22;q12), *PML-RARα*
With t(9;11)(p22;q23); *MLLT3-MLL*
With t(6;9)(p23;q34); *DEK-NUP214*
With inv(3)(q21q26.2) or t(3;3)(q21;q26.2); *RPN1-EVI1*
(Megakaryoblastic) with t(1;22)(p13;q13); *RBM15-MKL1*
Provisional entity: AML with mutated *NPM1*
Provisional entity: AML with mutated *CEBPA*
AML with myelodysplasia-related changes
Therapy-related myeloid neoplasms
AML not otherwise specified
AML, minimally differentiated
AML without maturation
AML with maturation
Acute myelomonocytic leukaemia
Acute monoblastic / monocytic leukaemia
Acute erythroid leukaemia
pure erythroid leukaemia
erythroleukaemia, erythroid / myeloid
Acute megakaryoblastic leukaemia
Acute basophilic leukaemia
Acute panmyelosis with myelofibrosis
Myeloid sarcoma
Myeloid proliferations related to Down syndrome
Transient abnormal myelopoiesis
Myeloid leukaemia associated with Down syndrome
Blastic plasmacytoid dendritic cell neoplasm

Table 11.4 WHO classification of acute leukaemias of ambiguous lineage. (NOS, not otherwise specified)

Acute leukaemias of ambiguous lineage
Acute undifferentiated leukaemia
Mixed phenotype acute leukaemia
with t(9;22)(q34;q11.2); (*BCR-ABL1*)
with t(v;11q23); MLL rearranged
Mixed phenotype acute leukaemia, B-myeloid, NOS
Mixed phenotype acute leukaemia, T-myeloid, NOS
Provisional entity: natural killer (NK) cell lymphoblastic leukaemia/lymphoma

Table 11.5 WHO classification of lymphoblastic leukaemia/lymphoma

B lymphoblastic leukaemia/lymphoma
B lymphoblastic leukaemia/lymphoma, NOS
B lymphoblastic leukaemia/lymphoma with recurrent genetic abnormalities
with t(9;22)(q34;q11.2); (*BCR-ABL1*)
with t(v;11q23); (*MLL* rearranged)
with t(12;21)(p13;q22); (*TEL-AML1*)
with hyperdiploidy
with hypodiploidy
with t(5;14)(q31;q32); (*IL3-IGH*)
with t(1;19)(q23;p13.3); (*TCF3-PBX1*)
T lymphoblastic leukaemia/lymphoma

(p13;q22); (*CBFB/MYH11*), t(15;17)(q22;q12); (PML/*RARα*). These all qualify for a diagnosis of AML regardless of bone marrow or circulating blast count. AML with t(9;11) (p22;q23); (*MLLT3-MLL*) also falls into this category, but a marrow or peripheral blood blast count of at least 20% is required for diagnosis. Newly-defined AML entities counted in this group include AML with t(6;9)(p23;q34); (*DEK-NUP214*), AML with inv(3) (q21q26.2) or t(3;3)(q21;q26.2); (*RPN1-EVI1*); and AML (megakaryoblastic) with t(1;22) (p13;q13); (*RBM15-MKL1*).

- **AML with myelodysplasia-related changes**, which incorporates cases of AML with a history of MDS or MDS/MPN that have evolved to AML (see *Chapter 14*), cases with an MDS-related cytogenetic abnormality (see *Chapter 13*), or that show ≥ 50% dysplastic cells involving two or more myeloid lineages.
- **Therapy-related myeloid neoplasms**, which usually have a history of treatment with alkylating agents (± radiation) or topoisomerase inhibitors. This form of AML is generally associated with a poor clinical outcome.
- **AML, not otherwise specified**: cases in this category are defined in a similar fashion to the FAB classification.
- **Myeloid proliferations related to Down syndrome**, which incorporates a condition known as transient abnormal myelopoiesis as well as MDS and AML associated with Down

syndrome. These latter two conditions can be grouped together as 'Myeloid leukaemia associated with Down syndrome'.

■ **Blastic plasmacytic dendritic cell neoplasm**, which is derived from a precursor of plasmacytoid dendritic cells.

Acute leukaemia of ambiguous lineage

A minority of acute leukaemias cannot be classified as belonging unequivocally to the myeloid or lymphoid lines. In some, there is an absence of lineage-specific markers (acute undifferentiated leukaemia, AUL) while in others the markers that are present suggest more than one lineage (mixed phenotype acute leukaemia, MPAL).

AUL is characterized by the presence of CD34, HLA-DR ± CD38 but an absence of specific myeloid or lymphoid antigens.

MPAL can be subdivided into B-myeloid or T-myeloid as follows:

■ markers of myeloid lineage or monocytic differentiation must be present. Myeloid lineage is defined as the presence of myeloperoxidase, while monocytic differentiation is present if at least two of the following markers are present: nonspecific esterase, CD11c, CD14, CD64 or lysozyme.
■ T lineage is defined by cytoplasmic CD3 or, rarely, surface CD3.
■ B lineage is defined by either strong CD19 with strong expression of at least one of CD79a, cytoplasmic CD22 or CD10, or alternatively, weak CD19 with strong expression of at least two of CD79a, cytoplasmic CD22 or CD10.

B/T lymphoblastic leukaemia / lymphoma

One of the most important changes in understanding of lymphoid neoplasms has been the recognition that lymphoid leukaemias and non-Hodgkin lymphomas are not truly distinct conditions, but represent different manifestations of the same diseases. The clinical distinction of whether a specific patient is diagnosed with a lymphoma is somewhat arbitrary and depends mainly on whether a mass is present and the extent of bone marrow involvement. By convention, most haematologists diagnose acute lymphoblastic leukaemia when the bone marrow lymphoblast count is 25% or more or when one of the cytogenetic abnormalities shown in *Table 11.5* is identified, even if a mass is present. Thus, lymphoma is characterized by the presence of a mass and a bone marrow lymphoblast count of less than 25%.

In this chapter, which focuses on acute leukaemias, the more common abbreviations B ALL and T ALL are used to denote the leukaemic presentations of B and T precursor leukaemia/ lymphoma.

11.2 ACUTE MYELOID LEUKAEMIA

Acute myeloid leukaemia (AML) is a malignant proliferation of early myeloid precursor cells and is universally fatal if untreated. It occurs at all ages but is most common in adults, with an exponential increase in incidence with age over 40 years. Only 10–15% of childhood leukaemias are AML. The disease can occur either as a primary disease or as a secondary progression from myelodysplastic syndrome (MDS), or following previous anti-neoplastic treatment.

AML is characterized by an accumulation of immature myeloid precursors (blasts) in the bone marrow, peripheral blood and other tissues (see also *Box 11.4*). Clinically, AML typically presents with a short history of illness. About one third of patients will present with bruising or haemorrhage and about one quarter of patients will have a serious infection involving the lung, soft tissues or skin. The leucocyte count is elevated above the normal range in half of patients.

> **Box 11.4 Tumour load in AML**
>
> A typical tumour cell load at diagnosis for AML is about 5×10^{11}–5×10^{12} cells: this compares to a total normal haemopoietic stem cell load of less than 1×10^9.

The peripheral blood contains leukaemic blast cells in almost all cases. A moderate degree of anaemia is common, and the neutrophil and platelet counts are typically reduced, sometimes severely.

AML is not limited to the bone marrow and peripheral blood. Abnormalities in one or more organ system(s) may result from leukaemia cell infiltration or metabolic complications related to leukaemia. Rarely, a patient with AML develops a solid mass of leukaemia cells called a granulocytic sarcoma or myeloblastoma.

Epidemiology of AML

Acute myeloid leukaemia accounts for nearly one third of all leukaemias in adults, and about 18 300 new cases of AML are diagnosed every year in Europe. Internationally, AML is more commonly diagnosed in developed countries. Across all age groups, AML occurs slightly less frequently than the most common leukaemia, chronic lymphocytic leukaemia (CLL).

Annual incidence rates range from 2–4 per 100 000 in Europe. In England and Wales, the incidence of AML has risen by 70% since 1971 in both sexes. AML-related mortality has also increased, although to a lesser degree, in both men and women. Similarly, the incidence of AML has been steadily increasing in the elderly and in patients previously treated for other malignancies.

AML is more common in adults than children (95% of patients are over the age of 20 years) with people over the age of 60 falling into the highest risk group. People over 60 years of age account for approximately two thirds of all AML patients diagnosed. The median age at the time of diagnosis of AML is 68 years. AML is slightly more common in men than in women, particularly in elderly patients. This may be explained by the male predominance in myelodysplastic syndrome or a greater likelihood of occupational exposure to chemicals or other factors associated with AML.

Aetiological factors

Several environmental factors have been implicated in the aetiology of AML. For example, long-term (primarily occupational) exposure to aromatic solvents such as benzene is associated with an increased risk of developing AML. Benzene is a volatile solvent that can be absorbed via the skin and lungs and gradually accumulates in body fat and neurological tissue. Prolonged exposure allows the concentration to exceed the threshold at which chromosomal damage is triggered. It is this secondary event that increases the risk of leukaemogenesis. Tobacco smoke contains benzene as well as several other known carcinogens such as urethane, nitrosamines and radioactive compounds, and also appears to be weakly leukaemogenic. The precise mechanisms involved are not well characterized, but the risk increases with both quantity and time of exposure. Heavy smokers who develop AML often have poor-risk cytogenetic abnormalities.

Perhaps the best-known risk factor for AML is exposure to ionizing radiation. The atomic bombs that were dropped on Hiroshima and Nagasaki have provided incontrovertible evidence that exposure to doses of ionizing radiation in excess of 1 Gray is leukaemogenic (see *Box 11.5* and *Box 11.6*). The excess risk of AML in those exposed (about × 20 overall) increased with

---

Box 11.5 Ionizing radiation dose

The biological damage inflicted by ionizing radiation is largely determined by the dosage, which is defined in terms of the amount of energy transferred to the irradiated tissue. Dosage is expressed in Gray, where 1 Gray is equivalent to the absorption of 1 joule of energy per kilogram of irradiated tissue. The older unit of dosage was the rad. 1 Gy = 100 rad.

Box 11.6 Leukaemia and the atomic bomb

Confirmatory evidence that the observed excess of leukaemia was attributable to the effects of the atomic bombs was provided by the dual observations that the leukaemia risk was inversely related to the distance from the hypocentre of the explosion and that survivors of the Hiroshima bomb, which emitted a greater level of neutron radiation than that dropped on Nagasaki, were more likely to develop leukaemia.

---

increasing age at the time of exposure, with a peak incidence about eight years afterwards. Chronic exposure to diagnostic or therapeutic irradiation has also been associated with an increased incidence of AML.

Non-ionizing radiation exposure has been implicated as a risk factor for AML in some studies, but others have failed to show an effect. If such an effect exists, it is likely to be small.

Treatment of established malignancy involves the administration of cytotoxic drugs. The use of alkylating agents is strongly associated with an increased incidence of therapy-related AML (t-AML). The median time from initiation of therapy to the development of t-AML is 3–10 years. Epipodophyllotoxin has also been implicated in the development of treatment-related AML, with a shorter latency period than alkylating agents (see *Box 11.7*). t-AML is typically associated with poor-risk cytogenetic abnormalities, treatment resistance and a poor prognosis. A subset of t-AML carries favourable-risk cytogenetic abnormalities and has a prognosis similar to *de novo* AML.

Box 11.7 Alkylating agents

Alkylating agents are polyfunctional molecules with highly reactive alkyl groups that form crosslinks between the side chains of proteins and nucleic acids. Alkylating agents are capable of alkylating the nitrogen and oxygen molecules of all four DNA bases, phosphodiester bonds and the 2' oxygen atom of ribose, resulting in inappropriate base pairing, strand breaks, complex rearrangements and the deletion of part or all of a chromosome. Mutations that alter the expression of normal cellular oncogenes can result in malignant change. Commonly prescribed alkylating agents include cyclophosphamide, chlorambucil, busulfan, melphalan, procarbazine and cisplatin.

A number of congenital conditions predispose to AML. The best characterized of these is Down syndrome (trisomy 21), which carries a 20-fold increased risk. Other associations include Turner (X0) and Klinefelter (XXY) syndromes.

Several rare inherited conditions also are associated with excess AML risk as summarized in *Table 11.6*.

Molecular basis of AML

Advances in the field of molecular genetics have led to the conclusion that all cancers are attributable to the accumulation of mutations in proto-oncogenes and tumour suppressor genes that lead to loss of control over cell growth, gene expression and apoptosis. In AML, the most common recurring cytogenetic abnormalities are translocations that create abnormal

Table 11.6 Inherited conditions that predispose to AML development

Condition	Genetic abnormality	Comments
Shwachman–Diamond syndrome	*SBDS* gene at 7q11	Autosomal recessive disorder with exocrine pancreatic insufficiency, bone marrow failure and skeletal abnormalities. > 50% develop MDS/AML, usually in the first decade of life.
Amegakaryocytic thombocytopenia	*MPL* gene at 1p34	Isolated thrombocytopenia and megakaryocytopenia. No physical abnormalities.
Diamond–Blackfan syndrome	Heterogeneous	Inherited pure red cell aplasia. Multiple malformations may be present.
Kostmann syndrome	Heterogeneous	Severe congenital neutropenia with maturation arrest of granulopoiesis.
Fanconi anaemia	mutations in 1 of 11 genes (*FANCA-FANCJ*)	Autosomal recessive or X-linked recessive disorder with multiple congenital anomalies, chromosomal instability and bone marrow failure. About 10% develop AML.
Bloom syndrome	*BLM* gene at 15q26	Autosomal recessive disorder with chromosomal instability, light sensitivity, growth retardation, immunodeficiency and mental retardation.
Ataxia telangiectasia	*ATM* gene at 11q22–23	Neurodegenerative disease with severe disability, immunodeficiency and characteristic blood vessel malformations. ATM gene is involved in DNA repair.
Familial platelet disorder	*CBFA2* at 21q22	Autosomal dominant disease with thrombocytopenia and platelet dysfunction. Up to two thirds develop MDS/AML.
Xeroderma pigmentosum	*XPA* gene at 9q22.3 (many variants exist)	Autosomal recessive disorder with ultraviolet light sensitivity and impaired DNA repair.
Li–Fraumeni syndrome	*P53* gene at 17p13	Autosomal dominant disorder with early onset of multiple cancers, including AML.

fusion genes, resulting in the expression of regulatory proteins with abnormal function. Several examples of this phenomenon are described below. In most cases of AML that appear to have no cytogenetic abnormality, point mutations or small deletions are present in genes that encode important regulatory proteins. Examples of this type of abnormality are also described below.

Mutations of the retinoic acid receptor α and APL
The t(15;17)(q22;q21) translocation characterizes acute promyelocytic leukaemia (APL). This subtype of AML has distinct morphology and requires different treatment to other forms of AML. For many years, the translocation was used simply as a diagnostic marker, but it is now known that the genes involved in the translocation play a central role in the pathogenesis of APL.

The gene at 15q22 that is disrupted in the translocation is the *PML* gene, which encodes a tumour suppressor protein that is involved in multiple cellular processes, including suppression of cell growth and apoptosis. The gene at 17q21 that is disrupted is the retinoic acid receptor α (*RARα*) gene, which encodes a ligand-dependent nuclear receptor that functions as a transcription factor for many genes, including genes important for myeloid differentiation such as *G-CSF* and its receptor *G-CSFR* (see also *Box 11.8*). The t(15;17)(q22;q21) translocation generates two abnormal fusion genes:

■ On the derivative chromosome 15, a fusion gene created from the 5′ end of the *PML* gene and the 3′ end of the *RARα* gene is created. This abnormal gene is transcribed and plays a key role in the arrest of myeloid differentiation that characterizes APL.

■ On the derivative chromosome 17, a fusion gene created from the 5′ end of the *RARα* gene and the 3′ end of the *PML* gene is created. This abnormal gene is sometimes transcribed and also appears to play a role in the pathogenesis of APL.

Box 11.8 t(15;17)(q22;q21) variants

There are three rare variants of the t(15;17)(q22;q21) translocation that may be present in APL. All involve the formation of fusion genes involving the RARα gene at 17q21:

• t(5;17)(q35;q21), which involves the nucleophosmin gene at 5q35. This form responds to ATRA therapy.
• t(11;17) (q13;q21), which involves the *NUMA* gene at 11q13. This form responds to ATRA therapy.
• t(11;17) (q23;q21), which involves the promyelocytic zinc finger (PLZF; a transcriptional repressor) gene at 11q23. This form is resistant to ATRA therapy.

The *RARα* gene is mainly expressed in haemopoietic cells and regulates gene expression and cellular differentiation. In the absence of retinoic acid, the RARα protein binds to the transcriptional co-regulatory protein nuclear corepressor factor, resulting in suppression of gene transcription and promyelocytic differentiation. Conversely, in the presence of retinoic acid, transcriptional suppression is removed, promoting terminal differentiation of promyelocytes. The PML-RARα fusion protein binds more tightly to the nuclear corepressor factor, with the result that physiological concentrations of retinoic acid no longer relieve the transcriptional suppression. This results in the promyelocytic differentiation block characteristic of APL.

The treatment of APL is very different to that of all other forms of AML. Most patients are treated with all-trans-retinoic acid (ATRA, a vitamin A derivative). The effect of ATRA in typical APL (see *Box 11.8*) is to induce terminal differentiation of the leukaemic cells. It is not cytotoxic. However, when combined with conventional cytotoxic chemotherapy, ATRA has helped to transform APL from a near-universally fatal disease to an eminently curable one.

Core binding factor translocations

Core binding factors (CBF) are a group of heterodimeric transcription factors. They are composed of two chains:

■ a variant chain, designated CBFα, that binds directly to enhancer elements on target genes. There are three variants of CBFα, each encoded by a distinct gene: *RUNX1* (also known as *AML1*) at 21q22, *RUNX2* at 6p21 and *RUNX3* at 1p36.

■ an invariant chain, designated CBFβ that does not bind to DNA directly but increases the affinity and stabilizes the binding of the CBFα chain. This chain is encoded by a gene at 16q22.

Core binding factors are critical for normal haemopoietic development. Deletion of either the *AML1* or the *CBFβ* genes in mice is incompatible with life due to total failure of haemopoiesis. Mutation of these genes is associated with the development of acute leukaemia, including two specific forms of AML:

- AML with t(8;21)(q22;q22); *(AML 1/ETO)*
- AML with inv(16)(p13q22) or t(16;16)(p13;q22), *(CBFβ/MYH 11)*

The t(8;21)(q22;q22) translocation is found in about 5–12% of AML patients, and is associated with a good prognosis. The translocation involves the *AML1* gene at 21q22 and the *ETO* gene at 8q22, and creates a chimeric *AML1/ETO* gene on the der8 chromosome and a reciprocal *ETO/AML1* gene on der21. The *AML1/ETO* gene is transcribed and it is the resultant fusion protein that plays a role in leukaemogenesis. The reciprocal *ETO/AML1* gene is not active. The AML1 protein normally acts as an activator of transcription in early haemopoietic stem cells. The ETO protein normally functions as a repressor of transcription. In the chimeric *AML1/ETO* gene, virtually the entire *ETO* gene is present and the result is a chimeric fusion protein that functions as a repressor of gene transcription and also of the tumour suppressor genes *P14^{ARF}* and *NF-1*.

Mutations of the *CBFβ* gene, including inv(16)(p13q22) and t(16;16)(p13;q22), are found in about 8% of cases of AML and are associated with acute myelomonocytic leukaemia with abnormal eosinophils. This form of AML has a good prognosis. In the t(16;16)(p13;q22) translocation, the gene for smooth muscle myosin heavy chain (*MYH11*) at 16p13 fuses with the *CBFβ* gene, resulting in a fusion protein that binds to AML1 and functions as a transcriptional repressor.

Core binding factor mutations contribute to leukaemogenesis but are not sufficient on their own to trigger the development of AML. There is strong experimental evidence for this assertion, but perhaps the most convincing evidence comes from study of patients with familial platelet disorder. This autosomal dominant condition is caused by *AML1* mutations. Affected individuals are strongly predisposed to the development of AML or MDS, but only in the presence of secondary mutations.

Translocation t(9;11)(p22;q23); MLLT3-MLL

Translocations involving the *MLL* gene at 11q23 are common in both AML and ALL and are the most common genetic mutation in infants with acute leukaemia, regardless of the phenotype. More than 80 different translocation partner genes have been identified. In the WHO classification system, only one specific rearrangement is considered to belong to the category of AML with recurrent genetic abnormalities. The other rearrangements are too diverse and are not sufficiently clinically distinct to warrant inclusion. The t(9;11)(p22;q23) translocation is associated with *de novo* AML, therapy-related AML (t-AML) and also, rarely, with ALL and is considered to be an intermediate prognosis form when associated with *de novo* disease. This abnormality is associated with monoblastic proliferation.

The *MLL* gene encodes a very large nuclear protein that acts as a histone methyltransferase and so is involved in epigenetic control of gene transcription. *MLL* plays a critical role in normal embryonic development and haemopoiesis via maintenance of *HOX* gene expression and appears to be a global transcriptional regulator.

The precise function of the *MLLT3* gene at 9p22 is unknown, but it is clear that the hybrid *MLLT3-MLL* gene confers a proliferative advantage to its host cell and plays a critical role in leukaemogenesis.

MLL rearrangements are seen more commonly in certain subtypes of leukaemia (60–80% of cases of acute leukaemia in infants, 70–90% of cases of acute leukaemias secondary to topoisomerase II inhibitor treatment). The most common cytogenetic abnormalities involving *MLL* gene rearrangement are shown in *Table 11.7*. Characteristically, MLL gene mutations

Table 11.7 Common MLL mutations in acute leukaemia

Karyotype	Gene affected	Comment
Normal		Partial tandem duplication of *MLL* in some cytogenetically normal cases of AML.
+11		1% of AML and MDS.
t(4;11)(q21;q23)	*AF4*	Mainly in B ALL, but also biphenotypic and AML. About half of cases are children and about one third are infants.
t(11;19)(q23;p13.3)	*ENL*	Both ALL and AML. Mostly seen in infants < 1 year. Most female cases are B ALL, most male cases are M4 or M5.
t(6;11)(q27;q23),	*AF6*	5% of cases of AML, some cases of T ALL, mostly children and young adults with a male predominance.
t(9;11)(p22;q23)	*AF9*	2–5% of AML cases, mainly M5 (70%), M4 (10%); also seen in ALL, *de novo* and therapy-related acute leukaemia; children (50%; infants 15%).
t(11;19)(q23;p13.1)	*ELL*	Mostly seen in M4 and M5 AML, but also other subtypes, including treatment-related AML. Biphenotypic expression may be present. Uncommon in infants.

(other than the t(9;11)(p22;q23) translocation) are associated with mixed myeloid and lymphoid marker expression and a uniformly poor prognosis (median survival typically less than one year), with hyperleucocytosis and early involvement of the central nervous system. The rare cases of T ALL in children that carry the t(11;19)(q23;p13.3) also carry a good prognosis.

Translocation t(6;9)(p23;q34); DEK-NUP214

AML with t(6;9)(p23;q34) is a rare disease with a poor prognosis. The translocation results in the formation of a chimeric fusion gene between *DEK* (located at 6p23) and *NUP214* (located at 9q34 and also known as *CAN*). This form of AML is associated with a younger age of presentation (median 25–30 years), shows marrow basophilia and myelodysplasia, and has been seen in *de novo* AML, AML with antecedent MDS and t-AML.

NUP214 encodes a 214 kDa component of the nuclear pore complex. The protein encoded by *DEK* is thought to be involved in nuclear transcription and signal transduction.

Inversion inv(3)(q21q26.2) or t(3;3)(q21;q26.2); RPN1-EVI1

The inversion inv(3)(q21q26.2) and similar rearrangements activate transcription of the *EVI1* gene by placing it in juxtaposition with the enhancer of the constitutively expressed housekeeping gene ribophorin 1 (*RPN1*) at 3q21. Rearrangements at 3q21 involving the *EVI1* and *RPN1* genes are associated with poor prognosis AML with abnormal megakaryocytes.

The *EVI1* gene encodes a protein with multiple functions critical to haemopoiesis, including direct interaction with the transcription factor GATA-2, which is crucial for haemopoietic stem cell development. *EVI1* knockout mice have defects in both the development and proliferation of haemopoietic stem cells. EVI1 has also been shown to prevent the terminal differentiation of bone marrow progenitor cells to granulocytes and erythroid cells, but to favour differentiation to megakaryocytes. *RPN-1* encodes a ribosome receptor involved in the binding of ribosomes to the rough endoplasmic reticulum.

Translocation t(1;22)(p13;q13); RBM15-MKL1

The translocation t(1;22)(p13;q13) is associated with a poor prognosis form of acute megakaryoblastic leukaemia in infants, with extensive organomegaly and marrow fibrosis. It is not seen in Down syndrome-associated megakaryoblastic leukaemia. The precise functions of the *RBM15* (also known as *OTT*) and *MKL1* (also known as *MAL*) genes is uncertain, but it is thought that they are involved in chromatin organization and *HOX* differentiation pathways.

AML with mutated NPM1

The WHO system includes a provisional entity of AML with mutated nucleophosmin gene (*NPM1*). Mutations of this gene are common in AML and have been seen in several subtypes of the disease. For example, the t(3;5)(q25.1;q35) translocation involves the *NPM1* gene at 5q35 and the *MLF1* gene at 3q25.1 and results in the formation of a fusion gene. Nucleophosmin acts as a nuclear-cytoplasmic shuttling protein that appears to regulate the p53 tumour suppressor. Mutations of *NPM1* are also found in other haematological malignancies, including APL and anaplastic large cell lymphoma.

AML with mutated CEBPα

A second provisional entity, AML with mutated *CEBPα* (CCAAT/enhancer-binding protein-α) gene at 19q13.1 is also included in the WHO system. This gene encodes a transcription factor that plays a critical role in haemopoietic lineage determination, cell cycle control and gene activation and is mutated in up to 8% of cases. *CEBPα* mutations are typically associated with a good prognosis form of AML.

Other common mutations in AML

The fact that the WHO system singles out certain AML-associated cytogenetic entities does not imply that these are the only non-random mutations seen in AML. On the contrary, AML is associated with a wide range of common, non-random mutations and most cases carry more than one mutation simultaneously. Currently, other mutations are not specifically represented because they do not produce a sufficiently clinically distinct AML phenotype.

For example, the *FLT-3* gene is the single most commonly mutated gene in AML, with about 24% of cases affected. Two types of *FLT-3* mutation are commonly observed: internal tandem repeat (ITD) mutations and point mutations in the activation loop. Both types of mutation result in constitutive activation of FLT-3 (i.e. continuous activation and signalling in the absence of ligand-binding). *FLT-3* ITD mutations have been demonstrated in all subtypes of AML, but are most commonly seen in APL.

The *FLT-3* gene encodes a receptor tyrosine kinase that is expressed on CD34+ haemopoietic progenitor cells, including multipotent progenitors and common lymphoid progenitors. The protein has been designated as CD135. Haemopoietic stem cells are CD135–. When FLT-3 binds to its ligand FLT-3L, it forms a homodimer, thereby activating intracellular signalling. FLT-3 signalling plays an important role in cell survival, proliferation, and differentiation.

FLT-3 mutations confer a poor prognosis in AML patients under the age of 60.

Clinical presentation of AML

Patients with AML present with signs and symptoms through three general mechanisms:

- bone marrow failure with deficiency of normal blood cells
- invasion of vital organs with impairment of organ function
- systemic disturbances with metabolic imbalance.

The treatment of leukaemia with cytotoxic chemotherapy is also associated with significant morbidity. In fact, it is often difficult to distinguish between the effects of treatment and the symptoms of the disease itself.

Symptoms arising from bone marrow failure

The dysregulated proliferation of leukaemic blasts in the bone marrow eventually displaces normal haemopoiesis and leads to a reduction in the counts of all normal blood cells. In addition, the leukaemic clone actively suppresses the proliferation of normal haemopoietic progenitor cells.

The most obvious consequences of bone marrow failure are anaemia, infection and haemorrhage. Some degree of normocytic, normochromic anaemia is extremely common at presentation in AML and is responsible for symptoms such as fatigue and a sense of ill health. The unregulated proliferation of leukaemic tissue results in the physical 'crowding out' of normal haemopoietic elements, leading to a reduction in erythropoiesis, thrombopoiesis and leucopoiesis. In some cases, ineffective erythropoiesis or, more rarely, haemolysis may exacerbate the anaemia. In most anaemic individuals, erythropoietin levels are raised in proportion to the degree of anaemia but the normal erythroid precursors show diminished responsiveness to this hormone. It is thought that leukaemic cells elaborate one or more inhibitors of normal haemopoiesis. The severity of the anaemia typically reflects the severity of the disease. In severe anaemia, symptoms such as breathlessness on exertion, dizziness, weakness and reduced exercise tolerance become apparent. In older patients, angina or myocardial infarction can often be the first indicator of a clinical problem.

Infection is one of the most common causes of death and a significant cause of morbidity in patients with AML. The increased infection risk is caused by impaired host defence due to neutropenia or neutrophil dysfunction. Neutropenia may be caused by the 'crowding out' of normal neutrophil production by leukaemic tissue in the bone marrow or cytoreductive therapy. The usual hallmark of infection is fever. Unfortunately, the leukaemic process itself can cause fever, leading to complications in the recognition of infection. Differentiation between fever caused by infection and fever caused by the leukaemia process itself is often difficult. Typically, humoral and cell-mediated immunity are normal in acute leukaemia but, as the disease progresses, immune function deteriorates and the frequency and severity of infection increase.

The prevention of infection is a vital part of the treatment of acute leukaemia. Antibiotic regimes are implemented at the first sign of fever because of the association of infection with mortality. In some cases, severely neutropenic patients are treated with prophylactic antibiotics, regardless of signs of infection.

Haemorrhage is a common problem in AML, both at presentation and during treatment. Usually it is the direct result of thrombocytopenia, but may be secondary to defective platelet function, disseminated intravascular coagulation (DIC), liver disease or, more rarely, hyperviscosity syndrome. Petechiae and ecchymoses are the most frequent clinical manifestations. Haemorrhage into the gut, subarachnoid space or lungs can be life- threatening. Disseminated intravascular coagulation is particularly troublesome in acute promyelocytic leukaemia due to the presence of thromboplastin-like substances in the abnormal granules of the leukaemic promyelocytes, but it may be seen in any form of acute leukaemia. Gram-negative septicaemia is associated with intractable DIC, which commonly results in death.

Symptoms arising from organ infiltration

The organs commonly infiltrated at presentation or during the course of AML include liver, spleen, gums and skin. In contrast to the solid tumours, the frequency of organ infiltration by acute leukaemia far exceeds the frequency of symptomatic complications associated with such infiltration. Broadly, there are three types of complication associated with organ infiltration in acute leukaemia:

■ **Hyperleucocytosis** – the extremely high white cell counts sometimes encountered at presentation in AML are associated with 'sludging' in the microcirculation, raised viscosity of the blood and the formation of microthrombi or acute haemorrhage. The organs most commonly involved are the brain, lungs and eyes. The increase in whole blood viscosity is usually partially offset by the presence of anaemia.

■ **Leucostatic tumours** – rarely, leukaemic blast cells may lodge in the vascular system of infiltrated organs and proliferate, forming macroscopic pseudotumours with haemorrhage, which is often severe. Leucostatic tumours are associated with hyperleucocytosis, particularly where expansion of the leukaemic cell load occurs rapidly. The organs most commonly affected are the brain, liver and lungs.

■ **Sanctuary site relapse** – infiltration of the testes and meninges is sometimes seen in AML. These organs provide an effective sanctuary for resident leukaemic blasts because cytotoxic drugs penetrate them poorly. In the absence of specific additional prophylactic therapy to these organs, they may provide a source for the resurgence of leukaemic proliferation, leading to relapse. Meningeal and testicular relapse are most commonly seen in childhood ALL.

Metabolic disturbances

Metabolic disturbances are common in acute leukaemia and may be caused by the disease process or by its treatment. For example, a reduction in plasma Na^+ and K^+ concentration is relatively common in AML. Breakdown of malignant cells causes release of large amounts of purines into the plasma, leading to hyperuricaemia. Left untreated, hyperuricaemia causes gouty arthritis and renal damage. Some degree of hepatic dysfunction is common in the course of AML and may result in deranged plasma concentrations of liver enzymes and lactic acidosis.

Several of the drugs used in the treatment of leukaemia are nephrotoxic and the resulting renal impairment may increase the severity of minor metabolic disturbances. When the presenting leukaemic cell count is high, therapy can induce massive cell lysis, leading to severe metabolic disturbance, increased plasma concentrations of K^+, phosphates, uric acid and a decreased plasma concentration of Ca^{2+}.

Diagnosis of AML

A definitive diagnosis of AML requires examination of a peripheral blood film and bone marrow smear. A battery of supplementary tests may be required to confirm and refine the diagnosis.

The major qualifying criterion for a diagnosis of AML is the presence of at least 20% blasts of myeloid origin in the bone marrow or peripheral blood. The identity of the blast cells should be confirmed by the presence of Auer rods (red rod-like structures in the cytoplasm), using myeloperoxidase, Sudan black B, chloroacetate esterase or nonspecific esterase staining or by immunophenotyping. AML blasts usually express CD34, HLA-DR, CD13, CD15, CD33, CD64, CD117 and myeloperoxidase and may also express the lymphoid antigens CD7, CD56, CD2 and CD19. The 20% blast count criterion is relaxed in the presence of the AML-specific cytogenetic abnormalities t(8;21)(q22;q22); (*AML1/ETO*), inv(16)(p13q22) or t(16;16)(p13;q22); (*CBFB/MYH11*), t(15;17)(q22;q12); (PML/*RARα*).

The peripheral blood film usually shows a variable normocytic, normochromic anaemia with a normal or reduced reticulocyte count. Most patients are thrombocytopenic at presentation, but platelet counts can also be normal or raised. The white cell count is markedly raised ($> 100 \times 10^9/l$) in about 20% of cases and reduced ($< 4.5 \times 10^9/l$) in up to 40% of cases. Blast cells are usually present. There may be signs of myelodysplasia.

The bone marrow smear typically shows a monotonous leukaemic blast proliferation, often in a hyperplastic setting. For the purposes of differential counting, blasts include myeloblasts, monoblasts, promonocytes, abnormal promyelocytes, megakaryoblasts and (only if erythroleukaemia is suspected) pronormoblasts.

About half of AML patients have one or more identifiable cytogenetic abnormality at diagnosis. Cytogenetic testing is important at diagnosis for confirmation of certain subtypes, for determination of prognosis and for later use in detection of minimal residual disease or relapse following treatment.

Molecular studies should also be performed to look for mutations of *FLT-3*, *NPM1*, *KIT* or *CEBPα*, which are also of prognostic significance.

Prognosis of AML

Of all of the leukaemias, AML has the poorest prognosis. There is no reported difference in survival between men and women, but there is a substantial reduction in five-year survival with age. Younger patients (15–45 years) have a five-year survival of 37%, whereas in older patients (75 years and above), five-year survival is only 2%.

Progress in treatment and supportive care in the past two decades has led to improvements in overall survival in children and adults under the age of 65 years, but has had little impact on the long-term survival of older AML patients who often present with unfavourable prognostic factors, and are less able to tolerate aggressive chemotherapy. Almost two thirds of AML patients over the age of 65 years at diagnosis will die within one year.

The prognostic factors in AML are summarized in *Table 11.8* and are discussed below. These factors interact with each other. For example, an elderly patient with MDR expression has a worse prognosis than one without, while a younger patient with a complex karyotype with *FLT-3* mutation has a poor prognosis.

Table 11.8 Summary of key prognostic factors for patients with AML. (KPS, Karnofsky performance score)

Prognostic factor	Good prognosis	Poor prognosis
Age	< 45 years	> 60 years
Disease	*De novo*	Antecedent haematological disorder
Performance status	KPS > 60%	KPS < 60%
Prior chemotherapy (t-AML)	No	Yes
White cell count	< 25 x 10⁹/l	> 100 x 10⁹/l
CNS disease	Absent	Present
Treatment response	Prompt	Slow
Auer rods	Present	Absent
FAB type	M2, M3, M4	M0, M6, M7
Immunophenotype	–	Biphenotypic or unclassifiable
MDR-1	Absent	Present
Cytogenetics	t(15;17), t(8;21), inv(16)	–7, del(7q), –5, del(5q), 3q21/3q26 abnormalities, complex karyotype
Gene mutation	*NPM1* or *CEBPA*	*FLT-3*

Age

Advanced age is one of the most important adverse prognostic factors in AML. Older age is associated with a poorer response to chemotherapy, a higher incidence of drug resistance (see *Box 11.9*), a higher incidence of unfavourable cytogenetics and a lower incidence of favourable

---

Box 11.9 Multi-drug resistance

One of the most important limitations to the successful use of cytotoxic chemotherapy is the development of multi-drug resistance. MDR is common in relapsed leukaemias and secondary AML and is associated with a poor prognosis. The development of the MDR phenotype is associated with the expression of a 170 kD transmembrane protein (P-glycoprotein), encoded by a gene located at 7q21-23 called *mdr*-1. A structurally related gene, *mdr*-2, is located nearby. P-glycoprotein acts as an energy-dependent efflux pump for a wide range of cytotoxic drugs, thereby reducing their toxic effects. The function of the *mdr*-2 gene product is unknown, but it does not act as an efflux pump. Atypical patterns of MDR have also been described, associated with alterations in topoisomerase activity, glutathione-S-transferase activity or CTP synthetase activity.

---

cytogenetics. Elderly patients also often present with a number of comorbid conditions including cardiovascular disease, kidney disease, diabetes, obstructive pulmonary disease, cerebrovascular disease and diseases of the gastrointestinal and urinary tracts. These conditions may affect the overall outcome of patients with AML because they reduce the capacity to tolerate chemotherapy. Elderly patients may also have a longer duration of bone marrow hypoplasia following treatment due to age-associated defects in haemopoiesis.

Response to therapy

Initial response to 1–2 courses of induction chemotherapy is also an important indicator of prognosis. More specifically, the time taken to clear leukaemic blasts from the peripheral blood or bone marrow can be used to indicate prognosis. The UK Medical Research Council (MRC) proposes that a blast count of > 15% after one course of chemotherapy, and > 5% after two courses of chemotherapy, is indicative of a poor prognosis. Similarly, the German AML Cooperative Group considers the failure to achieve complete blast clearance by day 16 a marker of poor prognosis.

Therapy-related AML

AML can develop following exposure to cytotoxic agents (t-AML), or as an evolution from an antecedent haematological disorder, most commonly myelodysplastic syndrome (MDS). Around one third of such cases are thought to be therapy-related and the remainder evolve from an AHD. These patients fare worse than those with *de novo* AML.

Cytogenetic abnormalities

Cytogenetic abnormalities are the most important prognostic factor in AML. The nature of the abnormality is predictive of remission, relapse and overall survival. Karyotypes associated with a better than average response to standard therapy include inv(16), t(16;16), t(8;21), and t(15;17) and variants. Patients with a normal karyotype, +8 or +21 or any other karyotype not considered to indicate good or high risk have an intermediate prognosis. Patients with –5, del(5q), –7, del(7q), inv(3p) most abnormalities of 11q, 20q, 21q, 17p, del(9q), t(9,22) or complex karyotypes, have a poor prognosis.

AML patients with 'favourable' cytogenetics have the best prognosis when treated with conventional doses of cytarabine and an anthracycline. In general, these patients are younger than the average patient with AML, and tend to have a lower incidence of AHD, and no prior exposure to cytotoxic therapy or radiation therapy (*de novo* AML). Complete response (CR) rates are as high as 91% for inv(16), 85% for t(8;21) and nearly 70% for t(15;17).

Patients with 'unfavourable' cytogenetics, on the other hand, have a very poor response to treatment with standard AML regimens. If patients are younger and have a good performance status, consolidation with stem cell transplant or experimental therapy is recommended after standard induction treatment. Older patients or those who cannot tolerate therapy are managed with best supportive care (prophylactic antibiotics, growth factors, blood products and cyclophosphamide or hydroxyurea).

Often cytogenetics are not available prior to the start of induction treatment. Therefore treatment decisions are frequently based on other prognostic factors including age, comorbidities and the existence of an antecedent haematological disorder. However, when APL is suspected, chemotherapy should be delayed until confirmation by cytogenetic testing, since treatment with specialized regimens improves outcome. Cytogenetic information is used primarily to determine the type of post-remission therapy that should be used.

Miscellaneous other factors

Clinical markers of a heavy tumour load, such as hepatosplenomegaly, raised serum lactate dehydrogenase (LDH) and high peripheral WBC counts are also associated with a worse prognosis, as are male sex and poor performance status.

Clinical management of AML

The treatment of AML may be divided into two general phases: remission induction and post-remission therapy. The principal aim of induction chemotherapy is the maximal destruction of the malignant cells to achieve a complete remission: a bone marrow with < 5% blasts, a platelet count > 100×10^9/l and a neutrophil count > 1.0×10^9/l in a bone marrow that is ≥ 20% cellular. The disappearance of a karyotype abnormality is not required for the definition of complete remission, but is an important prognostic factor. The achievement of complete remission translates into improved survival. Induction therapy must be accompanied by individually tailored best supportive care to manage the clinical consequences of the disease process, as well as the frequent side-effects of treatment.

Without post-remission therapy, the large majority of patients would relapse within four months. It is therefore standard practice to administer two courses of chemotherapy, similar to that used during the induction phase, after induction chemotherapy. The duration of this phase is largely determined by how well the treatment is tolerated; the benefits of treatment are balanced against its toxicity. Intensive chemotherapy given upon the achievement of complete remission is called consolidation therapy. Post-remission therapy that is less intense than that used in induction, but given following consolidation, is called maintenance therapy. If a complete remission is maintained for at least three years, long-term follow-up studies indicate subsequent relapse occurs in < 10% of patients.

Induction therapy

Standard therapy for patients with all subtypes of AML, except APL, is the 7+3 regimen. One cycle of therapy consists of three days of an anthracycline (usually daunorubicin or idarubicin, but the anthracenedione mitoxantrone may be as effective) on days 1–3 plus 7 days of cytosine arabinoside (ara-C) by continuous infusion on days 1–7. The 7+3 chemotherapy regimen is myelosuppressive so the patient's blood cell counts will fall during therapy.

During 7+3 induction, patients are monitored daily for [Hb], WBC and platelets. Neutrophil recovery generally occurs within 3–4 weeks. At some point during days 14–21 following the start of induction therapy, a bone marrow sample is obtained to assess the impact of treatment:

- If some leukaemic blasts remain but fewer than at presentation, a second course of the identical induction regimen or high-dose ara-C may be given.
- If the bone marrow is hypoplastic, a second course of chemotherapy should be delayed until the nature of recovery (leukaemic or normal) is clear.

■ If the number of leukaemic blasts has not reduced, the patient is considered to have failed induction chemotherapy and should be offered alternative therapy. Similarly, if blasts remain after the second course of chemotherapy, alternative therapy should be offered.

Using this approach, around half of patients achieve remission after the first course and a further 10–15% following the second course. In younger AML patients, complete remission rates are higher.

The CR rates achieved are strongly influenced by cytogenetic risk groups. The CR rate in patients with favourable cytogenetics is around 80–90%, while for unfavourable cytogenetics it is 50–60%.

Investigators have also attempted to improve induction therapy by increasing the Ara-C dose. This approach has increased toxicity so is only tolerable in younger patients. The results of high-dose Ara-C have been conflicting and so use of the approach outside of a clinical trial is controversial.

There have been a number of attempts at adding a third drug to the anthracycline and cytarabine combination. Both thioguanine and etoposide, for example, have been added to the standard 7+3 regimen. Thioguanine failed to offer any benefits in terms of remission induction, remission duration or overall survival. The addition of etoposide, on the other hand, improves remission duration, but has little effect on other outcomes.

Post-remission therapy

All patients who enter haematological remission are recommended to receive additional post-remission therapy in the hope of preventing relapse. Although the majority of patients with AML successfully enter remission with induction therapy, most will subsequently relapse and die from their disease. The choice of post-remission therapy is one of the most difficult and controversial topics for AML patients and their physicians. While induction therapy may not vary according to prognostic group, the choice of post-remission therapy should take both prognostic grouping and cytogenetic profile into account. The treatment options include:

■ high-dose Ara-C consolidation
■ autologous or allogeneic stem cell transplant
■ experimental therapy in the setting of a clinical trial.

Traditionally, patients were consolidated with the same agents administered in induction chemotherapy using a '5+2' regimen consisting of 5 days of standard dose Ara-C and 2 days of an anthracycline. Nowadays, however, high-dose Ara-C is considered a standard part of post-remission therapy for patients < 60 years, especially if stem cell transplant is not planned. Younger patients (< 60 years) have four courses of consolidation. Older patients are more difficult to treat because of comorbidities and higher sensitivity to treatment-related toxicity. A minority of elderly patients with good performance status and favourable cytogenetics benefit from standard therapy, perhaps with reduced-dose consolidation.

Haemopoietic stem cell transplantation is often employed in the treatment of AML as either intensive post-remission therapy for younger patients with intermediate- or poor-risk cytogenetics who are in CR, or as second-line therapy after failure for eligible patients. The source of stem cells can be either allogeneic or autologous.

Allogeneic transplants involve the infusion of haemopoietic stem cells from an HLA-matched donor following myeloablative chemoradiotherapy. Allogeneic transplants carry the advantage of providing a graft versus leukaemia effect but are associated with a high mortality and morbidity rate owing to infection, organ toxicity and life-threatening symptoms of graft versus host disease (GvHD). Up to 40% of patients who receive an allogeneic transplant die from complications. Non-myeloablative transplants, also known as 'mini-allo' transplants, are now being offered to older patients with greatly reduced risk from the preparative regimen.

Autologous transplantation of stem cells is an alternative approach for patients who lack a suitable HLA-matched allogeneic donor. The patient's own stem cells are harvested whilst the patient is in CR and reinfused after myeloablative therapy. The conditioning regimen does not need to be as severe as for allogeneic transplant. Autologous transplantation has the advantage of avoiding graft versus host disease but is limited by the fact that there is a potential to reintroduce malignant progenitor cells, and the additional benefit from the graft versus leukaemia effect is not present.

The results of studies of the role of stem cell transplantation have produced conflicting results, but there is wide agreement that:

■ patients with favourable cytogenetics typically respond well to standard chemotherapy, so allogeneic stem cell transplantation is usually reserved for treatment of relapse. Some centres use autologous SCT as intensification after standard consolidation in patients under 55 years.

■ younger patients with unfavourable cytogenetics are unlikely to be cured using chemotherapy so stem cell transplantation may be offered in first remission. Older patients are unable to withstand the rigours of this approach.

■ there is no universal agreement on the role of stem cell transplantation in patients with intermediate cytogenetics. Some centres opt for transplant in first remission, particularly in the youngest patients, while others reserve it for treatment of relapse.

Post-remission therapy of older patients (> 60 years)

The treatment of older AML patients presents a challenge. Such patients frequently present with multiple poor prognostic indicators and are often, because of other medical problems, frequently unable to tolerate intensive cytotoxic chemotherapy. Older AML patients without poor prognostic indicators and with a good performance status can be treated in the same way as younger patients and with similar outcomes. Little progress has been made in improving the long-term survival of older patients with AML.

Treatment of relapsed or refractory AML

Relapse is the most common cause of treatment failure, occurring in 50–80% of patients achieving CR. Treatment strategies for patients who relapse or are refractory (resistant) after first-line therapy are based on predicted outcome of salvage treatment. In general, however, the only therapy with curative potential in patients with recurrent/refractory AML is allogeneic stem cell transplantation. Therefore, the decision to offer aggressive salvage therapy (including debulking reinduction prior to transplant) or to pursue palliative strategies should be based largely on an assessment of the suitability of the patient for future transplantation. Additionally, since patients who respond to standard dose salvage therapy are likely to remain in remission only briefly, timely coordination with a transplant centre (preferably at the time of first relapse) is necessary to allow for a smooth transition between treatments.

The most important predictor of outcome following treatment with standard dose salvage therapy is the length of the initial CR. In addition, as the duration of the first CR decreases, the CR rate and disease-free survival following salvage therapy decreases continuously. Experimental therapy is appropriate for all patients relapsing, especially those patients with a short first remission.

Maintenance therapy

Following completion of consolidation treatment with intensive chemotherapy, some patients may be offered low dose prolonged treatment, known as maintenance therapy, in an attempt to further reduce the chance of relapse. The role of maintenance in AML is unclear because of conflicting trial results. Clinical trials with low dose Ara-C as maintenance therapy in patients with AML lasting for 1 or 2 years after initial remission induction did not reveal consistent benefits in either disease-free or overall survival. Recently, however, favourable results from a large German trial have revived this issue.

Maintenance therapy using ATRA, low-dose 6-mercaptopurine (6-MP) and methotrexate (MTX) is recommended for patients with APL because it has been shown to increase the duration of remission and to improve survival.

11.3   ACUTE LYMPHOBLASTIC LEUKAEMIA/LYMPHOMA IN CHILDREN

Acute leukaemia is the most common malignancy in children, accounting for just under a third of cases. About 80% of childhood leukaemia is acute lymphoblastic leukaemia/lymphoma (ALL), with most of the rest being AML. The treatment of ALL in children has improved markedly in the past few decades, mainly as a result of an intense international clinical trials programme. Currently, about 80% of children diagnosed with ALL will be alive five years later.

The incidence of ALL is about 3–4.5 cases per 100 000, but there is substantial geographic variation. It is unclear whether the incidence of childhood ALL is stable or rising as epidemiological studies have shown conflicting results. Overall, the incidence of childhood ALL is highest between the ages of 1 and 5 years, with a peak between the ages of 3 and 4 years. The disease is diagnosed more commonly in boys than girls and more commonly in white children than in those of African heritage. An increased incidence of ALL is seen in children with Down syndrome, neurofibromatosis type 1, Bloom syndrome and ataxia telangiectasia.

Many other epidemiological associations with childhood ALL have been proposed, such as exposure to ionizing or non-ionizing radiation, viral exposure *in utero*, parental tobacco and alcohol use and population density, but none are universally accepted as being clearly implicated because of inadequate or conflicting data.

Clinical presentation of childhood ALL

Childhood ALL is clinically heterogeneous. In some patients, there is a history of vague illness lasting from weeks to months before diagnosis while in others presentation is acute. The symptoms and signs are non-specific, but can all be traced to bone marrow failure and/or leukaemic cell infiltration. The most common presenting features attributable to bone marrow failure are abnormal bruising or bleeding secondary to thrombocytopenia, persistent fever, which is of non-infectious origin, fatigue and lethargy, which may be related to anaemia but can be more severe than the [Hb] suggests. Variable symptoms secondary to leukaemic infiltration include bone pain, lymphadenopathy, headache, testicular enlargement and mediastinal mass.

Bone pain, which is present in up to a third of cases, is typically caused by thinning of the long bones due to expansion of the marrow space and may present as a limp, avoidance of walking or even standing in infants. Less frequently, osteonecrosis may be seen. Sternal tenderness is a common finding.

Lymphadenopathy is seen in more than half of children with ALL at diagnosis and there may be a history of unsuccessful antibiotic therapy in the weeks leading to diagnosis. Typically, the enlarged nodes are non-tender and firm and rubbery on palpation.

Headache, sometimes with dizziness and vomiting, can indicate central nervous system (CNS) infiltration. Examination of cerebrospinal fluid shows the presence of leukaemic lymphoblasts. Many cases of ALL have CNS involvement without symptoms.

Painless testicular enlargement (usually involving only one testicle) is sometimes seen and indicates leukaemic infiltration.

A mediastinal mass may be present at diagnosis in cases of T ALL and, if large, can cause symptoms such as respiratory distress, pleural effusion and dysphagia.

Diagnosis of childhood ALL

Clinical examination usually reveals one or more clinical signs of marrow failure and leukaemic infiltration such as pallor due to anaemia, petechiae, purpura or mucous membrane bleeding due to thrombocytopenia, hepatomegaly and/or splenomegaly (which is usually asymptomatic), sternal and long bone tenderness and retinal haemorrhage.

Laboratory evaluation must include a bone marrow examination and full blood count with peripheral blood smear examination. A full blood count confirms the presence of anaemia, thrombocytopenia and, sometimes, an abnormal white cell count. There will frequently be an indication of white cell abnormalities such as atypical lymphoid cells or suspected blasts on the analyser report. The white cell count can be low, normal or high, but is raised in the majority of cases. Microscopic examination of a peripheral blood smear usually shows the presence of leukaemic lymphoblasts, particularly when the white cell count is raised. The leukaemic lymphoblasts can vary in appearance from small cells with scanty cytoplasm, condensed nuclear chromatin and indistinct nucleoli to larger cells with more abundant amounts of cytoplasm, dispersed chromatin and multiple nucleoli. Azurophilic granules may be present in the cytoplasm of some cells but the presence of Auer rods precludes a diagnosis of ALL. Markedly raised white cell counts at presentation are more commonly seen in cases of T ALL.

A bone marrow aspirate is required whenever possible to confirm diagnosis and also provides cells for cytogenetic and molecular genetic analysis and immunophenotyping, which form an important part of the diagnostic workup. The marrow smear is usually hypercellular with extensive infiltration by leukaemic lymphoblasts. Typically the morphology of the myeloid precursor cells is normal. Megakaryocytes are usually reduced in number, sometimes markedly so. Occasionally, the bone marrow may have the appearance of aplastic anaemia, but this is usually transient and is replaced by the typical findings of ALL within a few weeks or months. If a bone marrow aspirate is unobtainable, diagnosis can be made using leukaemic lymphoblasts from the cerebrospinal fluid or peripheral blood if the blast cell count is high.

Classification of childhood ALL

ALL in children is clinically and biologically heterogeneous. Characterization of the leukaemic blasts by cytogenetic, molecular and immunophenotypic analysis allows a more accurate subdivision of the disease that has prognostic significance (see *Box 11.10*).

Box 11.10 Flow cytometry

Flow cytometry involves the detection of particles such as cells, bacteria or chromosomes as they move in a liquid stream through a laser-controlled 'sensing' zone. The particles of interest are often rare 'events' in a mixture of normal or contaminating particles. As each particle passes through the laser beam, it scatters some of the light in all directions. If the particle has been marked with a fluorescent dye, the laser will cause it to fluoresce. The pattern of scattered and fluorescent light produced reveals much about the particle. For example, forward angle light scatter (FALS) gives an indication of cell size, while right angle light scatter (RALS) gives an indication of cell granularity. Modern flow cytometers can make several separate measurements on each particle, at the rate of several thousands of particles per second. The results can be displayed using single histograms or more complex multiparametric diagrams. Some flow cytometers are even capable of sorting particles of special interest out of the main particle stream, which can then be used in further experiments.

Immunophenotype

Using immunophenotype alone, 85–90% of cases of childhood ALL are of B-precursor lineage (Early pre-B ALL, common ALL or pre-B ALL). Early pre-B ALL is recognized by expression of CD19, CD79a, cytoplasmic CD22, TdT and HLA-DR and lack of expression of CD10, cytoplasmic or surface immunoglobulin. Common ALL is differentiated from early pre-B ALL by CD10 positivity and pre-B ALL is characterized by the emergence of cytoplasmic immunoglobulin and CD20 positivity (see *Box 11.11*).

Box 11.11 Common ALL and CD10

The discovery of Common ALL Antigen (CALLA) by Dr M Greaves in 1975 caused a great deal of excitement because it appeared to be the first leukaemia-specific marker to be identified. He produced a polyclonal antibody that reacted with up to 80% of cases of childhood ALL by immunization of a rabbit with ALL blast cells. However, as the use of monoclonal antibodies to type ALL progressed, it became apparent that there was no specific antibody to detect leukaemic cells: all antibodies produced to date detect a normal cell at some stage of differentiation. The structure and function of CALLA has been established, and it has been renamed CD10. It is a zinc metalloprotease of molecular weight 100 000 that hydrolyses peptide bonds, thereby reducing cellular responses to peptide hormones. Among the many biologically active peptides it cleaves are bradykinin, endothelin, angiotensin and oxytocin. CD10 is encoded by a gene on chromosome 3q21–q27. CD10 positivity is widely distributed in normal tissue: it is found in precursor T and B lymphocytes, granulocytes, brain, kidney and muscle, but its main diagnostic utility is as a marker of ALL.

About 20% of cases are shown to be pre-B cell ALL and this form has been associated with an unfavourable prognosis compared to early pre-B and common ALL, although it has recently been shown that the major determinant of the poor prognosis in this group is the presence of the t(1;19)(q23;q13) translocation.

About 1–2% of cases are of mature B cell origin (designated L3 in the FAB classification and Burkitt lymphoma / leukaemia in the WHO system). This condition is recognized by expression of CD10±, CD19, CD20, CD22, CD25 and surface immunoglobulin (sIg). This condition typically occurs in older children and CNS infiltration is common. Treatment with standard ALL therapy usually meets with limited success, but high-intensity NHL treatment is more successful.

Up to 15% of cases of childhood ALL are of T cell origin. This form is recognized by expression of CD7, surface or cytoplasmic CD3 and variable expression of CD1a, CD2, CD4, CD5 and CD8. As for B ALL, T ALL can be subdivided according to maturational stage of the leukaemic cells into early or pro-T (characterized by CD2, CD7, CD38 and cytoplasmic CD3 expression); common thymocyte (characterized by CD1a, sCD3, CD4/CD8 double positive expression) and late thymocyte (characterized by expression of either CD4 or CD8). The clinical significance of this division in children is doubtful. T ALL is most common in teenage years and is more common in boys. Common features of T ALL at diagnosis include high white cell count, a higher incidence of CNS involvement and an anterior mediastinal mass, often with pleural effusion. The prognosis for T ALL has been unfavourable, but this picture is changing.

About 10% of cases show mixed B cell and myeloid phenotype with the additional expression of the myeloid markers CD11, CD13, CD14, CD15, CD33, CD34, CD41 or CD42.

Care must be taken when interpreting the results of immunophenotyping because expression of markers is frequently aberrant and does not necessarily relate to expression on normal lymphoid counterparts.

Cytogenetics

Cytogenetic abnormalities are common in B ALL and many have prognostic significance. The incidence of the different types of cytogenetic abnormalities differs between adult and childhood B ALL.

> **Box 11.12 Fluorescent *in situ* hybridization**
>
> *In situ* hybridization is a technique by which specific portions of chromosomes can be marked by hybridization with a labelled nucleic acid probe. The label used can be a radioisotope, an enzyme or a fluorochrome. Fluorescent *in situ* hybridization (FISH) has revolutionized molecular cytogenetics. It is now possible to detect structural and numerical aberrations in disorders where conventional karyotyping is very difficult or impossible. The important feature of FISH is that the nucleic acid is retained *in situ*, and not degraded during processing. FISH techniques can be applied to most biological tissues, including whole cells, tissue sections, chromosomes and bare nuclei. The probes used are usually between 10 and 25 kilobases in length. Longer probes give weaker signals, probably because they penetrate less efficiently into cross-linked tissue and smaller probes may be difficult to visualize. Chromosome 'paints' which label complete chromosomes are useful in the detection of numerical abnormalities.

Numerical changes to chromosome number are classified as hyperdiploidy, when more than 50 chromosomes are present, and hypodiploidy, when fewer than 46 chromosomes are present in the leukaemic cells (see *Box 11.12*). Three groups are recognized: low hyperdiploidy (47–50 chromosomes), high hyperdiploidy (51–65 chromosomes) and extreme hyperdiploidy (65–84 chromosomes). Low and high hyperdiploidy are seen in about half of cases of B ALL and are associated with a favourable prognosis, most likely because of the association with the t(12;21) (p13;q22); (*TEL/AML1*) translocation and combined trisomy of chromosomes 4 and 10 or chromosomes 4, 10 and 17. Extreme hyperdiploidy (65–84 chromosomes) is associated with an unfavourable prognosis.

Hypodiploidy (fewer than 46 chromosomes) is also associated with an unfavourable prognosis. Three forms of hypodiploidy are recognized: near haploidy (23–29 chromosomes) is seen only in children and is associated with a very unfavourable prognosis; low hypodiploidy (30–39 chromosomes) is seen in older children and adults; and high hypodiploidy. Near haploidy and low hypodiploidy are clearly associated with an unfavourable prognosis; the impact of high hypodiploidy is less marked.

Important structural abnormalities include:

- t(9;22)(q34;q11.2); (*BCR-ABL1*) translocation (Philadelphia chromosome). This abnormality is seen most commonly in older children and adults and is not associated with a specific immunophenotype. The prognosis for patients with this rearrangement is adverse, although intensive chemotherapy and the addition of tyrosine kinase inhibitors to treatment is beginning to improve the picture.
- t(v;11q23); (*MLL* rearranged). These rearrangements, including t(4;11)(q21;q23), are associated with high-risk features including a high white cell count, presentation in infancy and mixed immunophenotype.
- t(12;21)(p13;q22); (*TEL/AML1*), which is seen in about one quarter of cases of B ALL with abnormalities involving 12p (about 10% of cases overall). This abnormality is associated with younger children and a favourable prognosis. On the other hand, intrachromosomal amplification of chromosome 21 with amplification of the *AML1* gene is associated with older children and a poor prognosis.
- t(5;14)(q31;q32); (*IL3-IGH*), is associated with a relatively rare form of B ALL with eosinophilia and sometimes basophilia, which is seen in children and young adults and is more common in males. The eosinophilia is reactive and not part of the malignant clone.
- t(1;19)(q23;p13.3); (*TCF3-PBX1*) is associated with a high white cell count and a pre-B cytoplasmic immunoglobulin positive phenotype. The earlier poor prognosis associated with this phenotype has been improved with current treatment. About 5% of patients carry this abnormality.

- t(8;14)(v;q24)(*MYC/IGH*). Rearrangements involving the immunoglobulin gene loci at 14q32, 2p12 or 2q11 with the *MYC* gene at 8q24 are associated with Burkitt lymphoma / leukaemia. The earlier poor prognosis associated with this rare subtype of ALL has been markedly improved by a switch to intensive NHL treatment regimens.
- t(1;14)(p32;q11.2)(*TAL1/TCR*) translocation is associated with T ALL, organomegaly and hyperleukocytosis. Rearrangements of the *TAL1* gene are present in up to 25% of cases of T ALL.
- Chromosome 9p deletions or translocations are found in up to 10% of both B and T ALL in children and are associated with high-risk disease and a decreased duration of remission. These abnormalities cause a variety of abnormalities including rearrangements involving the P16^{INK4A}, P15^{INK4B}, *PAX5* and *JAK2* genes.
- Mutations involving the *NOTCH1* gene at 9q34.3 are among the most common in T ALL. This gene is critical in T cell differentiation pathways.

Molecular basis of childhood ALL

t(9;22)(q34;q11.2); (BCR-ABL1)

The Philadelphia chromosome is seen in about 5% of cases of ALL in children and in up to 30% of cases in adults. The incidence is even higher in adults with B ALL (up to 50%). There are two forms of *BCR-ABL* rearrangements seen in ALL:

- in 30–50% of adult cases, the translocation is identical to that seen in chronic myeloid leukaemia (CML; see *Chapter 14*) and the result is an identical P210 BCR-ABL fusion protein. In these cases, the cytogenetic abnormality is present in both myeloid and lymphoid precursors, suggesting that these represent a lymphoblast transformation of undiagnosed CML.
- in the remaining cases, the breakpoint within the *BCR* gene differs and the resultant BCR-ABL fusion protein is smaller (p190). The cytogenetic abnormality in these cases is restricted to the lymphoblastic line, suggesting that these cases are a subtype of *de novo* B ALL.

t(v;11q23); (MLL rearranged)

The *MLL* gene is commonly rearranged in ALL, particularly in infants. The *MLL* gene encodes a histone methyltransferase and plays a critical role in normal embryonic development and haemopoiesis via maintenance of *HOX* gene expression. *IKAROS* is a lymphocyte-restricted gene that encodes a zinc finger DNA-binding protein that is crucial for regulation of lymphoid commitment and differentiation and appears to be regulated by MLL regulatory complexes. In the t(4;11)(q21;q23) rearrangement, the *MLL* gene is translocated to the *AF4* gene at 4q21, creating a fusion gene with altered properties.

Infants with ALL associated with *MLL* gene rearrangements have a particularly poor prognosis and require intensive therapy. They tend to respond well to primary therapy but relapse quickly and have a short median survival.

t(12;21)(p13;q22)(TEL-AML1)

The t(12;21)(p13;q22)(*TEL-AML1*) translocation is the most common cytogenetic abnormality in childhood ALL, with an incidence of 15–25% in precursor B ALL with rearrangements of 12p. It is most commonly seen in children aged 1–10 years and is uncommon in infants and in adults. The translocation relocates the *TEL* gene at 12p12 to the *AML1* gene at 21q22, resulting in a fusion protein. *AML1* encodes the variant core binding factor α chain, while *TEL* acts as a transcriptional repressor. The TEL-AML1 fusion protein inhibits the transactivation of gene expression by wild-type AML1. Patients with this translocation and ALL usually have a rearrangement or deletion of the other *TEL* allele. A *TEL-AML1* fusion gene is detectable in about 1% of fetuses, but does not cause progression to ALL in the vast majority, suggesting that the abnormality is insufficient in itself for ALL development.

Patients with ALL and t(12;21)(p13;q22)(*TEL-AML1*) usually have a favourable prognosis, even in the presence of some other high-risk factors.

t(1;19)(q23;p13.3); (TCF3-PBX1)

The t(1;19)(q23;p13.3); (*TCF3-PBX1*) translocation is associated with pre-B ALL with cytoplasmic immunoglobulin expression in children. It is seen in up to a third of cases of pre-B ALL in children, but less commonly in adults. The translocation occurs in two forms: a reciprocal translocation, t(1;19)(q23;p13.3) and, more commonly, an unbalanced form with a rearranged chromosome 19, der(19)t(1;19)(q23;p13.3).

The t(1;19)(q23;p13.3)(*TCF3-PBX1*) translocation involves the *TCF3* gene at 19p13.3 and the *PBX1* gene at 1q23, resulting in the creation of a fusion gene. *TCF3* is universally expressed and encodes two transcription factors, designated E12 and E47, that are involved in the regulation of immunoglobulin and other gene expression. *PBX1* is a *HOX* gene and is involved in the regulation of developmental processes and haemopoiesis, but is not normally expressed in lymphoid cells.

How the TCF3-PBX1 fusion protein contributes to leukaemogenesis is unknown, but it is thought to result in expression of genes that are normally silent in lymphoid tissues.

Prognosis of childhood ALL

One of the keys to the marked improvement in treatment outcomes in childhood ALL has been the ability to identify prognostic factors at diagnosis that permit a risk-adapted treatment strategy. This means that patients with a good prognosis can be offered less aggressive therapies with lower toxicities, while those with poor prognosis can be offered more aggressive treatment upfront, thereby maximizing the chance of treatment success.

Several laboratory and clinical characteristics have been identified that help to predict response to treatment and outcome in childhood ALL. However, as treatment has improved, many of these have become redundant. Factors that retain prognostic utility include:

- **white cell count**: children with a white cell count > 50×10^9/l at presentation are considered to have a higher risk than those with lower counts.
- **age at presentation**: infants (< 1 year old) and children aged > 10 years are considered to have a higher risk than children aged 1–9 years.
- **cytogenetics and ploidy**: the significance of cytogenetic and ploidy abnormalities is discussed above. In summary, high hyperdiploidy and trisomies of chromosomes 4, 10 and 17 are favourable prognostic indicators, whereas near haploidy and extreme hyperdiploidy are indicators of poor prognosis. Although many different cytogenetic abnormalities have been identified in childhood ALL, few have a clearly defined impact on prognosis. The t(12;21)(p13;q22); (*TEL/AML1*) translocation is a good prognostic indicator whereas t(9;22)(q34;q11.2); (*BCR-ABL1*), *MLL* rearrangements, iAMP21, del13q are associated with early relapse and thus poor prognosis.
- **immunophenotype**: the most important immunophenotypic indicators of prognosis are separation of cases of childhood ALL into precursor B types which are associated with a better prognosis and precursor T and mature B types that have historically been associated with poor prognosis.
- **response to induction therapy**: prompt and deep response to induction therapy is perhaps the most important indicator of good prognosis in childhood ALL. The depth of response is important because it has clearly been demonstrated that long-term relapse-free survival is related directly to the level of residual disease, both early and later during

the course of the disease. Failure of response or incompleteness of response to induction therapy are ominous signs in childhood ALL.

In addition to these factors, some studies have identified a subgroup of patients within the good prognosis group who respond less well to chemotherapy due to the presence of drug metabolism gene polymorphisms (e.g. cytochrome p450 gene polymorphisms).

Based on the presence of prognostic features at diagnosis, during and following induction therapy, several risk groups can be identified and used to guide treatment approaches in childhood ALL. Several such strategies exist and others are under investigation to try to define the optimum treatment for each individual child. This is important because patients with high-risk disease are treated more effectively if they are identified early and treated aggressively from the outset. However, children with low-risk disease treated too aggressively suffer unnecessarily from treatment-related morbidity (and even mortality) and can develop significant late effects of treatment. Clearly, for these children, a strategy that minimizes treatment consistent with optimal antileukaemic effectiveness represents an ideal approach.

Children's Cancer Group (CCG) and Pediatric Oncology Group (POG) studies currently use an initial risk assignment of children between the ages of one and nine years with a white cell count less than $50 \times 10^9/l$ as standard risk, with all others defined as high risk. These groupings are then refined based on cytogenetics, the presence of CNS disease and the kinetics of response to induction therapy as:

- **standard-risk low**, defined by the presence of trisomies of chromosomes 4, 10 and 17 or the t(12;21)(p13;q22); (*TEL/AML1*) translocation, coupled with an absence of leukaemic blasts in the cerebrospinal fluid, absence of testicular disease and a prompt and deep response to induction therapy assessed by < 5% leukaemic blasts in the bone marrow by day 8 or 15 of induction and < 0.1% residual disease by day 29.
- **standard-risk average**, defined in the same way as standard-risk low except that there are no combined trisomies or t(12;21)(p13;q22); (*TEL/AML1*) translocation.
- **standard-risk high**, defined by standard-risk disease with the presence of any of the following features
  - ☐ CNS disease with ≥ 5 leukaemic blast cells/μl
  - ☐ > 5% leukaemic blasts in the bone marrow on day 15 of induction therapy
  - ☐ residual disease > 0.1% but ≤ 1% on day 29 of induction therapy
  - ☐ *MLL* gene rearrangement.
- **high-risk 1**, defined as a high-risk patient with an absence of leukaemic blasts in the cerebrospinal fluid, absence of testicular disease and a prompt and deep response to induction therapy assessed by < 5% leukaemic blasts in the bone marrow by day 8 or 15 of induction and < 0.1% residual disease by day 29.
- **high-risk 2**, defined as a high-risk patient with the presence of any of the poor-risk indicators detailed for standard-risk high disease.
- **very high-risk**, defined as a high-risk patient with the presence of > 5% leukaemic blasts in the bone marrow on day 29 of induction therapy and > 1% on day 29 of induction therapy, Philadelphia translocation, hypodiploidy, residual *MLL* rearrangement or induction failure assessed by:
  - ☐ > 25% leukaemic blasts in the bone marrow on day 29
  - ☐ 5–25% leukaemic blasts or ≥ 1% residual disease on day 29 with > 5% leukaemic blasts or ≥ 1% residual disease on day 43.

Clinical management of childhood ALL

The treatment of childhood ALL (excluding B ALL, which is treated as an NHL) has four sequential components: remission induction, consolidation/intensification, CNS prophylaxis and maintenance. As for acute myeloid leukaemia, supportive therapy with transfusion of red cells and platelets as required, prompt treatment of suspected or confirmed infections and correction of metabolic imbalances play a critical role in the overall success of treatment. The full treatment takes 2–3 years to complete.

Remission induction

The goal of induction therapy is to achieve complete haematological remission (defined as < 5% blasts in the bone marrow, normal blood count and absence of leukaemic symptoms) as rapidly as possible. Induction therapy generally consists of a combination of weekly vincristine, daily corticosteroid such as prednisone, prednisolone or dexamethasone, and asparaginase. In high-risk patients, an anthracycline such as daunorubicin or doxorubicin may be added. This type of therapy induces complete remission in more than 90% of patients, irrespective of risk group (the differences in disease risk are manifest most obviously by risk of relapse rather than primary resistance to therapy).

The quality and speed of response to induction therapy is a major (perhaps the single most important) prognostic indicator. Prompt, complete response is an indicator of good prognosis. Complete haematological response assessed by examination of bone marrow morphology is a poor indicator of response because of its lack of sensitivity and the difficulty in distinguishing between leukaemic blast cells against a background of haemopoietic regeneration. Although patients in complete haematological remission have no apparent signs of residual disease, in fact they still carry a significant tumour burden (estimated as around 10^8–10^9 leukaemic blasts). If treatment is stopped at this stage, relapse is near-inevitable. A more sensitive indicator of response is to assess the presence of residual disease using the presence of 'markers' of the leukaemic blasts such as gene rearrangements identified at diagnosis, specific clonal T cell receptor or immunoglobulin heavy chain gene rearrangements or a distinct leukaemia-associated immunophenotype.

Patients who fail to achieve complete remission following induction therapy have a particularly bleak prognosis. Such patients seldom respond well to subsequent chemotherapy and may be offered stem cell transplantation.

Adverse effects associated with induction therapy include tumour lysis syndrome (in children with high blast cell counts), thrombosis (an adverse event associated with L-asparaginase therapy; see *Box 11.13*), bleeding (mainly due to thrombocytopenia), infection (mainly due to neutropenia), mucositis, pancreatitis and hyperglycaemia.

Box 11.13 Asparaginase and thrombosis

Asparaginase acts by depleting plasma asparagine, thereby inhibiting protein synthesis in leukaemic blasts but also synthesis of several plasma proteins, including albumin, thyroxine-binding globulin, prothrombin, coagulation factors V, VII, VIII, IX, X, XI and fibrinogen, protein C, protein S and plasminogen. Particularly in children with other prothrombotic features, the rapid fall in proteins C and S can trigger thrombotic complications. Typically, these coagulation abnormalities are reversed within 10–14 days of stopping asparaginase treatment.

Consolidation/intensification

Immediately following completion of induction therapy, patients are further stratified for consolidation, which is administered as soon after remission as possible. The rationale for consolidation is to reduce the risk of relapse by rapidly reducing any residual leukaemic blast burden. This reduces the risk of blast infiltration into sanctuary sites such as testicles or CNS and the emergence of drug resistance. Because consolidation chemotherapy is designed to maximize cell kill, it employs high doses of multidrug combinations with mechanisms of action that differ from those used during induction. Treatment-associated toxicity is significant and supportive therapy is required. Drugs often used include alkylating agents such as cyclophosphamide, antimetabolites such as methotrexate and cytarabine, anthracyclines such as daunorubicin and epipodophyllotoxins such as etoposide. Treatment is administered in blocks, with a recovery period in between. Standard-risk children typically receive 2–3 blocks of consolidation therapy.

High-risk patients can have their treatment intensity increased by increasing the doses of one or more of the drugs employed, by repeating the remission induction and consolidation/ intensification treatments or by haemopoietic stem cell transplantation.

CNS prophylaxis

The drugs used in remission induction and consolidation do not cross the blood–brain barrier, so the CNS provides a site where leukaemic blasts can avoid the effects of treatment. Unless specific therapy directed at the CNS is given, the risk of sanctuary site relapse is high. CNS prophylaxis usually begins during induction and continues until cessation of overall treatment and entails direct injection of methotrexate, cytarabine and hydrocortisone into the cerebrospinal fluid (intrathecal injection). Cranial irradiation is used less frequently than in the past because of its effects on cognition and brain development.

Maintenance

Maintenance therapy is designed to gradually kill residual leukaemic blasts over a protracted time-span of two to three years. In some centres, boys are generally treated for longer because of the risk of late testicular relapse. There is no benefit in prolonging therapy beyond three years.

Typically, maintenance consists of daily 6-mercaptopurine and weekly methotrexate with periodic intrathecal therapy for CNS prophylaxis. Some centres add intermittent pulses of vincristine-prednisone.

Although 6-mercaptopurine is generally well tolerated, children with an inherited deficiency of thiopurine S-methyltransferase, the enzyme responsible for mercaptopurine inactivation, may experience increased toxicity and so require dose reduction.

Relapsed disease

Around 25% of children with ALL will relapse, mostly with disease restricted to the bone marrow, although CNS and testicular infiltration are more common at relapse than at diagnosis. Relapsed disease is commonly drug-resistant and so requires aggressive re-induction with drugs not used previously. Patients with extramedullary involvement also require local radiotherapy to the relapse site. Relapse in a sanctuary site that has not spread to the bone marrow is often fairly amenable to treatment.

Induction of a second remission is fairly common, but is often short-lived. Early relapse (< 18 months) is associated with a bleak prognosis. Patients who attain a second remission may be considered for allogeneic stem cell transplantation.

11.4   ACUTE LYMPHOBLASTIC LEUKAEMIA/LYMPHOMA IN ADULTS

ALL in adults is biologically different to that in children. Adults usually present with a very short clinical history with symptoms reflecting bone marrow (and frequently extramedullary) leukaemic infiltration. There is a higher incidence of T ALL in adults (around 25%) and of myeloid antigen expression in adult ALL patients, both of which are associated with a poor prognosis. The favourable cytogenetic translocation t(12;21)(p13;q22); (*TEL-AML1*) is much less common and the unfavourable translocation t(9;22)(q34;q11.2); (*BCR-ABL1*) much more common in adults. Similarly, hyperdiploidy is much less common and hypodiploidy significantly more common in adults.

The great advances in treatment seen for children with ALL have not been mirrored for adults, where improvements have been more incremental.

Prognosis of adult ALL

As for children, certain features when present at diagnosis or in the early stages of treatment can be used as predictors of prognosis. In adults, age over 30 years, white cell count $> 30 \times 10^9/l$ (or $> 100 \times 10^9/l$ for T ALL) and the presence of t(9;22)(q34;q11.2); (*BCR-ABL1*), t(4;11)(q21;q23); (*AF4-MLL*), t(1;19)(q23;p13.3); (*TCF3-PBX1*) or hypodiploidy are all unfavourable indicators. In contrast to children, the T ALL immunophenotype is a favourable prognostic indicator in adults, probably because of its association with younger age at presentation and absence of unfavourable cytogenetic markers. The mature B ALL and early T ALL immunophenotypes are associated with a poor prognosis. Finally, achievement of complete remission within four weeks of induction therapy is a favourable prognostic indicator, whereas persistent residual disease at this time point is unfavourable.

Molecular basis of adult ALL

Up to a third of cases of adult ALL have a normal karyotype on conventional cytogenetic analysis, whereas this is much less common (< 10%) in children. However, this does not imply an absence of genetic abnormalities. Dysregulated expression of several T cell developmental regulatory genes, including *HOX11*, *TAL1* and *LYL1* has been demonstrated and associated with favourable (*HOX11*) or unfavourable (*TAL1* and *LYL1*) prognosis in T ALL.

A novel mechanism of oncogene activation that cannot be detected by cytogenetic analysis has been shown to be present in about 5–6% of cases of T ALL. In these cases, extrachromosomal (episomal) amplification of a chimeric *NUP214-ABL1* gene leads to constitutive expression of the aberrant tyrosine kinase. Because the mutation exists on an episome (a form of genetic material that can stably exist independently of chromosomal DNA), the abnormality is cytogenetically invisible. This form of T ALL, as well as those with *BCR-ABL* expression, need to be treated with tyrosine kinase inhibitors such as imatinib, dasatinib or nilotinib, rather than standard therapy.

Clinical management of adult ALL

The broad principles of treatment of adult ALL are similar to those for children: assess risk of relapse prior to treatment and offer more aggressive treatment to patients considered to be high risk.

In general, both standard and high-risk patients are offered remission induction therapy using vincristine, prednisone and an anthracycline such as daunorubicin, doxorubicin or the anthracenedione mitoxantrone. Some centres employ anthracycline dose escalation strategies. The addition of other drugs such as asparaginase or cyclophosphamide has not conclusively been shown to offer benefit. These strategies induce complete remission in up to 80% of cases.

The next phase of treatment for standard-risk adult ALL patients is consolidation/intensification using aggressive combinations of drugs not used during induction. A wide range of different combinations can be used and there is no universal agreement on the optimum content, sequencing or duration of consolidation/intensification therapy.

Maintenance therapy similar to that offered to children is administered to standard-risk adult patients, although its benefit has not been clearly established in clinical trials.

The higher incidence of CNS involvement in the course of adult ALL make CNS prophylaxis using a combination of intrathecal and high-dose chemotherapy mandatory. There is no clear agreement on the optimal combinations and schedule, but it is clear that up to a third of patients will experience CNS relapse without prophylaxis.

High-risk adult patients are offered allogeneic stem cell transplantation (allo-SCT) early in first remission wherever possible. Although procedure-related morbidity and mortality are high with allo-SCT, it offers the best prospect of long-term survival for these patients. Standard-risk patients can be offered autologous stem cell transplantation as an alternative to further chemotherapy, but this procedure is not effective in high-risk patients.

At some point, most adults with ALL undergo relapse. Re-induction of remission using chemotherapy is achievable in around half of cases, but responses are usually of short duration. Allo-SCT may be offered in second remission and has been shown to extend survival but, overall, the prognosis for relapsed adult ALL is very poor.

SUGGESTED FURTHER READING

Dunphy, C.H. (ed.) (2010) *Molecular Pathology of Hematolymphoid Diseases.* Springer.

Mughal, T.I., Goldman, J.M. & Mughal, S.T. (2010) *Understanding Leukemias, Lymphomas and Myelomas* (2nd ed). Informa Healthcare.

Pardee, A.B. & Stein, G.S (2009) *The Biology and Treatment of Cancer: Understanding Cancer.* Wiley-Blackwell.

Pecorino, L. (2008) *Molecular Biology of Cancer: Mechanisms, Targets and Therapeutics.* Oxford University Press.

Swerdlow, S.H., Campo, E., Harris, N.L. *et al.* (eds.) (2008) *WHO Classification of Tumours of Haematopoietic and Lymphoid Tissues, Volume 2.* WHO Press.

SELF-ASSESSMENT QUESTIONS

1. With which FAB type acute leukaemia are the following associated?
   a. bundles of Auer rods
   b. poorly differentiated monoblasts
   c. vacuolated lymphoblasts with deeply basophilic cytoplasm
2. Which of the following cytogenetic abnormalities is commonly associated with AML?
   a. t(8;21)(q22;q22); (*AML1/ETO*)
   b. t(12;21)(p13;q22); (*TEL-AML1*)
   c. t(15;17)(q22;q12); (PML/*RARα*)
   d. t(1;19)(q23;p13.3); (*TCF3-PBX1*)
3. Which of the following are poor prognostic indicators in AML?
   a. age > 60 years
   b. antecedent haematological disorder
   c. FAB type M2
   d. absent Auer rods
   e. CEBPA mutation
4. Which form of AML is most closely associated with disseminated intravascular coagulation?
5. Which acute leukaemia is more common in children, AML or ALL?
6. Which form of ALL is associated with the presence of a mediastinal mass?
7. Which historically poor prognosis form of ALL is recognized by the presence of surface immunoglobulin on the leukaemic blasts?

8. Which of the following numerical chromosomal changes is associated with an unfavourable prognosis in childhood ALL?
   a. hyperdiploidy in the range 51–65 chromosomes
   b. extreme hyperdiploidy (65–84 chromosomes)
   c. near haploidy (23–29 chromosomes)
9. Which of the following cytogenetic abnormalities is associated with a good prognosis in children with ALL?
   a. t(9;22)(q34;q11.2); (*BCR-ABL1*)
   b. t(4;11)(q21;q23); (*AF4-MLL*)
   c. t(12;21)(p13;q22); (*TEL/AML1*)
   d. t(8;14)(v;q24); (*MYC/IGH*)
10. Which drug used in induction therapy of ALL in children is most associated with a temporary increase in thrombotic risk?
11. Is the Philadelphia chromosome more common in adults or children with ALL?

Chronic lymphoid leukaemias

Learning objectives

After studying this chapter you should confidently be able to:

■ **Review the epidemiology, pathophysiology, clinical presentation and diagnosis of the chronic lymphoid leukaemias**
The chronic lymphoid leukaemias (CLL, HCL and PLL) are predominantly diseases of the elderly and share many clinical and biological features. Differential diagnosis of these conditions relies on a combination of clinical and laboratory features such as blood and bone marrow examination, immunophenotyping, cytogenetics and molecular analysis. These features are all reviewed in this chapter.

■ **Outline the staging of CLL**
Although CLL is a relatively indolent disease in many cases, it can follow a more aggressive course from the outset while in others it can transform into a more aggressive terminal phase. This raises the dilemma of when to initiate treatment and how aggressively to treat. Aggressive treatments are associated with significant toxicity and should be administered only where the clinical benefit outweighs the risk. The use of clinical staging and other prognostic indicators offers a mechanism for treatment decisions in CLL. There have been many staging systems proposed in CLL, but only two are widely used, the Rai and Binet systems.

■ **Outline the approaches to treatment of the chronic lymphoid leukaemias**
The first clinical decisions in the management of CLL are whether and when to, rather than how to treat. In contrast to many other haematological malignancies, there is no universally agreed standard treatment for CLL, although certain approaches have been shown to be effective.

The lymphoid neoplasms are derived from cells that normally develop into the different forms of T and B cells, and are further subdivided into neoplasms derived from T and B lymphoid precursors and those derived from mature T and B cells and plasma cells. The traditional clear separation of lymphoid leukaemias and lymphomas into distinct diseases has recently blurred as it has become increasingly clear that this separation is artificial. Indeed, it is now recognized that chronic lymphocytic leukaemia (CLL) and small lymphocytic lymphoma (SLL) are different manifestations of the same disease (see also *Box 12.1*).

Chronic lymphoid leukaemia can be subdivided into three main subtypes: chronic lymphocytic leukaemia (CLL), prolymphocytic leukaemia (PLL) and hairy cell leukaemia (HCL). All are mature B cell neoplasms, although a rare T cell variant of PLL exists.

Box 12.1 Early leukaemia classification

It was Virchow who first proposed that there was more than one form of leukaemia. He suggested that one form was characterized by massive splenomegaly and marked expansion of the numbers of one type of colourless cells in the blood while the other was characterized by swelling of the lymph nodes and an increase in the other main type of colourless blood cells (remember that Romanowsky staining was not yet available and the distinctions between the types of leucocyte were far from clear). Virchow coined the terms 'splenic leukaemia' and 'lymphatic leukaemia' to describe these two types. Several years later, in 1879, it was suggested that the predominant cells in the splenic form of leukaemia emanated from the bone marrow and so the term 'myeloid leukaemia' was coined and gradually came to replace the term 'splenic leukaemia'.

12.1   CHRONIC LYMPHOCYTIC LEUKAEMIA

Chronic lymphocytic leukaemia (CLL) is characterized by a progressive accumulation in the peripheral blood, bone marrow, lymph nodes and spleen of monoclonal, mature-looking, functionally incompetent memory B cells. The disease is the most common of the lymphoid neoplasms and typically follows a relatively indolent course. Because of this it is certainly the most prevalent adult leukaemia in the western world, representing almost a third of cases. There is a marked geographic disparity in CLL incidence; the disease is relatively uncommon in Asian countries, particularly China and Japan. Interestingly, there appears to be a genetic basis for this disparity because CLL remains uncommon in Asian migrants to the West.

CLL is somewhat more common in men than women, with a male:female ratio of about 1.7–2.1:1 (see also *Box 12.2*). The incidence of CLL increases with increasing age; the median age at diagnosis is about 72 years. The disease can occur at any age, but fewer than 3% of cases are diagnosed below the age of 35 years and more than 80% over the age of 60 years.

Box 12.2 Early cases of leukaemia

The earliest known cases of leukaemia involved a 28-year-old slater called John Menteith and a 50-year-old cook called Marie Straide. Menteith was admitted to the Edinburgh Royal Infirmary on 27 February 1845 and Straide was admitted two days later to the Charité Hospital in Berlin. Both succumbed shortly after admission and were examined *post mortem* by Drs Bennett and Virchow respectively. With the benefit of hindsight, it seems likely that both were suffering from CML. Both complained of progressive lethargy and a painful, swollen abdomen, probably reflecting anaemia and massive splenomegaly. Straide also had a severe cough and Menteith had numerous solid tumours scattered about his body, a classical feature of end-stage untreated CML. Ironically, CML is no longer classified as a leukaemia, but as a myeloproliferative disorder (see *Chapter 14*).

There are no definite risk factors for CLL; studies have failed to show any association with exposure to ionizing radiation or antineoplastic drugs. No genes have been definitively identified that predispose to CLL, although a familial association has been identified and there is an over-representation of *ATM* gene mutations and 13q21.33–22.2 abnormalities. First-degree relatives of patients with CLL have a much higher than expected risk of developing the disease, perhaps as much as 30-fold. Studies of some families where CLL incidence is higher than expected across several generations have suggested that a degree of genetic anticipation may be present, with the age at onset being 10–15 years younger than average. The genetic basis for these observations remains obscure.

Pathophysiology of CLL

The cell of origin in CLL has been the subject of debate, but is now definitively known to be an antigen-exposed memory B cell. However, there are two different cell types involved: pre-germinal centre cells that do not have somatic rearrangement of the immunoglobulin heavy chain variable gene complex and post-germinal cells that carry such rearrangements. The CLL cells in individual patients are of one or other type. The presence of a germline immunoglobulin heavy chain variable gene complex is associated with an unfavourable prognosis.

One of the hallmark features of CLL cells is that they are less susceptible to apoptosis than their normal counterparts. This is due to up-regulation of anti-apoptotic proteins of the BCL-2 family (primarily BCL-2, BAX and BAK) and down-regulation of pro-apoptotic proteins including BCL-XL and BAD. Additional abnormalities that impair apoptosis may be present in some cases. For example, *TP53* mutations are present in 10–15% of cases of CLL.

There is evidence that CLL cells can modulate their micro-environment to promote their own growth and survival in a manner analogous to that of myeloma cells (see *Chapter 16*).

Cytogenetics in CLL

Because CLL typically has a very low proliferative index, conventional cytogenetic analysis has been difficult, but suggests that karyotypic abnormalities are present in about half of cases. Using the more sensitive fluorescent *in situ* hybridization (FISH) technique, abnormalities are found in more than 75% of cases, with del13q14 (~55% of cases), del11q22–23 (~18% of cases), trisomy 12q13 (~16% of cases), del17p13 (~7% of cases), del6q21 (~6 of cases) and translocations involving the immunoglobulin heavy chain locus at 14q32 (~7% of cases) being most commonly seen. Individual patients frequently carry more than one cytogenetic abnormality.

The presence of particular cytogenetic abnormalities has prognostic significance. For example, an 11q22–23 deletion is associated with increased lymphadenopathy, splenomegaly, an increased incidence of lymphoma B symptoms (see *Box 12.3*) and is an indicator of unfavourable prognosis, particularly in younger patients. Chromosome 11q also contains the ataxia telangiectasia (*ATM*) gene and loss or mutation of both copies of this gene is an additional indicator of poor prognosis.

Box 12.3 B symptoms

B symptoms are constitutional symptoms (fever, night sweats and unexplained weight loss) that are widely used as markers of advanced disease in lymphoma (see *Chapter 15*). When used in the staging of lymphoma, B symptoms are defined as a fever > 38 °C, severe, drenching night sweats or unexplained loss of at least 10% of body weight in the six months prior to diagnosis.

Deletions involving 17p13 are associated with loss of *TP53* and aggressive, drug-resistant disease with marked lymphocytosis and a shortened survival.

Deletion or rearrangement of 13q14, sometimes with loss of the retinoblastoma (*RB*) tumour suppressor gene, is associated with classical CLL presentation and a favourable prognosis. The deleted region contains two other CLL-related tumour suppressor genes in addition to *RB* (see the section on molecular abnormalities in CLL, below*).

Trisomy 12q13 is associated with atypical CLL features and overexpression of the *MDM-2* at 12q13–15. The prognostic significance of trisomy 12q13 is indeterminate.

Translocations involving the immunoglobulin heavy chain gene locus at 14q32 are fairly common in lymphoproliferative disorders. Common translocation partners include the *BCL-1* gene at 11q13, the cyclin D1 (*CCND1*) at 11q13, the *BCL-2* gene at 18q21 and the *BCL-3* gene at 19q13.1.

Clonal progression occurs in around a third of cases of CLL and is associated with disease progression.

Molecular abnormalities in CLL

BCL-2 is an anti-apoptotic protein whose presence within the cell promotes survival. One of the characteristics of several lymphoproliferative disorders, including CLL, follicular lymphoma (FL) and some cases of diffuse large B cell lymphoma (DLBCL), is overexpression of *BCL-2* (see *Chapter 15*). In FL and DLBCL the mechanism underlying *BCL-2* overexpression is a translocation t(14;18)(q32;q21) that brings the BCL-2 gene in juxtaposition with the immunoglobulin heavy chain gene locus. However, this translocation is found in only about 5% of cases of CLL.

The mechanism of *BCL-2* overexpression in CLL cells is distinct. The common deletion at 13q14 deletes the *RB* tumour suppressor gene only in about half of cases, suggesting that other tumour suppressor genes must be involved. A determined search for protein-coding genes in this region proved fruitless. It is now known that the culprit genes located in this region that lead to *BCL-2* overexpression, *miR-15* and *miR-16-1*, do not encode protein. Instead, they encode two microRNAs, short sequences of RNA that are critically important negative regulators of protein-coding genes. Their deletion or down-regulation in 13q14 mutations leads to *BCL-2* overexpression and is thought to be the key leukaemogenic event in CLL.

Other anti-apoptotic mechanisms operate in many cases of CLL. For example, the tumour suppressor gene *TP53* at 17p13 encodes a protein with multiple cellular roles. p53 acts as a mechanism to prevent cells with damaged DNA from reproducing; it can arrest cells at the G_1-S cell cycle checkpoint and activate DNA repair mechanisms before allowing cell cycle progression. Where DNA damage is severe or irreparable, p53 can initiate apoptosis. Inactivation of *TP53* by deletion or mutation is seen in up to 45% of cases of CLL. P53 protein is negatively regulated by MDM-2, which is overexpressed in the common CLL-associated cytogenetic abnormality trisomy 12q13. Deletion of *TP53* is associated with shorter survival in CLL.

Clinical presentation of CLL

CLL is an indolent disease and patients present with a range of non-specific symptoms, often with a protracted history leading to diagnosis. The most common presenting symptom is painless lymphadenopathy, often in the cervical supraclavicular or axillary regions. Most patients do not feel unwell and the lymph node swelling may tend to wax and wane over time, causing delay in presentation. It is quite common for cases of CLL to be picked up during investigations for another condition or as part of a routine 'wellness' screen.

Less commonly, patients present with symptoms typical of lymphoma 'B symptoms' (see *Chapter 15*). Occasionally, the immune disturbances that accompany CLL can cause autoimmune-mediated haemolysis, thrombocytopenia or pure red cell aplasia and a diagnosis of CLL is made during investigation of these secondary phenomena.

Clinical examination usually reveals generalized or localized lymphadenopathy with firm, non-tender and mobile lymph nodes. Some degree of painless splenomegaly is present in up to half of cases. This may be accompanied by mild hepatomegaly in about a quarter of cases. Skin infiltration by leukaemic cells is sometimes noted.

Diagnosis of CLL

The diagnosis of CLL requires a full blood count with differential, examination of a peripheral blood film and immunophenotyping of the circulating lymphocytes. A bone marrow aspirate and lymph node biopsy are not an absolute requirement but may help to confirm the diagnosis.

The full blood count shows an absolute lymphocytosis, which can be marked, and variable degrees of anaemia and thrombocytopenia. Lymphocyte counts at presentation range widely but most commonly lie between 20 and $50 \times 10^9/l$.

The peripheral blood film confirms the lymphocytosis and characteristically shows small, mature-looking lymphocytes with a narrow rim of featureless, sky blue cytoplasm, moderately condensed nuclear chromatin and an absence of obvious nucleoli. There is usually a second minority population of larger lymphocytes with large nuclei, 'lace-like' nuclear chromatin and obvious nucleoli. The film also often contains 'smudge' or 'smear' cells (lymphocytes disrupted during blood film preparation).

A bone marrow aspirate is normo- or hypercellular, with prominent lymphocytosis (typically > 30%). Erythroid hyperplasia in the bone marrow is strongly indicative of the presence of autoimmune haemolysis, a common complication of CLL. Pure red cell aplasia may also be seen, although much less frequently.

A bone marrow biopsy shows nodular, interstitial or diffuse infiltration by small lymphocytes. Diffuse infiltration is a marker of advanced disease and a poorer prognosis.

Immunophenotyping demonstrates that, contrary to their appearance, CLL cells are functionally and developmentally immature. Characteristically, CLL cells express the B cell associated antigens CD19, CD20 (weak), and CD23, the T cell associated antigen CD5, and show low levels of surface membrane immunoglobulin. Clonality is established by the expression of only one immunoglobulin light chain (i.e. κ or λ but not both). CLL cells are normally negative for cyclin D1 and CD10. FMC7, CD22 and CD79b are also commonly negative or weakly expressed.

A lymph node biopsy is not required for a diagnosis of CLL, but is still a common component of diagnosis of suspected cases of small lymphocytic lymphoma (SLL) when peripheral lymphocytosis, neutropenia and thrombocytopenia are absent. Typically, the lymph node biopsy shows diffuse infiltration with mature-looking, small lymphocytes with effacement of the nodal architecture. There may be a variable population of prolymphocytes and paraimmunoblasts.

Clinical staging and prognosis of CLL

Although CLL is a relatively indolent disease in many cases, it can follow a more aggressive course from the outset while in others it can transform into a more aggressive terminal phase. This raises the dilemma of when to initiate treatment and how aggressively to treat. Aggressive treatments are associated with significant toxicity and should be administered only where the clinical benefit outweighs the risk. The use of clinical staging and other prognostic indicators offers a mechanism for treatment decisions in CLL.

There have been many staging systems proposed in CLL, but only two are widely used, the Rai and Binet systems.

The Rai staging system for CLL

The Rai staging system is based on the assumption that the natural history of CLL is a gradual and progressive accumulation of leukaemic cells with increasingly widespread infiltration involving extramedullary tissues and eventually leading to bone marrow failure. Rai originally proposed a five-stage system as shown in *Table 12.1*.

In practice, the Rai system is simplified to three stages:

■   low-risk disease (Rai stage 0), which accounts for about 25% of cases
■   intermediate-risk disease (Rai stages I and II), which accounts for about 50% of cases
■   high-risk disease (Rai stages III and IV), which accounts for the remaining 25% of cases.

Table 12.1 Rai classification system for CLL

Stage	Definition	Median survival
0	Lymphocytosis*	150 months
I	Lymphocytosis + lymphadenopathy	101 months
II	Lymphocytosis + splenomegaly ± lymphadenopathy	71 months
III	Lymphocytosis + anaemia* ± lymphadenopathy or splenomegaly	19 months
IV	Lymphocytosis + thrombocytopenia* ± anaemia ± splenomegaly ± lymphadenopathy	19 months
*Lymphocytosis defined as $15 \times 10^9/l$ for more than four weeks; anaemia defined as [Hb] < 11.0 g/dl; thrombocytopenia defined as platelet count < $100 \times 10^9/l$		

The Binet staging system for CLL

The Binet staging system is based on similar principles to those of Rai, i.e. that more advanced disease is more widespread. This system uses the number of involved sites and the presence of bone marrow failure to divide patients with CLL into three risk groups. The Binet system recognizes five sites of disease infiltration: the cervical lymph nodes, the axillary lymph nodes, the inguinal lymph nodes, the spleen and the liver. The Binet system is shown in *Table 12.2*.

The Rai and Binet staging systems are most accurate for identifying high-risk disease. The disease course in Rai stage III–IV and Binet stage C is relatively uniformly poor. Within the intermediate and low-risk categories, there remains significant variation in prognosis. There is currently no prognostic indicator that can be used to satisfactorily subdivide these groups, although studies have suggested that two additional markers may be useful:

■ The lymphocyte doubling time (LDT, the time taken for the peripheral blood lymphocyte count to double) provides a useful measure of the aggressiveness of the disease, although its usefulness is limited by the often protracted time required to measure it. In general, an LDT longer than 12 months is an indicator of indolent disease.
■ The pattern of infiltration seen on a bone marrow biopsy has been associated with prognosis, with diffuse infiltration indicating more advanced or more aggressive disease and nodular or interstitial infiltration representing indolent or early disease.

If both of these additional indicators suggest indolent disease, they may identify a subset of patients with low-risk disease in whom the prognosis is no different to that of the general age-matched population.

As in myeloma, the serum β_2-microglobulin level is correlated with tumour burden. This measure is probably more suited to assessment of treatment response rather than prognosis.

The impact of cytogenetic abnormalities and the presence of a germline or rearranged immunoglobulin heavy chain variable gene complex is discussed above.

Table 12.2 Binet classification system for CLL

Stage	Definition	Median survival
A	< 3 involved lymphoid sites	Comparable to age-matched controls
B	≥ 3 involved lymphoid sites	84 months
C	Presence of anaemia and/or thrombocytopenia*	24 months
*Anaemia defined as [Hb] < 10.0 g/dl; thrombocytopenia defined as platelet count < $100 \times 10^9/l$ Some studies have suggested that autoimmune haemolytic anaemia should be excluded from Stage C because it does not confer high risk.		

Transformation of CLL

In a minority of cases, either CLL undergoes transformation to a different lymphoproliferative disorder or the patient develops a second lymphoid malignancy. The most common transformation (about 10% of cases) is into prolymphocytic leukaemia (PLL), but cases of aggressive lymphoma (Richter's transformation), Hodgkin lymphoma and myeloma have all been reported.

Transformation into PLL is accompanied by a change in the morphological appearance of the peripheral blood lymphocytes to larger cells with distinct nucleoli and less dense nuclear chromatin. This phenomenon is a relatively slow process and may take several years. Transformed disease is clinically and immunophenotypically distinct from *de novo* PLL and is typically refractory to treatment.

Richter's transformation is clinically distinct from prolymphocytic transformation in that it follows a more acute course. The first signs of Richter's transformation are usually an acute onset of increasing lymphadenopathy, splenomegaly and appearance or worsening of B symptoms. The clinical course is usually highly aggressive, with a median survival of only a few months.

CLL patients are also at increased risk of developing a second malignancy, most commonly involving bone, skin, thyroid, kidney, mouth or lung.

Clinical management of CLL

The first clinical decisions in the management of CLL are whether and when to treat rather than how to treat. CLL is a heterogeneous disease, affecting a predominantly elderly population. Patients with low-risk indolent disease may have a prognosis similar to age-matched controls, even without treatment. Additionally, current treatment options do not offer the prospect of a cure. Allogeneic stem cell transplantation may be curative, but this option is only available to a tiny minority of patients due to age and comorbidity. Clinical studies have failed to show any benefit of early treatment for Rai stage I/II or Binet stage A disease, and it may actually reduce 10-year overall survival.

Conversely, symptomatic CLL patients and those with advanced stage or progressive disease have a median survival without treatment of 18–36 months. Treatment is indicated for patients with B symptoms, painful lymphadenopathy, symptomatic anaemia and/or thrombocytopenia or progressive disease with an LTD of < 6 months.

As many as one third of CLL patients may never require treatment and will die of unrelated causes. Another third do not require treatment at presentation, but at some stage progress to the point where treatment is indicated. The remaining one third of patients require immediate treatment.

Unlike many other haematological malignancies, there is no single standard treatment for CLL. Treatment options include the alkylating agents chlorambucil or cyclophosphamide, either alone or with concomitant prednisone; purine analogues such as 2′-deoxycoformycin, 2-chlorodeoxyadenosine or fludarabine; monoclonal antibodies such as rituximab (anti-CD20) or alemtuzumab (anti-CD52) or various combinations of these, including fludarabine + cyclophosphamide (FC), fludarabine + rituximab (FR) and fludarabine + cyclophosphamide + rituximab (FCR).

There have been few comparative studies conducted to select the most effective regimen. In general, although there are differences in response rates and toxicities between regimens, overall survival appears to be similar for each of these approaches.

There is no conclusive evidence that consolidation/intensification or maintenance therapy improves outcomes in CLL. Typically then, front-line treatment is continued until a complete response or disease stabilization is obtained or toxicity becomes unacceptable.

A complete response requires all of the following to be present at least three months after completion of treatment:

- absence of constitutional symptoms attributable to CLL
- no lymph nodes > 1.5 cm in diameter on physical examination
- no hepatomegaly or splenomegaly by physical examination
- absolute neutrophil count > $1.5 \times 10^9/l$
- platelet count > $100 \times 10^9/l$
- untransfused [Hb] > 11 g/dl
- absence of clonal lymphocytes in the peripheral blood by immunophenotyping.

Patients with the high-risk cytogenetic abnormalities del17p13 or del11q22–23 are at high risk of treatment failure, either by lack of response to treatment or a short-lived response. It is unclear what the best treatment approach is for such patients. Common approaches include fludarabine-based combination therapy followed by alemtuzumab or non-myeloablative allogeneic haemopoietic stem cell transplantation (mini-allo). The latter option is reserved for younger, fitter patients with a matched related or matched unrelated donor.

12.2 HAIRY CELL LEUKAEMIA

Hairy cell leukaemia (HCL) is an uncommon B lymphoid disorder, accounting for no more than 10% of cases of chronic lymphoid leukaemia. The median age at presentation of HCL is about 52 years. There is a strong male predominance of about 5:1 and the disease is about three times more common in Caucasians than in black people (see also *Box 12.4*).

Box 12.4 Naming hairy cell leukaemia

The name 'hairy cell leukaemia' was coined by Schrek and Donnelly in 1966, but the disease was first described by Bouroncle in 1958 and was then called 'leukaemic reticuloendotheliosis'. The lineage and normal counterpart of the hairy cell was the subject of heated scientific debate for many years, but it is now definitively proven that HCL is a B cell disease.

The normal counterpart of the leukaemic cell in HCL has not been definitively identified, but after many years of controversy, it is clear that this is a B cell disorder. HCL cells typically show clonal rearrangements of immunoglobulin light and heavy chain genes and express monoclonal surface immunoglobulin, CD19, CD20, and CD22, as well as the early plasma cell marker PCA-1. Additionally, non-B cell markers are commonly expressed, including CD11c (a monocyte and neutrophil marker), CD25 (an activated T cell marker) and CD103 (an intraepithelial T cell marker). These findings are consistent with the normal counterpart being pre-plasma cell or a post-germinal centre memory B cell.

Cytogenetic abnormalities are found in about 60–70% of cases of HCL, with trisomy 5, rearrangements involving 5q13, 15p13 deletion, 14q32 rearrangements and 12p abnormalities being relatively common. Abnormalities involving 5q13 are not commonly found in other B cell malignancies.

In most cases of HCL, the immunoglobulin heavy chain variable genes are rearranged. In a minority of cases, germline arrangement is seen, and this is associated with an unfavourable prognosis.

Clinical presentation of HCL

There are few characteristic presenting features of HCL, although most symptoms are attributable to cytopenias (weakness, fatigue, bruising or bleeding and recurrent infection) and splenomegaly (abdominal fullness or discomfort). Many patients are asymptomatic at diagnosis. Classical

B symptoms are rare in HCL. About a quarter of patients have hepatomegaly. Peripheral lymphadenopathy is seen in less than 10% of cases, although deep abdominal and mediastinal lymphadenopathy may be present.

Diagnosis of HCL

About three quarters of cases present with moderate pancytopenia. Examination of a peripheral blood film reveals the presence of the eponymous 'hairy' cells. These are mononuclear cells, typically larger than normal small lymphocytes, with eccentric nuclei of variable appearance, reticular chromatin and indistinct nucleoli. The defining feature of these cells is the abundant, pale cytoplasm with multiple projections that give the cell its 'hairy' appearance. These projections are often indistinct on light microscopy, but are more obvious on phase contrast or scanning electron microscopy. Often, the typical hairy cells represent less than 10% of the mononuclear cells. Set against a reduced white cell count, this can mean that a determined search is required to identify these cells on a blood film. Occasionally, a patient presents with a leucocytosis, with hairy cells being the predominant cell type.

Attempts to obtain a bone marrow aspirate frequently result in a 'dry tap' due to marrow fibrosis. A bone marrow trephine biopsy is an important component of the diagnosis of HCL and is usually hypercellular with leukaemic infiltration best seen using immunohistochemical staining for B cell markers such as CD20. The pattern of infiltration may be diffuse, focal or interstitial. Less commonly, the marrow may be hypocellular, with smaller numbers of leukaemic cells. There is usually moderate to severe fibrosis of the marrow, with reticulin fibres associated with leukaemic cells, but extending into normal haemopoietic tissue.

In the past, the diagnosis of HCL would be clinched by the demonstration of tartrate-resistant acid phosphatase in the leukaemic cells. However, this test is no longer widely used and has been replaced by immunophenotyping.

The typical pattern of expression of the leukaemic cells in HCL is strong positivity for surface immunoglobulin and the pan-B cell antigens CD19, CD20, CD22 and CD25, negativity for CD5, CD10, CD21 and CD23 and positivity for the non-B cell markers CD11c (a monocyte and neutrophil marker), CD25 (an activated T cell marker) and CD103 (an intraepithelial T cell marker). A marker that is useful to differentiate HCL from other B cell leukaemia / lymphomas is overexpression of the annexin1 (*ANXA1*) gene. Annexin1 overexpression can easily be assessed immunohistochemically.

Variant HCL

A variant of HCL exists (about 10% of cases) that is clinically and biologically distinct. This form often presents with marked leucocytosis and is associated with an older median age at diagnosis (about 70 years). Morphologically, the leukaemic cells have a more prolymphocytic or blastic appearance and prominent nucleoli. Marrow fibrosis is less obvious and the immunophenotype is distinct (negative for CD25, HC-2, and CD123, and positive for CD27; CD103 can be negative or positive). Cytogenetic abnormalities of chromosome 5 are typically absent.

The treatment required for variant HCL is different: responses to interferon and purine analogues are poor, with monoclonal antibody-based therapy (rituximab or alemtuzumab), with or without concomitant chemotherapy, proving more useful. The prognosis for variant HCL is shorter, with a median overall survival of 9 years compared to more than 12 years for classical HCL.

Clinical management of HCL

HCL is typically an indolent disease and many patients do not require treatment at presentation. There is no clear benefit to early intervention, so most physicians adopt a 'watch and wait' policy until patients develop significant cytopenias, symptomatic splenomegaly or symptomatic lymphadenopathy or B symptoms.

The treatment options available for frontline treatment of HCL include splenectomy, interferon α, and the purine analogues 2′-deoxycoformycin or 2-chlorodeoxyadenosine. Most physicians employ cytotoxic chemotherapy with either of the purine analogues. Using these agents, complete response rates of 80–90% are attainable, with four-year disease-free survival rates of more than 90%.

Interferon α is best reserved for patients who fail to respond to purine analogues, but long-term maintenance therapy may be required.

Splenectomy is offered much less commonly nowadays, but may still be an option where splenomegaly is troublesome or where cytotoxic chemotherapy is best avoided, e.g. during pregnancy.

Up to half of HCL patients who respond to purine analogues will relapse within 10 years. Second, and even third, responses to purine analogues can be obtained in the great majority of patients, although the duration of response is shorter. Patients who fail reinduction with purine analogues are offered interferon α or monoclonal antibody-based treatment.

12.3 B-PROLYMPHOCYTIC LEUKAEMIA

B-prolymphocytic leukaemia (B-PLL) is a rare condition that primarily affects the elderly, with a median age at presentation of around 65–70 years. The leukaemic cell is a mature, activated B cell (see *Box 12.5*). The male:female ratio is close to 1:1. B-PLL is seen most commonly in Caucasians.

Box 12.5 Naming PLL

Prolymphocytic leukaemia was originally thought to be a variant of CLL. The term 'prolymphocytic' was used to signify the immaturity of the leukaemic cells relative to those of CLL, which were thought to be mature. However, the judgement on the relative maturity of the leukaemic cells in PLL was based entirely on morphological grounds and was incorrect. In fact, B-PLL is a malignancy of mature B cells.

Typical presenting features include weakness and fatigue due to anaemia, abnormal bruising due to thrombocytopenia, abdominal discomfort due to marked splenomegaly and constitutional B symptoms are common. Peripheral lymphadenopathy is usually absent or minor.

Marked lymphocytosis is usually present and the blood film shows that more than half (often up to 90%) of the mononuclear cells are leukaemic cells. Morphologically, B-PLL cells are larger than a typical small lymphocyte with a round or oval nucleus that contains moderately condensed chromatin and a prominent nucleolus. The cytoplasm is abundant and mildly basophilic. The bone marrow smear shows extensive infiltration with these leukaemic cells and the biopsy typically shows a nodular or interstitial pattern of infiltration.

The immunophenotype of B-PLL shows strong surface immunoglobulin (IgM ± IgD, monoclonal κ or λ light chain), strong CD20 (a useful differentiator from CLL, which usually shows dim expression of surface immunoglobulin and CD20), CD19, CD22, CD79a, and FMC7 with an absence of CD11c, CD103, CD10, CD25, and cyclin D1. About half of cases express ZAP-70 and CD38 and about 30% express CD5 and CD23.

In common with other B cell malignancies, deletions of 17p, p53 mutations and rearrangements involving 13q14 are common. Patients with B-PLL morphology and t(11;14) (q13;q32) involving the *CCND1* gene are classified as having a leukaemic variant of mantle cell lymphoma (MCL). The molecular basis of B-PLL is poorly characterized but overexpression of *MYC* and *AKT* genes and down-regulation of *P53* are common.

There is no standard treatment approach for B-PLL, although most patients receive some combination of purine analogue and monoclonal antibody-based therapy. Median survival is about three years.

12.4   T-PROLYMPHOCYTIC LEUKAEMIA

T-PLL is an extremely rare condition with a median age at diagnosis of 65 years and a male:female ratio of about 1.3:1. There is an association between T-PLL and patients with ataxia telangiectasia. The presentation of T-PLL is similar to that of B-PLL, although skin involvement and serous effusions are more common. The morphology of the leukaemic cells is similar to that of B-PLL cells in the majority of cases, although variant morphology also exists.

T-PLL is distinguished by strong expression of CD52 and the pan-T cell markers CD2, CD3 and CD7. Terminal deoxynucleotidyl transferase (TdT) is absent. About 25% of cases coexpress CD4 and CD8, a useful marker of T-PLL.

Cytogenetic abnormalities are common in T-PLL and particularly include abnormalities of chromosome 14 (e.g. inv(14), t(14;14)(q11;q32) and t(X;14)(q28;q11) with overexpression of the *TCL1* or *MTCP1* genes). Other abnormalities associated with T-PLL include: idic(8p11), t(8;8), and trisomy 8q, del(12p13), abnormalities in chromosome 6 and 17, P53 deletion and deletions or missense mutations of the *ATM* gene.

T-PLL is a highly aggressive condition with a median survival of only a few months.

SUGGESTED FURTHER READING

Dunphy, C.H. (ed.) (2010) *Molecular Pathology of Hematolymphoid Diseases.* Springer.

Mughal, T.I., Goldman, J.M. & Mughal, S.T. (2010) *Understanding Leukemias, Lymphomas and Myelomas* (2nd ed). Informa Healthcare.

Swerdlow, S.H., Campo, E., Harris, N.L. *et al.* (eds.) (2008) *WHO Classification of Tumours of Haematopoietic and Lymphoid Tissues, Volume 2.* WHO Press.

Tuffaha, M.S.A. (2008) *Phenotypic and Genotypic Diagnosis of Malignancies: An Immunohistochemical and Molecular Approach.* WileyVCH.

SELF-ASSESSMENT QUESTIONS

1. Which of the following cytogenetic abnormalities is seen most commonly in CLL?
    a.   del17p13
    b.   del11q22–23
    c.   del13q14
    d.   trisomy 12q13
    e.   del6q21

2. Which of the following cytogenetic abnormalities is associated with younger patients, increased lymphadenopathy, splenomegaly and an increased incidence of lymphoma B symptoms, and is an indicator of unfavourable prognosis in CLL?
    a.   del17p13
    b.   del11q22–23
    c.   del13q14

  d. trisomy 12q13

  e. del6q21

3. Name the two genes located at 13q14 that encode microRNAs and regulate *BCL-2* expression.

4. Three patterns of marrow infiltration can be seen in CLL; nodular, interstitial or diffuse. Which is indicative of more advanced disease?

5. A case of CLL has a lymphocyte count of $23.0 \times 10^9/l$ and lymphadenopathy but no splenomegaly, thrombocytopenia or anaemia. What is the Rai stage?

6. If in the case above, the lymphadenopathy involves three sites, what is the Binet stage?

7. Name the monocyte / neutrophil marker, activated T cell marker and intraepithelial T cell marker characteristically expressed on HCL cells.

8. Which of the following are purine analogues?

  a. interferon α

  b. 2′-deoxycoformycin

  c. methotrexate

  d. busulfan

  e. 2-chlorodeoxyadenosine

CHAPTER 13

The myelodysplastic syndromes

> **Learning objectives**
> *After studying this chapter you should confidently be able to:*
>
> ■ **Define myelodysplastic syndromes**
> Myelodysplastic syndromes (MDS) are a clinically diverse group of malignant diseases characterized by marrow hypercellularity and ineffective haemopoiesis with consequent peripheral blood cytopenia and dysplasia / dysfunction of one or more cell lines.
>
> ■ **Outline the FAB and WHO classification systems for the myelodysplastic syndromes**
> The FAB classification scheme divides the MDS into five subgroups, based on morphological findings in blood and bone marrow: refractory anaemia, refractory anaemia with ring sideroblasts, refractory anaemia with excess blasts, refractory anaemia with excess blasts in transformation and chronic myelomonocytic leukaemia. This system is widely used in clinical practice. The WHO system differentiates between dysplasia of one or more cell lines and takes account of cytogenetic abnormalities. This system does not recognize refractory anaemia with excess blasts in transformation or chronic myelomonocytic leukaemia as forms of MDS.
>
> ■ **Outline the diagnostic criteria for the myelodysplastic syndromes**
> Anaemia or cytopenia that does not respond to haematinics in an elderly patient raises the clinical suspicion of MDS. There may be a history of bruising or recurrent infection. Splenomegaly is typically absent. Laboratory investigation confirms the peripheral cytopenia(s) and any of a wide range of dysplastic features. The bone marrow aspirate is typically hypercellular, with ineffective haemopoiesis and variable ring sideroblasts. Cytogenetic analysis is an important facet of determining the prognosis and treatment plan and abnormalities are demonstrable in about half of MDS patients.
>
> ■ **Outline the approaches to treatment of the myelodysplastic syndromes**
> The treatment options for MDS include supportive care, low-intensity therapy, and high-intensity therapy. The decision on treatment approach is usually based on prognostic score and the patient's ability to tolerate treatment.

13.1   WHAT ARE MYELODYSPLASTIC SYNDROMES?

Myelodysplastic syndromes (MDS) are a group of diseases that are characterized by marrow hypercellularity and ineffective haemopoiesis with consequent peripheral blood cytopenia. There is clear evidence of dysplasia and dysfunction of one or more cell lines, although lymphocytes are unaffected.

The underlying cause of MDS is a chromosomal abnormality that develops in a multipotent haemopoietic stem cell that triggers increased haemopoietic proliferation but abnormal haemopoietic maturation. There is a markedly increased rate of apoptosis in haemopoietic precursor cells. The result is the apparent contradiction of a highly haemopoietically active bone marrow, but a lack of mature circulating blood cells. In some cases, there may be immune-mediated suppression of normal haemopoiesis.

The myelodysplastic syndromes are clinically diverse, with a median survival ranging from one to more than 10 years. There is a tendency for progression to acute myeloid leukaemia (AML), and MDS is sometimes thought of as a preleukaemic condition. However, many patients will succumb to the effects of bone marrow failure, including infection and bleeding, before transformation.

MDS is classified by bone marrow and peripheral blood counts and morphology, but there is also a clinically important distinction between 'primary' or '*de novo*' MDS where the cause is unknown and 'secondary' MDS which results from prior cancer chemotherapy or exposure to an environmental toxin. About 60–70% of MDS is of the primary type. This distinction is clinically important because patients with secondary MDS are typically much less likely to respond to treatment.

13.2   EPIDEMIOLOGY

MDS is predominantly a disease of older adults. About 80–90% of all patients are older than 60 years. The reported incidence of MDS varies from 2.1 to 12.6 cases per 100 000 population per year, but approaches 50 cases per 100 000 population per year in patients over the age of 70 years. The exact incidence of MDS is difficult to quantify because of the complexity of diagnosis and classification. Furthermore, until 2001, MDS was not a reportable condition, so precise incidence data were not included in most population-based cancer registries (see also *Box 13.1*).

Box 13.1 Reportable cancers

A reportable cancer is one that doctors are required to report to their local or national cancer registry. Most cancer registries consider cancers listed in the International Classification of Diseases for Oncology, Third Edition (ICD-O-3) to be reportable. The purpose of designating a disease as reportable or notifiable is to permit surveillance and determination of incidence and prevalence data that can be used for epidemiological and outcomes research.

The most important risk factors for MDS are advancing age and male gender. Other important risk factors for the development of MDS are listed in *Table 13.1*.

Previous cancer chemotherapy predisposes to MDS development because of the genotoxic nature of many cytotoxic agents. In particular, exposure to mechlorethamine, procarbazine, chlorambucil, etoposide, teniposide, and to a certain extent, cyclophosphamide or doxorubicin, is associated with an increased risk. The risk is further increased by combination chemotherapy and radiation treatment. Secondary MDS commonly occurs in patients who have been treated for Hodgkin's disease, non-Hodgkin's lymphoma, or childhood acute lymphoblastic leukaemia (ALL). About 10–20% of MDS cases are secondary to previous cancer chemotherapy. Typically, secondary MDS is more difficult to treat than *de novo* MDS.

Prolonged or heavy exposure to environmental toxins, such as benzene, organic solvents, certain pesticides or ionizing radiation has also been linked to secondary MDS. Cigarette smoking is the only known lifestyle-related risk factor for secondary MDS and is also a known risk factor for AML. Certain rare congenital diseases such as Fanconi anaemia are also associated with secondary MDS.

Table 13.1 Risk factors for MDS

Previous cancer therapy
Mechlorethamine
Procarbazine
Chlorambucil
Etoposide
Teniposide (with or without concomitant radiation therapy)
Other chemotherapy agents
Exposure to environmental toxins
Benzene and other organic solvents
Pesticides
Ionizing radiation
Cigarette smoking
Congenital disorders
Familial disorder
Advanced age
Male gender

13.3   CLASSIFICATION OF MDS

The presentation of MDS is highly variable, but about 90% of cases are anaemic and up to 50% are pancytopenic. In addition, a wide range of dysplastic and dysfunctional states may be present. None of these features are, in themselves, diagnostic of MDS. Rather, it is the pattern of refractory cytopenia with dysplastic features affecting all three cell lines in an elderly person which suggests the diagnosis. However, before a diagnosis of MDS can be made, it is important to exclude all other potential causes of cytopenia or dysplasia.

The FAB classification system

The FAB classification scheme divides the MDS into five subgroups, based on morphological findings in blood and bone marrow (see *Box 13.2*). This system is widely used in clinical practice and has been validated as having prognostic significance, as described below.

The FAB classification scheme is shown in *Table 13.2*.

Box 13.2 FAB and MDS

When the original FAB classification scheme for acute leukaemia was proposed in 1976, a group of conditions called the dysmyelopoietic syndromes were defined, but were not included in the scheme. At this stage two types of dysmyelopoietic syndrome were recognized; refractory anaemia with excess blasts (RAEB) and chronic myelomonocytic leukaemia (CMML). In the years that followed, it rapidly became apparent that the range of morphological appearances in the MDS was very wide and that there was some correlation between morphological subtypes and the risk of transformation to AML. In 1982, a more detailed FAB classification scheme for the MDS was proposed which took account of these findings.

Table 13.2 FAB classification system for MDS

MDS subtype	Bone marrow			Blood		
	% blasts	Auer rods	Ring sideroblasts	% blasts	% monocytes	% MDS diagnoses
RA	< 5%	No	< 15%	< 1%	–	10–40%
RARS	< 5%	No	> 15%	< 1%	–	10–35%
RAEB	5–20%	No	–	< 5%	–	25–30%
RAEB-t	21–29%	Yes/No	–	> 5%	–	10–30%
CMML	< 20%	No	–	< 5%	> 1x10⁹/l	10–20%

RA, refractory anaemia; RARS, refractory anaemia with ring sideroblasts; RAEB, refractory anaemia with excess blasts; RAEB-t, refractory anaemia with excess blasts in transformation; CMML, chronic myelomonocytic leukaemia.

Refractory anaemia (RA)

Up to 40% of MDS cases are classified as RA. The typical picture includes a macrocytic or, less commonly, normocytic anaemia and reticulocytopenia which does not respond to haematinic therapy. Basophilic stippling is commonly present (see *Box 13.3*). In some cases, dysplastic features are restricted to the red cells but, typically, features such as neutropenia with hypogranular and hypolobulated neutrophils and thrombocytopenia with large, agranular platelets also are present. Up to 90% of cases of RA at presentation are pancytopenic. Bone marrow examination typically reveals hypercellularity with dysplastic, normoblastic or megaloblastic erythropoiesis. Ring sideroblasts are present but do not exceed 15% of the erythroblasts present. The blast cell count is always less than 5% of the total nucleated cells. Fewer than 10% of the patients with RA develop AML. Eventually succumbing to complications associated with having a low blood count (such as infection) or unrelated disease, patients with RA have a median survival of about 4 years. Some patients will live longer than 10 years. RA is the most benign form of MDS.

Box 13.3 Basophilic stippling

The term basophilic stippling describes red cell inclusions, which are composed of ribonucleoprotein and mitochondrial remnants. They are seen on Romanowsky stained blood films as diffuse or punctate cytoplasmic granules. These inclusions are not specific for MDS. They are also seen in toxic states such as lead poisoning.

Refractory anaemia with ring sideroblasts (RARS)

RARS constitutes about 20% of cases of MDS. It is characterized at presentation by the presence of anaemia and a dual red cell population: a major population of normochromic macrocytes and a minor population of hypochromic microcytes. Typically, the serum iron, ferritin concentration and transferrin saturation are all raised and Pappenheimer bodies and basophilic stippling are present. Neutropenia, thrombocytopenia and trilineage dysplasia are much less common than in RA. The bone marrow is typically hypercellular with prominent normoblastic or megaloblastic erythroid hyperplasia and dysplasia. The defining feature for a diagnosis of RARS is that ring sideroblasts should comprise at least 15% of the erythroblasts present and that blast cells should comprise less than 5% of the total of nucleated cells in the bone marrow (see *Box 13.4*). Fewer than 5% of patients with RARS develop AML, and the median survival is about 4½ years.

> **Box 13.4 Sideroblasts and siderocytes**
>
> A sideroblast is a nucleated red cell that contains stainable iron granules. These granules are iron-laden mitochondria. A ring sideroblast occurs when the poisoned mitochondria encircle the nucleus, forming a necklace-like appearance. Ring sideroblasts are not specific to MDS (see *Chapter 4*, sideroblastic anaemias). They are seen in a wide range of haematological conditions but are usually relatively few in number. A mature red cell with stainable iron granules (Pappenheimer bodies) is known as a siderocyte.

Refractory anaemia with excess blasts (RAEB)

RAEB constitutes up to 25% of MDS and is a much more aggressive disease than RA or RARS. It is characterized at presentation by symptomatic anaemia, neutropenia and thrombocytopenia. Trilineage dysplasia is more common and tends to be more severe than in the relatively benign forms of the MDS. Blast cells are typically present in the peripheral blood but do not exceed 5% of the total of nucleated cells. Bone marrow examination reveals a variable number of ring sideroblasts and a blast cell count of between 5 and 20% of the total nucleated cell count. This is a more serious form of the disease in which patients have a 20–30% chance of developing AML and a median survival of only about two years.

Refractory anaemia with excess blasts in transformation

A case of RAEB is said to be in transformation to acute leukaemia (RAEB-t) when any of three markers are present:

- A peripheral blood blast cell count that exceeds 5% of the total of nucleated cells
- Auer rods in the blast cells in the peripheral blood
- A bone marrow blast cell population that exceeds 20% of the total of nucleated cells.

If blast cells exceed 30% of the total nucleated cells in the bone marrow, transformation to acute leukaemia is complete. Typically, such cases are profoundly neutropenic and thrombocytopenic and trilineage dysplasia is almost universal. Some degree of hepatosplenomegaly is commonly present.

Auer rods may or may not be present. About 75% of the patients with this condition develop AML, and in the newer WHO classification system RAEBt is classified as AML rather than as a subtype of MDS. The median survival of patients with this disorder is only about six months. The high mortality rate of this disorder results from not only the proliferative advantage of the malignant cells, but also their ability to suppress the growth and maturation of normal blood cells, by mechanisms not fully understood, resulting in anaemia, neutropenia and thrombocytopenia.

Although both RAEB and AML are associated with peripheral blood cytopenia despite the presence of a hypercellular bone marrow, the mechanisms involved are quite different. In acute leukaemia, the pancytopenia is directly related to the dominance of leukaemic blast cells in the marrow, whereas in RAEB it is the result of ineffective haemopoiesis, i.e. a large proportion of the cells produced are morphologically and functionally defective and are doomed to die in the bone marrow. Further, trilineage dysplasia is invariably present in RAEB while it is infrequent in *de novo* AML.

Chronic myelomonocytic leukaemia

CMML is characterized at presentation by hepatosplenomegaly, a peripheral blood monocyte count that exceeds $1 \times 10^9/l$ and monocytic dysplasia. Anaemia and thrombocytopenia are much less common than in other types of the MDS. Where present, the anaemia is usually normocytic and normochromic but macrocytes, microcytes and siderocytes may all be present. Dysplastic features are commonly present but trilineage dysplasia is not as common as in other types of the MDS. Typically, the bone marrow is hypercellular with dysplastic promonocytes being especially prominent. The blast and ring sideroblast counts vary but seldom exceed 20% of the total. The median survival is about three years.

The WHO classification system

Since 1982, the FAB classification of MDS had been the universal standard and had been validated as having clinical relevance. However, FAB does not differentiate between dysplasia of one or more cell lines and does not take account of cytogenetic abnormalities. The subgroups can include patients with widely different clinical outcomes. The WHO system was designed to overcome these criticisms by relying more heavily on evidence of dysplasia, and taking account of the number of cell lines affected. *Table 13.3* summarizes the WHO classification system.

Refractory cytopenia with unilineage dysplasia (RCUD)

The WHO system recognizes a category of MDS within which the dysplasia is restricted to a single cell line. By far the most common member of this group is refractory anaemia (RA), which is described in both the FAB and WHO classification systems as primarily affecting the red cell line, having no detectable blasts in the peripheral blood and less than 5% blasts in the marrow. The other members of this group are designated as refractory neutropenia (RN), which is characterized by unilineage granulocytic dysplasia and neutropenia and refractory thrombocytopenia (RT), which is characterized by unilineage megakaryocytic dysplasia and thrombocytopenia.

The WHO classification system specifically states that the marrow contains less than 15% ring sideroblasts.

Refractory anaemia with ring sideroblasts (RARS)

The criteria for refractory anaemia with ring sideroblasts (RARS) are the same as those for RA except that the bone marrow contains at least 15% ring sideroblasts.

Refractory cytopenia with multilineage dysplasia (RCMD)

The WHO system contains two categories of MDS that are similar to RA and RARS, except that the dysplasia is not limited to the red cell line. In RCMD and RCMD-RS, there is a deficiency in more than one cell line and dysplasia is present in at least 10% of the bone marrow cells in at least two cell lines. In an earlier iteration of the WHO classification system, two distinct RCMD entities were defined: RCMD and RCMD-RS in which there were ≥ 15% ring sideroblasts in the bone marrow. These two entities have been merged in the latest iteration.

RAEB-1 and RAEB-2

Refractory anaemia with excess blasts is subdivided into two categories, designated RAEB-1 and RAEB-2 in the WHO system. Both involve unilineage or multilineage dysplasia and deficiencies in one or more types of circulating blood cell. In RAEB-1, 5–9% of the cells in the marrow are blasts and the peripheral blood contains up to 4% blasts. Auer rods (typically seen in patients with AML) are generally absent. There is a 25% risk for disease progression to AML. In RAEB-2, the marrow contains 10–19% blasts, and the peripheral blood contains 5–19% blasts. Auer rods may or may not be present and the risk of developing AML increases to about 33%.

MDS with isolated del(5q)

Patients designated as MDS with isolated del(5q) have a deletion in the q arm of chromosome 5, which contains genes that code for several important haemopoietic growth factors, and typically

Table 13.3 WHO classification system for MDS

MDS subtype	Blood findings	Bone marrow findings
RCUD		
RA	Anaemia	Erythroid dysplasia only (≥ 10% of cells)
RN	No or rare blasts	< 5% blasts
RT	Neutropenia	< 15% ring sideroblasts
	No or rare blasts	Granulocytic dysplasia
	Thrombocytopenia	< 5% blasts
	No or rare blasts	Megakaryocytic dysplasia
		< 5% blasts
RARS	Anaemia	Erythroid dysplasia only
	No blasts	< 5% blasts
		≥ 15% ring sideroblasts
RCMD	Bi- or pancytopenia	Dysplasia in ≥ 10% of cells in two or more myeloid cell lines ± ring sideroblasts
	No or rare blasts	< 5% blasts
	No Auer rods	No Auer rods
RAEB-1	Cytopenias	Unilineage or multilineage dysplasia
	< 5% blasts	5–9% blasts
	No Auer rods	No Auer rods
RAEB-2	Cytopenias	Unilineage or multilineage dysplasia
	5–19% blasts	10–19% blasts
	± Auer rods	± Auer rods
MDS-U	Cytopenias	Does not fit other categories
	No or rare blasts	Dysplasia and < 5% blasts OR
		Absence of dysplasia with MDS-associated karyotype
MDS with del(5q)	Anaemia	Normal to increased megakaryocytes with hypolobated nuclei
	< 1% blasts	< 5% blasts
	Platelets normal/ increased	No Auer rods
		Isolated del(5q)

RCUD, refractory cytopenia with unilineage dysplasia; RA, refractory anaemia; RN, refractory neutropenia; RT, refractory thrombocytopenia; RARS, refractory anaemia with ring sideroblasts; RCMD, refractory cytopenia with multilineage dysplasia; RCMD-RS, refractory cytopenia with multilineage dysplasia and ring sideroblasts; RAEB-1, refractory anaemia with excess blasts-1; RAEB-2, refractory anaemia with excess blasts-2; MDS-U, myelodysplastic syndrome, unclassified.

Box 13.5 Recognition of 5q– syndrome

Van den Berghe *et al.* first described refractory macrocytic anaemia associated with deletion of the long arm of chromosome 5, in 1974. The condition was originally known as Belgian disease or *'anémie refractaire de type belge'*, and is characterized clinically by a higher female preponderance, refractory macrocytic anaemia, normal or high platelet counts, hypolobulated megakaryocytes and slight leucopenia. Although the limits of 5q deletions vary among patients with 5q– syndrome, the most frequent deletion is del(5)(q13q33) and, in nearly all cases studied, the critical region of deletion includes 5q31.

have less than 5% blasts in the bone marrow and up to 4% blasts in the peripheral blood (see also Box 13.5). Anaemia is common and the platelet count may be normal or increased. Marrow megakaryocytes may be increased. Patients with this subgroup have a relatively good prognosis compared to those with other forms of MDS.

Myelodysplastic syndrome, unclassifiable (MDS-U)

A small minority of cases of MDS do not fit neatly into any of the established categories and so are grouped together as MDS-U. To qualify for this classification, all other possible diagnoses should be carefully excluded. Cases of refractory cytopenia that lack a high enough blast count or sufficient signs of dysplasia can be accorded a presumptive diagnosis of MDS-U if any of the following cytogenetic abnormalities are also present: -7, del(7q), -5, del(5q), i(17q), t(17p), -13, del(13q), del(11q), del(12p) or t(12p), del(9q), idic(X)(q13), t(11;16)(q23;p13.3), t(3;21) (q26;q22.1), t(1;3)(p36.3;q21.2), t(2;11)(p21;q23), inv(3)(q21q26.2), t(6;9)(p23;q34). This listing of cytogenetic abnormalities that allow a diagnosis of MDS-U excludes some abnormalities that are commonly seen in MDS, such as +8, -Y and del(20q).

Table 13.4 shows the median survival for patients within each of the WHO classification categories.

Table 13.4 Median survival for WHO classification system MDS subgroups

MDS subtype	Median survival (years)
Refractory anaemia (RA)	5.5
Refractory anaemia with ring sideroblasts (RARS)	5.5
Refractory cytopenia with multilineage dysplasia (RCMD)	3
Refractory cytopenia with multilineage dysplasia and ring sideroblasts (RCMD-RS)	3
Refractory anaemia with excess blasts-1 (RAEB-1)	1.5
Refractory anaemia with excess blasts-2 (RAEB-2)	1
Myelodysplastic syndrome, unclassified (MDS-U)	3.7
MDS associated with isolated del(5q)	10

Risk levels and prognosis

The myelodysplastic syndromes are clinically diverse, ranging from a relatively benign condition to aggressive malignancy with a short median survival. Even within subgroups, survival can vary significantly. Identifying the likely prognosis of individual patients aids therapeutic decision-making.

In 1996, a group of MDS experts developed the International Prognostic Scoring System (IPSS) in an attempt to standardize risk assessment. IPSS is now the *de facto* standard for risk assessment in MDS. The system assigns a risk level to each case of MDS based on three major factors:

- the bone marrow blast count
- the cytogenetic risk profile
- the number of cytopenias.

In the IPSS:

- the greater the number of blasts present in the bone marrow, the higher the score
- cytogenetic profile is categorized as 'good' if the chromosomes are normal, or if the only abnormality is an absent Y chromosome, del(5q) or del(20q). Abnormalities in chromosome 7 or a combination of three or more abnormalities are characterized as 'poor'. Any other type of chromosome abnormality is characterized as 'intermediate'
- cytopenias are defined as a haemoglobin level of < 10.0 g/dl, a platelet count < 100 × 10^9/l and an absolute neutrophil count < 1.5 × 10^9/l.

Tables 13.5 and *13.6* show how the IPSS scoring system works. The first step is to obtain a score value, based on the factors listed above (see *Table 13.5*). For example, a patient presenting with a marrow blast count of 6%, normal cytogenetics and isolated neutropenia would have scores of 0.5 + 0 + 0. The patient's condition is then categorized as low, intermediate or high risk, based on the total score (see *Table 13.6*).

Table 13.5 The International Prognostic Scoring System (IPSS) for MDS

Score value					
Prognostic variable	**IPSS score**				
	0	0.5	1.0	1.5	2.0
Bone marrow blasts	< 5%	5–10%	—	11–20%	21–30%
Cytogenetic risk	Good	Intermediate	Poor	—	—
Cytopenias	0 or 1 lineage	2 or 3 lineages	—	—	—

Table 13.6 IPSS risk group scores

Risk group	Score
Low	0
Intermediate-1	0.5–1.0
Intermediate-2	1.5–2.0
High	≥ 2.5

The lifetime risk of evolution to AML can be estimated using the IPSS (see *Table 13.7*). For low-risk patients, median survival is 5.7 years, while for high-risk patients median survival is only about 5 months.

In 2005, a new prognostic scoring system that utilizes the WHO classification system (the WPSS) was proposed. The WPSS includes three variables:

- WHO subtype, replacing the blast percentage in the IPSS
- blood transfusion requirements, defined as none or regular if one or more unit of blood is needed every eight weeks. This replaces the cytopenia category in the IPSS
- cytogenetics as defined by the IPSS.

Table 13.7 Median survival and risk of AML evolution by IPSS score

	IPSS risk group			
	Low	**Intermediate-1**	**Intermediate-2**	**High**
Score	0	0.5–1.0	1.5–2.0	≥ 2.5
Lifetime AML evolution	19%	30%	33%	45%
Median years to AML	9.4	3.3	1.1	0.2
Median survival (years)	5.7	3.5	1.2	0.4

In a similar way to the IPSS, each of these variables is associated with a score, allowing patients to be grouped into five risk groups. *Tables 13.8* and *13.9* summarize the WPSS.

Table 13.8 The WHO prognostic scoring system (WPSS) for MDS

	Points			
	0	**1**	**2**	**3**
WHO subtype	RA, RARS, 5q–	RCMD, RCMD-RS	RAEB-1	RAEB-2
Transfusion needs	None	Regular*		
IPSS cytogenetic risk	Good	Intermediate	Poor	

RA, refractory anaemia; RARS, refractory anaemia with ring sideroblasts; RCMD, refractory cytopenia with multilineage dysplasia; RCMD-RS, refractory cytopenia with multilineage dysplasia and ring sideroblasts; RAEB, refractory anaemia with excess blasts

* Defined as one unit blood transfusion in eight weeks

Table 13.9 The impact of WPSS score on median survival

WPSS category	WPSS score	Median survival (months)
Very low	0	138
Low	1	63
Intermediate	2	44
High	3–4	19
Very high	5–6	8

13.4 THE DIAGNOSIS OF MDS

The finding of anaemia or cytopenia in an elderly patient often raises the clinical suspicion of MDS. There may be a history of bruising or recurrent infection. Splenomegaly is typically absent.

Laboratory investigation confirms the suspicion by demonstrating one or more peripheral cytopenias and any of a wide range of dysplastic features (*Table 13.10*).

A bone marrow aspirate and biopsy are required for a definitive diagnosis of MDS. The aspirate is most useful for determining the differential cell count (including the % blasts and ring sideroblasts) and examination of the morphology of the cells present to define dysplastic features. The biopsy provides more reliable information on marrow architecture and cellularity. MDS typically demonstrates a hypercellular marrow with peripheral blood cytopenia as a result

Table 13.10 Commonly observed abnormal and dysplastic features in MDS

Red cells	White cells	Platelets
Ovalomacrocytosis	Hypogranularity	Micromegakaryocytes
Dimorphic population	Abnormal granulation	Megakaryocyte fragments in peripheral blood
Megaloblastic change	Pseudo Pelger–Huët	Platelet dysfunction
Gross poikilocytosis	Nuclear appendages	Agranular platelets
Multinuclearity	Gross hypersegmentation	Giant platelet granules
Nuclear budding	Decreased MPO	
Ring sideroblasts	Abnormal esterase activity	
Raised HbF	Neutrophil dysfunction	
Raised HbH	ALIP in marrow**	
Reticulocytopenia	Monocytosis	
Howell Jolly bodies	Abnormal monocytes	
Pappenheimer bodies		
Basophilic stippling		
Decreased PK activity*		
*PK – pyruvate kinase **ALIP – abnormally localized immature myeloid precursors		

of ineffective haemopoiesis. Ring sideroblasts are demonstrable in the bone marrow aspirate using Perls' Prussian blue stain to identify the iron-laden mitochondria that encircle their nuclei.

Cytogenetic analysis is an important facet of determining the prognosis and treatment plan. Because certain chromosomal abnormalities are associated with a poor prognosis, more aggressive treatment may be justified (*Table 13.11*). Cytogenetic abnormalities are demonstrable in about half of MDS patients, most commonly deletions on chromosomes 5 or 7, or the addition of an extra chromosome 8 (see *Box 13.6*).

Table 13.11 Prognosis associated with cytogenetic abnormalities in MDS

Prognosis		
Good	**Intermediate**	**Poor**
del(5q)	del(11q)	t(1;3)(p36;q21)
del(20q)	del(13q)	inv(3)(q21;q26)
+21	del(12q)	t(3;3)(q21;q26)
	+8	t(6;9)(p23;q34)
		combined –7 and del(5q)
		combined –5 and del(5q)

Box 13.6 5q– syndrome

Chromosome 5q– contains many genes that are involved in the regulation of haemopoiesis, including cytokines and their receptors, cell cycle regulators, transcription factors, and signalling molecules. The region of chromosome 5q that is always deleted in 5q– syndrome (the common deleted region or CDR) contains 40 identified genes, 33 of which are expressed in haemopoietic stem cells. No single gene has been identified as critical to the development of 5q– syndrome. The CDR in 5q– syndrome is distinct from the deleted region in most in AML patients with 5q–, implying a different pathogenesis.

About 15–20% of patients with MDS have some degree of hypocellularity in the bone marrow, and so can be misdiagnosed as having hypoplastic anaemia. Cytogenetic abnormalities common in MDS are unusual in hypoplastic anaemia and so can help in the differential diagnosis.

13.5   TREATMENT AND MANAGEMENT OF MDS

The treatment options for MDS include supportive care, low-intensity therapy and high-intensity therapy. The decision on treatment approach is usually based on IPSS score and the patient's ability to tolerate treatment.

Supportive care

Progression to AML is not the dominant concern in IPSS low-risk and intermediate-1-risk patients. Instead, prevention and treatment of cytopenias and their sequelae drive treatment decisions. Supportive care is intended to address symptoms and does not alter the course of the disease. Treatment typically includes regular red cell transfusion for anaemia, platelet transfusion for thrombocytopenia and antibiotics to treat infections (see also *Box 13.7*).

Box 13.7 Growth factors and MDS

Recombinant human erythropoietin has been used in the therapy of MDS for many years. Initially, the erythroid response rates obtained were modest (15–20%), as EPO was used in all subgroups of MDS patients without discretion. However, with increased sophistication in patient selection and response evaluation criteria, there has been a significant improvement in the response rates to EPO therapy. Selection of patients with lower-risk disease who have low endogenous serum EPO levels and a low transfusion requirement has more than doubled response rates. Evidence suggests that G-CSF may have a synergistic effect on red cell production, especially in patients with ring sideroblasts.

Low-intensity therapy

In some patients, for example those with high transfusion needs, the administration of haemopoietic growth factors such as recombinant erythropoietin and granulocyte colony-stimulating factor (G-CSF) can be effective. Novel approaches in this group of patients include the use of hypomethylating agents, antiangiogenic agents, and histone deacetylase inhibitors. In patients with hypoplastic MDS, immunosuppressive agents can be useful (see *Box 13.8*).

Box 13.8 Hypermethylation and MDS

Methylation of genes is an important physiological mechanism for deciding which genes are expressed and which are silenced. Excess methylation (hypermethylation) of genes that encode oncoproteins has been shown to be important in MDS. For example, the gene that encodes the cell cycle regulatory protein p15 is hypermethylated in up to half of all patients with MDS, and up to 83% in patients with more severe disease. Hypomethylating agents such as DACOGEN™ and VIDAZA™ have been shown to reverse the silencing of hypermethylated genes and show promise in the treatment of MDS.

High-intensity therapy

High-intensity therapy for MDS patients is generally reserved for patients with high-risk disease who can tolerate the rigours of aggressive chemotherapy. AML-like chemotherapy is used and induces a remission, which is typically short-lived in many patients. Intensive chemotherapy carries a high risk of prolonged pancytopenia because the MDS marrow regenerates slowly.

A minority of patients may be suitable for allogeneic stem cell transplants. This procedure offers the prospect of cure, but is associated with high morbidity and mortality. Reduced intensity conditioning transplants (mini-allografts) carry a lower procedural toxicity and can be offered to a wider range of patients.

SUGGESTED FURTHER READING

Catenacci, D.V. & Schiller, G.J. (2005) Myelodysplastic syndromes: a comprehensive review. *Blood Rev.* **19**: 301–319.

Giagounidis, A.A. & Aul, C. (2008) The 5q– syndrome. *Cancer Treat. Res.* **142**: 133–148.

Jädersten, M. & Hellström-Lindberg, E. (2009) Myelodysplastic syndromes: biology and treatment. *J. Intern. Med.* **265**: 307–328.

Komrokji, R.S. & Bennett, J.M. (2007) Evolving classifications of the myelodysplastic syndromes. *Curr. Opin. Hematol.* **14**: 98–105.

Shadduck, R.K., *et al.* (2007) Recent advances in myelodysplastic syndromes. *Exp. Hematol.* **35**: 137–143.

Steensma, D.P. & Tefferi, A. (2007) Risk-based management of myelodysplastic syndrome. *Oncology (Williston Park)*, **21**: 43–62 (including discussion).

SELF-ASSESSMENT QUESTIONS

1. List the five different subtypes of myelodysplastic syndrome in the FAB classification system.
2. Which FAB subtypes of MDS do the following results suggest?
    a. > 5% blasts in the peripheral blood
    b. a blood monocyte count of $> 1.0 \times 10^9/l$
    c. 10% blasts in the marrow, < 5% blasts in the peripheral blood
3. Which of the following is associated with a poor prognosis in MDS?
    a. abnormalities of chromosome 7
    b. > 15% ring sideroblasts in the marrow
    c. complex or multiple cytogenetic abnormalities
    d. a neutrophil count at presentation of $3.4 \times 10^9/l$
    e. abnormal localized immature myeloid precursors
4. Which FAB subtypes are the most likely and the least likely to transform into AML?
5. Differentiate between the WHO subtypes of MDS known as RA and RCMD.
6. Which WHO subtype of MDS is being described here?
    Dysplasia in all three cell lines, anaemia and thrombocytopenia with 3% blasts in the peripheral blood and 7% blasts in the bone marrow. Auer rods are absent.
7. To which IPSS risk group does a score of 2.0 belong?
8. To which WHO risk group does a score of 3 belong?

The chronic myelo-proliferative neoplasms

Learning objectives
After studying this chapter you should confidently be able to:

■ Outline the WHO classification system for chronic myeloproliferative and myelodysplastic/myeloproliferative neoplasms
The WHO classification of haematological malignancies includes sections devoted to chronic myeloproliferative neoplasms (MPN), myelodysplastic syndromes (MDS) and myelodysplastic / myeloproliferative neoplasms (MDS/MPN). These are all clonal, neoplastic disorders of haemopoiesis, but are distinguished from each other by the degree of dysplasia present and the extent to which haemopoiesis is effective.

■ Demonstrate knowledge of the distinguishing features of the different forms of polycythaemia
The defining criterion of polycythaemia is a rise in the venous PCV to more than 0.53 in males or more than 0.51 in females, reflecting an increase, real or apparent, in the circulating red cell mass. Polycythaemia vera is the only malignant form. Other forms are caused by a secondary increase in red cell mass (appropriate or inappropriate) or a reduction in plasma volume.

■ Outline the defining features of polycythaemia vera, essential thrombocythaemia and primary myelofibrosis
Polycythaemia vera is a malignant disorder characterized by absolute erythrocytosis in the absence of a physiological cause and the presence of a mutated JAK2 signalling molecule. Essential thrombocythaemia is a malignant clonal disorder characterized by megakaryocytic hyperplasia with marked thrombocytosis, progressive collagen fibrosis of bone marrow and massive splenomegaly secondary to extramedullary haemopoiesis. Primary myelofibrosis is characterized by anaemia, metabolic derangement, platelet dysfunction, fibrotic overgrowth of marrow and splenomegaly.

■ Review the pathogenesis, pathophysiology and treatment for chronic myeloid leukaemia
Chronic myeloid leukaemia (CML) is characterized by malignant proliferation of granulocyte precursors and accounts for about one fifth of all adult leukaemias. Most commonly, CML affects the middle-aged, although it can strike at any age. Classic CML is marked by the presence of the Philadelphia chromosome, a reciprocal translocation between chromosomes 9 and 22 that creates a novel hybrid gene called *BCR–ABL*. It is this mutant gene that is responsible for driving the leukaemic proliferation in CML. CML is a disease of three phases, known as the chronic, accelerated and blast phases. Most patients present in the chronic phase. The standard treatment for CML is drugs that specifically inhibit the aberrant *BCR–ABL* gene, thereby blocking the intracellular signals that drive the malignant proliferation.

The WHO classification of haematological malignancies includes sections devoted to chronic myeloproliferative neoplasms (MPN), myelodysplastic syndromes (MDS), and myelodysplastic/

myeloproliferative neoplasms (MDS/MPN). These are all clonal, neoplastic disorders of haemopoiesis, but are distinguished from each other by the degree of dysplasia present and the extent to which haemopoiesis is effective. The myelodysplastic syndromes are characterized by ineffective haemopoiesis and the presence of variable dysplastic features in haemopoietic cells. In contrast, the chronic myeloproliferative neoplasms typically lack dysplastic features and haemopoiesis is effective, resulting in overproduction of mature blood cells. However, the distinction between these two groups is not always clear-cut, so the myelodysplastic/ myeloproliferative neoplasms category includes a group of diseases where the characteristics overlap and so do not belong clearly to either the myelodysplastic syndrome or myeloproliferative neoplasm category. The diseases included in these three categories are summarized in *Figure 14.1*.

The myelodysplastic syndromes are discussed in detail in *Chapter 13* and the chronic leukaemias are discussed in *Chapter 12*. This chapter focuses on polycythaemia vera (and non-malignant forms of polycythaemia), essential thrombocythaemia and primary myelofibrosis.

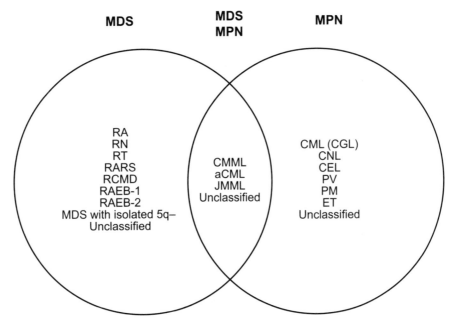

Figure 14.1
WHO classification of the chronic myeloproliferative neoplasms (MPN), myelodysplastic syndromes (MDS), and myelodysplastic / myeloproliferative neoplasms (MDS/ MPN). CML, chronic myeloid leukaemia; CNL, chronic neutrophilic leukaemia; CEL, chronic eosinophilic leukaemia; PV, polycythaemia vera; PM, primary myelofibrosis; ET, essential thrombocythaemia; CMML, chronic myelomonocytic leukaemia; aCML, atypical chronic myeloid leukaemia; JMML, juvenile myelomonocytic leukaemia (see *Chapter 13* for MDS abbreviations).

14.1 POLYCYTHAEMIA

The defining criterion of polycythaemia is a rise in the venous PCV (packed cell volume) to more than 0.53 in males or more than 0.51 in females, reflecting an increase, real or apparent, in the circulating red cell mass (see *Box 14.1*). Although this is a useful way of easily spotting polycythaemia, it is imperfect. For example, if a rise in circulating RBC mass is accompanied

---

Box 14.1 Venous haematocrit

The reference ranges for venous haematocrit (PCV) are as follows:

Cord blood	0.44–0.62
Child (10 years)	0.37–0.44
Adult male	0.40–0.54
Adult female	0.36–0.47

The venous haematocrit overestimates the whole body haematocrit (WBPCV) because of normal changes in the ratio of plasma to cells in arterial and venous blood. As a general guide, the WBPCV is about 91% of the venous PCV, but this value varies considerably, for example in pregnancy, splenomegaly and congestive cardiac failure.

---

by a rise in plasma volume, the expected rise in PCV may not occur and the existence of polycythaemia may be masked.

Normally, the red cell count is under tight hormonal control and is maintained within remarkably narrow limits. Alterations in the venous PCV can be caused by a reduction in plasma volume or by a true increase in red cell numbers. An absolute increase in the rate of erythropoiesis can be caused by malignant transformation, which frees the haemopoietic stem cells from hormonal control, via hypoxic or physiologically inappropriate stimulation of erythropoietin release or, rarely, by ectopic hormone production. Thus, the polycythaemias are a large and diverse group of disorders, only one member of which, polycythaemia vera (also known as polycythaemia rubra vera or primary proliferative polycythaemia), is a malignant disorder. However, an understanding of the aetiology and classification of all types of polycythaemia is essential because recognition of polycythaemia vera is based partly upon exclusion of the other types. The classification of the polycythaemias is illustrated schematically in *Figure 14.2*.

Polycythaemia vera

Polycythaemia vera (PV) is a malignant disorder of haemopoietic stem cells, and is characterized by absolute erythrocytosis and, commonly, a moderately increased granulocyte count and platelet count. It is predominantly a disease of late middle-age: the median age at diagnosis is 55 years. Males are affected slightly more commonly than females.

The presenting features of PV are related to the hypervolaemia and hyperviscosity that accompanies the absolute increase in red cell mass. Typical complaints include ruddiness of the complexion, headaches, blurred vision, dizziness, mental impairment and a feeling of congestion in the head. Splenomegaly secondary to vascular engorgement, extramedullary haemopoiesis and fibrosis are common. Hyperviscosity causes an increased incidence of arterial and venous thrombosis (see *Box 14.2*). Paradoxically, platelet dysfunction with a tendency to bruise and bleed excessively following trauma is also common in all of the non-leukaemic myeloproliferative disorders. The laboratory characteristics of PV are shown in *Table 14.1*.

Box 14.2 Polycythaemia vera

Thrombotic complications in PV are manifest as an increased incidence of:
- **transient ischaemic attacks** (TIAs) which are secondary to emboli in the cerebral circulation and show as sudden neurological deficit. The neurological deficits in TIAs normally resolve completely within 24 hours.
- **intermittent claudication**, which is secondary to atherosclerosis of the arteries of the lower limbs and shows as painful cramping of the legs and feet following exercise.

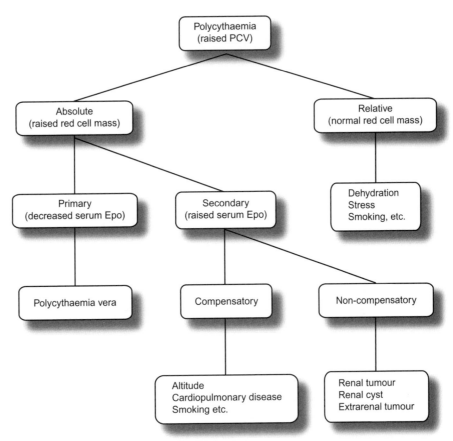

Figure 14.2
Classification of the polycythaemias.

Diagnosis of PV is made using the WHO criteria shown in *Table 14.2*. A diagnosis of PV can be made when the first two A criteria are present, together with either any one other A criterion or two B criteria.

Another useful marker in differentiating PV from other causes of polycythaemia is the presence of a specific mutation in the signalling molecule JAK2 in a haemopoietic stem cell. Substitution of a phenylalanine for a valine at position 617 of the JAK2 (JAK2 V617F) molecule appears to cause permanent activation of the mutated JAK2, resulting in increased proliferation and prolonged survival of the stem cell and its progeny. This mutation is identifiable in almost 100% of cases of PV and around half of cases of essential thrombocythaemia and primary myelofibrosis. Non-malignant forms of polycythaemia will be negative for this mutation.

Treatment options for PV include regular venesection to reduce the red cell mass, myelosuppression using hydroxyurea, busulfan or radioactive phosphorus and α-interferon to suppress haemopoietic proliferation. Aspirin can be used to reduce the thrombotic risk.

The median survival of PV patients is 10–16 years. The most important problems affecting survival are thrombosis and haemorrhage. Up to 30% of cases of PV transform to chronic myelofibrosis and of these, up to one-third eventually progress to acute myeloid leukaemia (AML). The duration of PV prior to transformation in these cases has varied from less than 2 years to more than 20 years. Treatment with alkylating agents such as busulfan and radioactive

Table 14.1 Differential diagnosis of the polycythaemias

Laboratory/clinical variable	Polycythaemia vera	Relative polycythaemia	Compensatory polycythaemia	Non-compensatory polycythaemia
Packed cell volume	↑	↑	↑	↑
Red cell mass	↑	N	↑	↑
Serum erythropoietin	↓	N	↑	↑
White cell count	↑	N or ↑	N	N
Platelet count	↑	N	N	N
Bone marrow	Hyperplastic	N	Erythroid hyperplasia	Erythroid hyperplasia
Spleen	Enlarged	N	N	N
Arterial pO$_2$	N	N	↓	N
Serum erythropoietin	↓	N	↑	↑
Serum ferritin	↓	N	N	N
Serum vitamin B$_{12}$	↑	N	N	N
Leucocyte alkaline phosphatase	↑	N	N	N
Serum lysozyme	↑	N	N	N

N, normal; ↑ raised; ↓ decreased.

Table 14.2 Diagnosis of polycythaemia vera

A Criteria
1. Elevated red cell mass > 25% above mean normal predicted value, or Hb > 18.5 g/dl in men, 16.5 g/dl in women, or > 99th percentile of method-specific reference range for age, sex, altitude of residence
2. No cause of secondary erythrocytosis, including: absence of familial erythrocytosis   no elevation of erythropoietin due to hypoxia (arterial pO$_2$ > 92%)   high oxygen affinity haemoglobin   truncated erythropoietin receptor   inappropriate erythropoietin production by tumour
3. Splenomegaly
4. Clonal genetic abnormality other than Philadelphia chromosome or *BCR–ABL* fusion gene in marrow cells
5. Endogenous erythroid colony formation *in vitro*
B Criteria
1. Platelet count > 400 x 10⁹/l
2. White blood cell count >12 x 10⁹/l
3. Bone marrow biopsy showing panhyperplasia with prominent erythroid and megakaryocytic proliferation
4. Low serum erythropoietin level

phosphorus is associated with a higher rate of progression to AML, so is avoided where possible, particularly in younger patients.

Primary familial polycythaemia

A rare congenital polycythaemia exists, which appears to be caused by mutations in the von Hippel–Lindau gene (see *Box 14.3*). The VHL protein has been found to regulate the cellular response to hypoxia via its interaction with the hypoxia-inducible factors HIF1α and HIF2α. Mutations in the *VHL* gene interfere with normal sensing of hypoxia and lead to inappropriate erythropoietin production and polycythaemia. The mutations involved in familial polycythaemia are distinct from those that cause von Hippel–Lindau syndrome, a disorder that predisposes strongly to a variety of cancers including haemangioblastomas of the central nervous system, renal and pancreatic cysts, phaeochromocytomas, clear cell renal cell carcinomas and epididymal cystadenomas.

Box 14.3 Primary familial polycythaemia

Primary familial polycythaemia is inherited as an autosomal recessive disorder, and is particularly common in the Chuvash Autonomous Republic of Russia. The VHL gene mutation in this region is a 598C→T VHL mutation. Affected individuals are homozygous for this mutation. Primary familial polycythaemia is sometimes known as Chuvash polycythaemia. A number of other mutations in the VHL gene have been identified sporadically in other parts of the world.

Relative (apparent) polycythaemia

Apparent polycythaemia occurs where an increased venous PCV is explained by a reduction in the plasma volume. Alternative names for this condition include relative polycythaemia, pseudopolycythaemia, stress polycythaemia, spurious polycythaemia and Gaisböck's syndrome. Red cell mass and plasma volume are under separate physiological control and so may vary independently of each other. Plasma volume may fall as a result of dehydration secondary to diuretic therapy, severe diarrhoea and vomiting, excess sweating, burns or alcohol ingestion. Prolonged stress, hypertension and smoking have a similar effect. Other clinical and laboratory signs that can be used to differentiate between apparent polycythaemia and the other forms are summarized in *Table 14.1* (see also *Box 14.4*).

Box 14.4 Adaptation to high altitude

Animal species that are indigenous to high altitudes, such as llama and vicuña, do not normally have high red cell counts. They have adapted to the low oxygen tension of their environment by synthesizing a form of haemoglobin with an extraordinarily high oxygen affinity. This helps to maximize the extraction of atmospheric oxygen in the lungs but the mechanisms involved in maintaining optimal oxygen delivery to the tissues in these animals are much less clear.

Secondary polycythaemias

The secondary polycythaemias are the result of increased stimulation of erythropoiesis, either in response to hypoxia or to another, physiologically inappropriate, stimulus, for example ectopic production of erythropoietin. Those secondary to reduced oxygen delivery are much more common than PV, and leucocytes and platelets are not involved in any secondary polycythaemias. Physiologically appropriate release of erythropoietin occurs in response to tissue hypoxia, which results from persistently low atmospheric oxygen tension, inadequate uptake of atmospheric oxygen due to cardiovascular or respiratory disease, or to defective transport of absorbed oxygen from the lungs. This leads to the compensatory forms of secondary polycythaemia (see also *Box 14.5*).

A variety of disorders are associated with the inappropriate (ectopic) synthesis and release of erythropoietin, for example polycystic kidneys and renal tumours, leading to the non-compensatory forms of secondary polycythaemia.

Box 14.5 Erythrocytosis

Congenital cardiac malformations which are associated with erythrocytosis include:
- **ventricular septal defect** (hole in the heart), where malformation of the septum permits shunting of blood from the left to the right ventricle. VSD is frequently accompanied by other congenital cardiovascular abnormalities such as persistence of the ductus arteriosus.
- **transposition of the great vessels**, where the aorta and pulmonary artery are linked to the opposite ventricles, leading to dyspnoea (shortness of breath) and a grey complexion (cyanosis) due to suboptimal oxygenation of the arterial blood.

14.2   ESSENTIAL THROMBOCYTHAEMIA

Essential thrombocythaemia (ET) is a malignant clonal disorder that is characterized by megakaryocytic hyperplasia and a markedly increased circulating platelet count. Alternative names for this disorder include primary thrombocythaemia, idiopathic thrombocythaemia and primary haemorrhagic thrombocythaemia. The median age at diagnosis is 60 years; essential thrombocythaemia is rare in children and young adults. Men and women appear to be affected with equal frequency.

ET characteristically presents with a platelet count greater than $1000 \times 10^9/l$ but platelet counts as high as $10\,000 \times 10^9/l$ are not rare. Examination of a blood film reveals the presence of platelet clumping and bizarre morphological abnormalities of the platelets with marked variation in size, shape and granulation. Megakaryocyte fragments may be present in the peripheral blood. Typically, a moderate neutrophilia is present, but the white cell count seldom exceeds $35 \times 10^9/l$. The red cell count and haemoglobin concentration are normal in most cases but some degree of iron deficiency may be present, secondary to chronic blood loss. Examination of the bone marrow reveals hypercellularity with pronounced megakaryocytic hyperplasia, granulocytic hyperplasia and, sometimes, erythroid hyperplasia. Up to half of cases have the JAK2 V617F mutation described above for PV.

In close to 50% of cases the discovery of ET is fortuitous, revealed by the finding of thrombocytosis during investigations for other purposes. Presenting features of ET include a spectrum of microvascular symptoms (e.g. headaches, visual symptoms, atypical chest pains, etc.), but the major clinical problems of ET are thrombo-embolic complications secondary to the extremely high platelet count and haemorrhagic complications secondary to platelet dysfunction. The thrombotic tendency is of uncertain mechanism, and may involve abnormal thromboxane A_2 generation and abnormal interaction between platelets and small blood vessel endothelium. There is, however, increasing evidence that the thrombotic tendency may be due in some way to granulocytes in this disorder. Whatever the mechanism, aspirin therapy, which interferes with thromboxane production, may be found useful to alleviate symptoms. The haemorrhagic tendencies are believed to be due to proteolysis of high molecular weight von Willebrand factor, leading to acquired von Willebrand's syndrome consequent on the thrombocytosis. The thrombocytosis may be modulated by the use of cytoreductive agents, such as hydroxyurea. Paradoxically, both thrombo-embolic and haemorrhagic complications may be present in the same individual. Significant splenomegaly is present in up to 80% of cases and some degree of hepatomegaly is also common.

Up to 25% of cases of ET transform to myelofibrosis or, rarely, PV or AML. By far the most common cause of death in this disorder is thrombo-embolic complications. The median duration of survival with essential thrombocythaemia is about 10 years.

14.3 PRIMARY MYELOFIBROSIS

This condition is predominantly a disease of the middle-aged and elderly. It is characterized by progressive collagen fibrosis of the bone marrow spaces, megakaryocytic hyperplasia and massive splenomegaly secondary to extramedullary haemopoiesis (see also *Box 14.6*). Primary myelofibrosis affects men and women equally.

Box 14.6 Naming of chronic primary myelofibrosis

Primary myelofibrosis is also known as chronic idiopathic myelofibrosis, agnogenic myeloid metaplasia, myelosclerosis and myeloid fibrosis with myeloid metaplasia.

The onset of primary myelofibrosis is insidious. Typical complaints at presentation include lethargy and exercise intolerance secondary to anaemia, weight loss and night sweats secondary to metabolic derangement, bruising secondary to platelet dysfunction, and splenomegaly secondary to extramedullary haemopoiesis. Marked splenomegaly is present at diagnosis in at least 50% of cases.

Examination of the blood reveals leucoerythroblastic anaemia with prominent polychromasia, anisocytosis and 'tear-drop' poikilocytosis. The white cell count and platelet count are variable but are frequently raised. Platelet morphology is frequently grossly atypical, suggesting overlap with essential thrombocythaemia. Attempts to aspirate bone marrow frequently fail because of the fibrotic overgrowth of the marrow space. This is known as a 'dry tap'. Trephine biopsy typically reveals large areas of fibrosis with patchy areas of hypercellularity, which contain prominent clusters of dysplastic megakaryocytes. Up to half of cases have the JAK2 V617F mutation described above for PV.

The median survival in primary myelofibrosis from diagnosis is about 3.5 years. About 10% of cases progress to AML.

14.4 CHRONIC MYELOID LEUKAEMIA

Chronic myeloid leukaemia (CML) occurs with an annual incidence of about 1 per 100 000 of the population with no apparent geographic variation. There is a slight excess incidence of CML in males. There was a significant increase in the incidence of CML in survivors of the atomic explosions in Hiroshima and Nagasaki, but no other universally accepted predisposing factors have been identified.

CML is characterized by an insidious onset of ill health and is associated with a massive increase in the circulating granulocyte count and with splenomegaly. The condition affects all age groups, but is seen most frequently in middle age, with a median age at presentation of about 53 years. Until recently, the prognosis of patients with CML was poor, with a median survival of around 4 years. However, the recent use of novel specific therapies has transformed the outlook for CML patients.

CML was the first leukaemia in which a specific chromosomal abnormality, the Philadelphia chromosome (see *Box 14.7*), proved to be a consistent finding. The chromosome is not, however, pathognomonic of CML since it may be found in around 20% of adult cases and 2–5% of paediatric cases of acute lymphoblastic leukaemia (ALL) and also in some cases of AML.

Clinically, the natural history of CML includes three phases, named the chronic, accelerated and blast phases. Typically, the disease evolves from chronic, through accelerated to blast phase. The clinical picture on presentation is dependent on the phase of disease.

Box 14.7 The Philadelphia chromosome

The name Philadelphia chromosome, for the characteristic chromosomal abnormality in CML, derives from the city in which it was discovered in 1960. Peter Nowell worked at the University of Pennsylvania School of Medicine, while David Hungerford worked at the Fox Chase Cancer Center. Both are located in Philadelphia.

The nature of the reciprocal translocation in the Philadelphia chromosome was first identified by Janet D. Rowley from the University of Chicago.

Chronic phase CML

Most CML patients are first diagnosed in the chronic phase. Presenting features at this stage are variable because of the insidious nature of chronic phase disease, but mainly reflect derangement of cell counts and increased cell turnover:

- shortness of breath on exertion, lethargy, loss of energy due to anaemia
- sternal tenderness due to hypercellularity of the bone marrow
- increased sweating and fever due to hypermetabolism
- weight loss, sometimes with anorexia and a feeling of abdominal fullness due to variable splenomegaly with or without hepatomegaly (both the result of extramedullary haemopoiesis)
- petechiae, bruising or haemorrhage due to thrombocytopenia; paradoxically, haemorrhagic symptoms may also be present when the platelet count is raised and in such cases, a defect of platelet function may be present.

Less common presenting features, almost invariably seen alongside the more common ones, include:

- visual disturbances, due to retinal haemorrhages or leukaemic infiltration
- gout, due to increased cell turnover
- symptoms associated with extreme elevation of the white cell count such as hyperviscosity or priapism.

The three defining features of typical chronic phase CML are a raised granulocyte count, the presence of the Philadelphia chromosome and splenomegaly. The total WBC at presentation often exceeds $100 \times 10^9/l$ and may be as high as $1000 \times 10^9/l$ although, with increasing access to health care in the developed world, it is becoming increasingly frequent for CML to be discovered when the total WBC is much lower. Typically, all stages of granulocyte differentiation are present in the peripheral blood but a rise in the level of circulating myelocytes and mature neutrophils is especially prominent. Typically, the proportion of myeloblasts and promyelocytes is low during chronic phase. The absolute basophil, eosinophil and monocyte count may all be increased. The cells of the leukaemic clone have been shown to have an increased rate of cytoplasmic maturation relative to nuclear maturation. This is most obviously manifest as an increased number of cytoplasmic granules in CML promyelocytes. A variety of functional abnormalities have also been noted in the leukaemic clone including defects of chemotaxis and phagocytosis and deficiency of granule contents such as lactoferrin, myeloperoxidase and alkaline phosphatase. This last observation is exploited in the differentiation of early CML from other causes of leucocytosis where the level of alkaline phosphatase is normal or increased.

The Philadelphia chromosome

The absolute requirement for a diagnosis of CML is demonstration of the Philadelphia chromosome (see *Box 14.7*) or its molecular marker *BCR–ABL*. This disease marker can be found in all blood cells, including B and, less frequently, T cells. This strongly suggests that the abnormality first arises in a pluripotent stem cell. The Philadelphia chromosome is manifest as a minute chromosome 22 and results from the reciprocal translocation t(9;22)(q34;q11).

The chromosome 9 breakpoint (9q34) involves the *ABL* gene. This gene contains two alternative first exons (designated 1a and 1b) and is therefore capable of producing two distinct mature mRNA transcripts. This requires that the splice acceptor site of exon 2 is capable of binding to a variety of splice donor sites. This promiscuity is crucial to the malignant potential of the *ABL* gene because it also permits the binding of non-*ABL* sequences. The precise location of the breakpoint varies from case to case, but always lies within a 200 kb region 5′ to exon 2 of the *ABL* gene. Thus, the *ABL* gene is translocated to chromosome 22, complete with exons 2–11. The normal ABL protein (p145[abl]) is a cytoplasmic and nuclear protein tyrosine kinase that is involved in the processes of cell division, differentiation, adhesion and stress response.

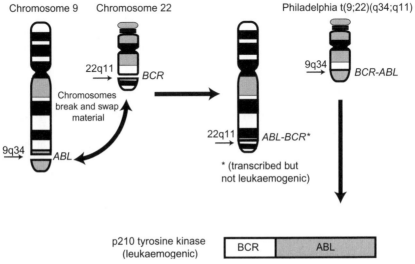

Figure 14.3
The Philadelphia chromosome.

The chromosome 22 breakpoint (22q11) in CML always lies within a 5.8 kb region of the *BCR* gene called the breakpoint cluster region. The normal BCR protein (p160^{bcr}) is known to have serine / threonine kinase activity and is involved in the activation of GTP-binding proteins within cells. Three different breakpoint areas in the *BCR* gene have been identified and designated major (M-bcr), minor (m-bcr) and μ-bcr. Translocation between *BCR* broken at one of these three areas and the second exon of *ABL* results in three different sized hybrid proteins: p210 (M-bcr breakpoint), p190 (m-bcr breakpoint) p230 (μ-bcr breakpoint).

Sometimes, the *BCR–ABL* gene results from a more complex rearrangement of three or more chromosomes.

In almost all cases of CML, in 1–2% of AML and in up to 5% of children and 15–30% of adults with ALL, the p210 BCR–ABL hybrid is demonstrable. Conversely, the p190 BCR–ABL hybrid is found in about half of adult Philadelphia positive ALL cases and about 80% of childhood cases, but rarely in CML. The p230 BCR–ABL hybrid has been associated with neutrophilic CML, and suggested to have a more benign clinical course.

The creation of a hybrid *BCR–ABL* gene is required, but is not sufficient, for the development of CML. There is strong evidence that the acquisition of this abnormality is a relatively late step in CML leukaemogenesis.

Accelerated phase CML

Eventually, despite treatment, most patients with chronic phase CML slowly transition into the accelerated phase, which is marked by a gradual accumulation of blast cells in the peripheral blood and bone marrow, the development of basophilia in the peripheral blood, worsening thrombocytopenia, increasing splenomegaly and cytogenetic evidence of clonal evolution. About 10% of CML patients who present are already in accelerated phase.

According to the WHO criteria, accelerated phase is established if any of the following are present:

- 10–19% myeloblasts in the peripheral blood or bone marrow
- > 20% basophils in the blood or bone marrow
- thrombocytopenia (platelet count < 100 × 10^9/l), unrelated to therapy
- thrombocytosis (platelet count > 1000 × 10^9/l) unresponsive to treatment
- cytogenetic evidence of clonal evolution in addition to the Philadelphia chromosome (commonly isochromosome 17q, an additional Philadelphia chromosome, +19 or trisomy 8)
- increasing splenomegaly or white cell count, unresponsive to treatment.

Blast phase CML

The development of blast phase is typically a terminal event in CML, with resistance to treatment and short survival.

According to the WHO criteria, blast phase is established if any of the following are present in a patient with CML:

- > 20% myeloblasts or lymphoblasts in the blood or bone marrow
- extramedullary blast proliferation, with development of a pseudotumour (chloroma)
- bone marrow biopsy demonstrating large clusters or foci of blasts.

About 10% of patients present in accelerated phase and another 10% present already in blast phase. The major change that accompanies transition to the blast phase is transformation from a chronic to an acute leukaemia. In about two-thirds of cases, CML transforms into an acute myeloid, promyelocytic, myelomonocytic, erythroblastic or megakaryoblastic leukaemia. In the remaining cases, the disease transforms into an ALL, most commonly precursor B-cell type, although rare cases of precursor T-cell type have been reported.

Treatment of CML

The treatment of CML has undergone a revolution since the introduction of imatinib, the first clinically useful tyrosine kinase inhibitor. Prior to the launch of imatinib, the standard treatment of CML included hydroxyurea, recombinant interferon-α and allogeneic haemopoietic stem cell transplantation. The median survival using these approaches was about 5 years.

Imatinib specifically inhibits the BCR–ABL tyrosine kinase, thereby inhibiting leukaemic cell proliferation and promoting apoptosis in BCR–ABL-positive cells. The pivotal clinical study that established the superiority of imatinib monotherapy in chronic phase CML is known as the IRIS study. A recent, 7-year follow-up showed that the 75% of patients with complete cytogenetic response (see *Table 14.3*) have maintained that response and that the estimated 6-year event-free survival (EFS), progression-free survival (PFS) and overall survival (OS) rates were 83%, 93% and 88%, respectively.

The greatly improved results seen following the introduction of imatinib therapy changed the treatment goals in chronic phase CML. The aims of treatment are to sequentially attain complete haematological response, complete cytogenetic response and complete molecular response. Data have shown that the time taken to achieve these treatment milestones is associated with likely outcome and can be used to determine second-line treatments (see *Table 14.4*).

Hydroxyurea remains an option for patients who cannot tolerate imatinib therapy. Recombinant interferon therapy is recommended for patients who are pregnant or contemplating pregnancy; imatinib is not recommended during pregnancy.

Table 14.3. Definitions of haematological, cytogenetic, and molecular response in CML

Response type	Definition
Complete haematological response (CHR)	WBC <10 x 10^9/l
	Basophils <5%
	No myelocytes, promyelocytes, myeloblasts in the differential count
	Platelet count <450 x 10^9/l
	Spleen non-palpable
Cytogenetic response	
Complete (CCgR)	No Ph+ metaphases
Partial (PCgR)	1–35% Ph+ metaphases
Minor (mCgR)	36–65% Ph+ metaphases
Minimal (minCgR)	66–95% Ph+ metaphases
None (noCgR)	<95% Ph+ metaphases
Molecular	
Complete (CMolR)	Undetectable *BCR–ABL* mRNA transcripts by RTQ-PCR and/or nested PCR in two
Major (MMolR)	consecutive blood samples of adequate quality (sensitivity >10^4)
	Ratio of *BCR–ABL* to *ABL* (or other housekeeping genes) $\leq$ 0.1% on the international scale
RTQ-PCR, real-time quantitative PCR	

Table 14.4 Evaluation of overall response to frontline imatinib therapy in chronic phase CML

Time (months)	Optimal response	Suboptimal response	Treatment failure	Warnings
Baseline	—	—	—	High risk; clonal chromosome abnormalities (CCA/Ph+)
3	CHR and at least minor CgR	No CgR	Less than CHR	—
6	At least PCgR	Less than PCgR	No CgR	—
12	CCgR	PCgR	Less than PCgR	Less than MMolR
18	MMolR	Less than MMolR	Less than CCgR	—
Any time during treatment	Stable or improving MMolR	Loss of MMolR; new BCR–ABL kinase domain mutations still sensitive to imatinib	Loss of CHR; new BCR–ABL kinase domain mutations poorly sensitive to imatinib; CCA/Ph+	Increase in BCR–ABL transcript levels; CCA/Ph+

Patients who fail therapy or acquire resistance to imatinib are offered second-line treatment with the newer tyrosine kinase inhibitors dasatinib or nilotinib.

Allogeneic haemopoietic stem cell transplant is recommended as the best available option for patients who progress to accelerated or blast phase CML and also in patients who acquire mutations that confer insensitivity to tyrosine kinase inhibitors. For example, a single nucleotide C→T change results in a threonine to isoleucine substitution at position 315 of ABL and alters the binding site for imatinib. Unless the patient is resistant to tyrosine kinase inhibitors, treatment with imatinib, dasatinib or nilotinib is recommended as preparation for transplant. Unfortunately, the outcomes for patients in blast phase CML are poor, with long-term survival rates of <10%. Outcomes for those in accelerated phase are somewhat better, but still poor compared to those in chronic phase CML.

14.5   PHILADELPHIA CHROMOSOME-NEGATIVE CHRONIC MYELOID DISORDERS

There is a group of disorders that show similarities to aspects of CML, but which are negative for the Philadelphia chromosome. These include chronic neutrophilic leukaemia, atypical (Ph-negative) CML, chronic myelomonocytic leukaemia, eosinophilic leukaemia and juvenile myelomonocytic leukaemia.

Chronic neutrophilic leukaemia

Chronic neutrophilic leukaemia (CNL) is an extremely rare condition. Patients with CNL typically present with persistent leucocytosis (>25 × 10^9/l), which comprises mainly mature neutrophils and band forms. The bone marrow is hypercellular with a predominance of granulocytes. Blast cells are rarely seen in the peripheral blood. Hepatosplenomegaly is sometimes present.

It is important to exclude the possibility of an extreme leukaemoid reaction as an alternative diagnosis. CNL is, by definition, negative for the Philadelphia chromosome and the *BCR–ABL* translocation. Suspected cases of CNL in which the *BCR–ABL* translocation is present are classified as neutrophilic CML, rather than CNL.

Atypical CML

Atypical CML (aCML) is a rare malignancy that shows both myelodysplastic and myeloproliferative features at diagnosis and typically affects older patients than classical CML, with people in their 60s and 70s being most commonly affected. By definition, aCML is negative for both the Philadelphia chromosome and the *BCR–ABL* translocation. Cases in which there is no conventional cytogenetic evidence of Philadelphia chromosome, but in which molecular techniques have demonstrated a *BCR–ABL* rearrangement (about 1% of cases of CML), are no longer considered to have aCML.

The typical presenting features of aCML include:

Peripheral blood
- leucocytosis with prominent increase in the neutrophil series. Promyelocytes, myelocytes, and metamyelocytes typically represent >10% of leucocytes. Severe basophilia is not a feature of aCML. Mild monocytosis may be present.
- prominent dysgranulopoiesis and other signs of myelodysplasia such as pseudo-Pelger–Huët changes.
- thrombocytopenia is common.
- cytogenetic abnormalities are found in most cases, but none are specific. All cases are negative for the Philadelphia chromosome and the *BCR–ABL* translocation.
- around one third of cases show mutations of *NRAS* or *KRAS*.

Bone marrow
- hypercellular bone marrow with prominent, dysplastic granulopoiesis. A variety of other dysplastic features may be present and may affect all cell lines.
- blast cells < 20%.

Clinical
- fatigue, shortness of breath and other symptoms related to anaemia.
- bruising due to thrombocytopenia.
- recurrent or unusually severe infection.
- splenomegaly.

Treatment for aCML is largely ineffective, achieving at best short-lived partial remissions. Overall, the prognosis for aCML is poor, with median survival of less than 20 months. The presence of thrombocytopenia and/or marked anaemia is a poor prognostic indicator. Evolution to acute leukaemia as a terminal event occurs in up to 40% of cases.

Chronic myelomonocytic leukaemia

Chronic myelomonocytic leukaemia (CMML) is a malignant condition most common in older people, with a median age at diagnosis of 65–75 years. In common with juvenile myelomonocytic leukaemia (JMML), there is a male predominance of around 2:1, but the reason for this is unknown. Clinical presentation is non-specific, with most symptoms reflecting abnormal blood counts, i.e. weakness and fatigue secondary to anaemia, petechiae, bruising and bleeding due to thrombocytopenia, and infections due to leucopenia. Splenomegaly and hepatomegaly may also be present.

The WHO diagnostic criteria for CMML include:

- a persistent peripheral blood monocytosis ($>1 \times 10^9$/l)
- absence of the Philadelphia chromosome or the BCR–ABL fusion gene
- < 20% myeloblasts or monoblasts in the peripheral blood or the bone marrow
- evidence of dysplasia in one or more myeloid lineages.

In cases that fulfil the first three criteria but show minimal myelodysplasia, the diagnosis can still be made if there is clear evidence of an acquired, clonal cytogenetic abnormality (not Philadelphia) in marrow cells, persistent monocytosis for at least 3 months and if all other causes of monocytosis have been excluded. Mutations of the *NRAS* or *KRAS* genes can be demonstrated in up to 60% of cases and cytogenetic abnormalities are demonstrable in up to 40% of cases, but none are specific for the condition.

The WHO criteria also permit distinction between two subtypes, based on the percentage of blasts and promonocytes in the peripheral blood and bone marrow. CMML-1 is defined by the above criteria plus <5% blasts in the peripheral blood and <10% in the bone marrow, while CMML-2 has 5–19% blasts in the peripheral blood and 10–19% in the bone marrow.

Cases that resemble CMML with eosinophilia should be investigated for mutation of the *PDGFRB* (see below) gene and, where present, classified as a myeloid neoplasm with eosinophilia associated with PDGFRB rearrangement.

The prognosis for CMML is highly variable. The optimal treatment for this condition remains to be defined, although hypomethylating agents such as decitabine and azacytidine have shown promise. The only prospect of cure for CMML is offered by allogeneic haemopoietic stem cell transplantation, although this rigorous treatment is only available to younger patients.

Chronic eosinophilic leukaemia

The WHO classification system recognizes two forms of neoplasm with a prominent eosinophilia:

- myeloid and lymphoid neoplasms associated with eosinophilia and abnormalities of the genes *PDGFRA*, *PDGFRB* or *FGFR1*
- chronic eosinophilic leukaemia (CEL), not otherwise specified.

In all cases of severe, persistent eosinophilia, it is important to exclude other possible causes before considering a diagnosis of eosinophilic malignancy.

The myeloid and lymphoid neoplasms with eosinophilia and abnormalities of the growth factor receptor genes *PDGFRA*, *PDGFRB* or *FGFR1* are a diverse group of conditions that previously may have been diagnosed with CMML, CEL, hypereosinophilic syndrome or T or B lymphoblastic leukaemia / lymphoma. Confusion can arise because sometimes such cases evolve from pre-existing malignancies without an eosinophilic component.

The most commonly seen abnormality of the platelet-derived growth factor receptor-A gene (*PDGFRA*) involves an interstitial deletion at 4q12, which creates a *FIP1L1–PDGFRA* fusion gene that encodes the first 233 amino acids of FIP1L1 to the last 523 amino acids of PDGFRA. The fusion protein is a constitutively activated tyrosine kinase that drives the malignant eosinophilic growth. The normal product of the *FIP1L1* gene is a component of the cleavage and polyadenylation specificity factor (CPSF) complex that polyadenylates the 3′ end of mRNA precursors. Most such cases would previously have been diagnosed as CEL. Because of the nature of the molecular defect underlying this condition, it is susceptible to treatment with imatinib.

The most common rearrangement involving the platelet-derived growth factor receptor-B (*PDGFRB*) gene is a reciprocal translocation t(5;12)(q33;p13) that involves the *ETV6* (*TEL*) transcription factor gene at 12p13. Again, the result is a constitutively activated tyrosine kinase. The resultant condition resembles CMML with eosinophilia and is sensitive to tyrosine kinase inhibitors such as imatinib.

Translocations involving the fibroblast growth factor 1 (*FGFR1*) gene at 8p11 have been known to be associated with haematological malignancy for some years. Several different translocation partners have been identified but the most common involves the zinc finger gene *ZNF198* located at 13q11. The t(8;13)(p11;q11) translocation creates a novel gene that encodes a fusion protein that contains proline-rich and zinc finger domains from ZNF198 and the cytoplasmic tyrosine kinase domain of FGFR1. This protein oligomerizes and causes constitutive activation of downstream signal transduction pathways that drive both myeloid and lymphoid growth pathways. This perhaps explains the unusual presentation of an associated myeloproliferative condition and a lymphoma, most commonly T lymphoblastic lymphoma.

CEL, not otherwise specified, is partly a diagnosis of exclusion. By definition, CEL is a persistent clonal eosinophilia that is both negative for the Philadelphia chromosome and lacks rearrangement of the *PDGFRA*, *PDGFRB* or *FGFR1* genes. The peripheral blood shows > 2% blast cells and morphological abnormalities such as decreased (patchy) granulation and cytoplasmic vacuolation, nuclear hypersegmentation or hyposegmentation of the eosinophils, although none of these changes is specific. The bone marrow is typically hypercellular with prominent eosinophil maturation. Again, there are no specific morphological stigmata. Some cases of CEL have been reported to undergo an accelerated / blast phase similar to that seen with CML.

Juvenile myelomonocytic leukaemia

Most cases of juvenile myelomonocytic leukaemia (JMML; formerly known as juvenile CML) present in early childhood, with a median age at presentation of about 2 years. The condition affects boys more often than girls, with a sex ratio of 2.5:1. There is a wide range of non-specific presenting features, including: pallor, failure to thrive, decreased appetite, irritability, swollen abdomen (secondary to hepatosplenomegaly), dry cough, skin rash, lymphadenopathy, diarrhoea and lung abnormalities.

The minimum diagnostic criteria are a peripheral blood monocyte count $>1.0 \times 10^9/l$, negative for the Philadelphia chromosome and the BCR–ABL translocation, bone marrow blasts <20%, hepatosplenomegaly, lymphadenopathy, pallor, fever, and skin rash.

There are no specific cytogenetic abnormalities, although monosomy 7, del7q and other chromosome 7 abnormalities are present in around one-quarter of cases. The underlying pathogenetic mechanism in JMML appears to be constitutive activation of the ras signalling pathway. There are three lines of evidence supporting this contention:

- children with neurofibromatosis type 1 have a heterozygous abnormality of the *NF1* gene, which encodes a negative regulator of the ras signalling pathway called neurofibromin. Affected children have been estimated to be about 500 times more likely to develop JMML or other myeloid disorders. The mechanism appears to be acquisition of a mutation of the other *NF1* gene, which leads to constitutive activation of the ras signalling pathway. About 15% of cases of JMML have *NF1* mutations.
- point mutations of the NRAS or KRAS (but not HRAS) genes are present in around one-quarter of JMML patients.
- children with Noonan syndrome, which is caused by mutation of the *PTPN11* gene are at a much greater risk of developing JMML. *PTPN11* encodes the signalling molecule shp-2. About 35% of cases of JMML have somatic mutations involving this gene, with consequent hyperactivation of the ras signalling pathway.

The clinical course of JMML is variable, but the prognosis is frequently poor. Indicators of a poor prognosis include age < 2 years, thrombocytopenia and increased HbF concentration. Responses to chemotherapy are typically suboptimal and, currently, allogeneic haemopoietic stem cell transplantation offers the only prospect of cure. Splenectomy may be indicated in some cases.

SUGGESTED FURTHER READING

Ahmed, A. and Chang, C.C. (2006) Chronic idiopathic myelofibrosis: clinicopathologic features, pathogenesis, and prognosis. *Arch. Pathol. Lab. Med.* **130:** 1133–1143.

Cao, M., Olsen, R.J. and Zu, Y. (2006) Polycythemia vera: new clinicopathologic perspectives. *Arch. Pathol. Lab. Med.* **130:** 1126–1132.

Fava, C., Cortés, J.E., Kantarjian, H. and Jabbour, E. (2009) Standard management of patients with chronic myeloid leukemia. *Clin. Lymphoma Myeloma Leuk.* **9:** S382–S390.

Levine, R.L. and Gilliland, D.G. (2007) JAK-2 mutations and their relevance to myeloproliferative disease. *Curr. Opin. Hematol.* **14:** 43–47.

Michiels, J.J., Bernema, Z., Van Bockstaele, D., De Raeve, H. and Schroyens, W. (2007) Current diagnostic criteria for the chronic myeloproliferative disorders (MPD) essential thrombocythemia (ET), polycythemia vera (PV) and chronic idiopathic myelofibrosis (CIMF). *Pathol. Biol. (Paris)* **55:** 92–104.

Penninga, E.I. and Bjerrum, O.W. (2006) Polycythaemia vera and essential thrombocythaemia: current treatment strategies. *Drugs,* **66:** 2173–2187.

Sanchez, S. and Ewton, A. (2006) Essential thrombocythemia: a review of diagnostic and pathologic features. *Arch. Pathol. Lab. Med.* **30:** 1144–1150.

Santos, F.P.S. and Ravandi, F. (2009) Advances in treatment of chronic myelogenous leukemia – new treatment options with tyrosine kinase inhibitors. *Leuk. Lymphoma,* **50:** 16–26.

SELF-ASSESSMENT QUESTIONS

1. Which of the following is a malignant disease?
   a. Relative polycythaemia
   b. Compensatory polycythaemia
   c. Polycythaemia vera
   d. Non-compensated polycythaemia
2. In which form of polycythaemia is the serum erythropoietin level characteristically normal?
3. Which gene is mutated in primary familial (Chuvash) polycythaemia?
4. Which mutation is identifiable in almost 100% of cases of polycythaemia vera and around half of cases of essential thrombocythaemia and primary myelofibrosis?
5. Which myeloproliferative neoplasm is most closely associated with the presence of 'tear-drop' poikilocytosis on the peripheral blood film?
6. What is the most likely cause of the splenomegaly commonly seen in chronic myeloid leukaemia?
7. Which two chromosomes are involved in the reciprocal translocation that creates the Philadelphia chromosome?
8. What are the specific chromosomal locations of the two genes that are rearranged in the formation of the Philadelphia chromosome?
9. Which of the following neoplasms are characteristically Philadelphia negative?
   a. blast phase chronic myeloid leukaemia
   b. chronic neutrophilic leukaemia
   c. atypical chronic myeloid leukaemia
   d. juvenile myelomonocytic leukaemia
   e. chronic eosinophilic leukaemia

The lymphomas

Learning objectives
After studying this chapter you should confidently be able to:

■ **Outline the classification of HD and NHL**
Both Hodgkin disease (HD) and non-Hodgkin lymphoma (NHL) are lymphoid neoplasms, but many different subtypes exist. The current standard for classification is the WHO system, which employs a combination of morphological, immunophenotypic, genetic and clinical features to define distinct disease entities. Broadly, HD is divided into classical and nodular lymphocyte-predominant forms, and the various forms of NHL are grouped into precursor lymphoid neoplasms, mature B cell neoplasms and mature T cell and NK cell neoplasms. Numerous subtypes exist.

■ **Outline the staging and prognosis of HD and NHL**
Staging is a formal procedure that identifies and classifies the extent and location of disease and is used to assess prognosis and to inform treatment selection. The most commonly used staging system for both HD and NHL is the Ann Arbor Staging System. In patients with advanced HD, prognosis can be predicted using the IPFP score. The equivalent system for NHL is the IPI. Both prognostic scoring systems are based on the presence of easily measured baseline factors.

■ **Discuss the aetiology of HD and NHL**
The causes of NHL are not well understood. No single factor is responsible, but rather multiple factors interact to promote a multistep transformation process. Three main mechanisms of lymphomagenesis have been described, although these may overlap and interact: viral-induced survival and genetic instability, chronic immune stimulation by antigen and chronic immunosuppression. EBV is implicated in the aetiology of both HD and NHL.

■ **Review the treatment approaches for HD and NHL**
HD is considered a curable disease, but this needs to be balanced against the need to minimize long-term toxicities. This is achieved using multidrug combination chemotherapy supplemented by radiotherapy. Treatment of resistant or relapsed disease is more aggressive. The appropriate choice of treatment for a patient with NHL is a key determinant of success and is based on a combination of disease subtype, stage, and patient factors such as age and co-morbidity. The types of treatment options currently used for NHL include: 'watch and wait'; radiotherapy; single agent or combination chemotherapy; immunotherapy; radioimmunotherapy; high-dose chemotherapy followed by stem cell transplantation.

The lymphomas are a heterogenous group of malignant diseases, each with differing biology and prognosis. In general, the lymphomas are divided into two groups: Hodgkin disease and non-Hodgkin lymphoma. About 85% of all malignant lymphomas are non-Hodgkin lymphoma (see also *Box 15.1*).

Box 15.1 Hodgkin disease

Hodgkin disease was first described by Thomas Hodgkin of Guy's Hospital, London in 1832. His report was based on seven cases with massive lymphadenopathy and splenomegaly. Most of his colleagues thought that these were cases of tuberculosis but Hodgkin, with remarkable prescience, thought that they were clinically distinct. The name was not given to the disease by Hodgkin himself – he was a modest and unassuming man. Samuel Wilks, also of Guy's, coined the eponymous title 33 years later when he published a more detailed account of several cases of this condition.

15.1 HODGKIN DISEASE

Hodgkin disease (HD) is a malignant lymphoma of B cell origin that first affects the reticuloendothelial and lymphatic systems, but frequently spreads to involve other organs including the lungs, bone, bone marrow, liver and, rarely, the central nervous system. According to the WHO classification system, five types of HD exist:

- **nodular sclerosis classical HD** accounts for around 60–80% of cases and is frequently seen in young adults. It is characterized histologically by a nodular pattern of growth, with prominent bands of fibrosis dividing the lymph node into affected nodules and a thickened capsule. The malignant cell is the lacunar Reed–Sternberg (R–S) cell, which is a large cell with plentiful pale cytoplasm and multiple lobulated nuclei with prominent eosinophil nucleoli (see also *Box 15.2*). R–S cells are present in a mixed cellular background of mature T and B cells, plasma cells, macrophages and eosinophils.
- **mixed cellularity classical HD** accounts for 15–30% of cases and is characterized histologically by a diffuse infiltrate of R–S cells against a mixed cellular background of lymphocytes, eosinophils and macrophages. This form of HD commonly infiltrates abdominal lymph nodes and the spleen and is the form of HD most commonly seen in HIV patients.
- **lymphocyte-depleted classical HD** accounts for less than 1% of cases and is characterized by a diffuse, hypocellular infiltrate with prominent, often morphologically bizarre R–S cells and areas of fibrosis or necrosis. This form of HD is seen most commonly in elderly patients or those with HIV, and often presents at an advanced stage.
- **lymphocyte-rich classical HD** accounts for about 5% of cases and is characterized by scanty R–S cells of classical morphology against a background of lymphocytes with occasional eosinophils and plasma cells.
- **nodular lymphocyte-predominant HD** accounts for about 5% of cases and is characterized by the presence of a specific cell known as an LP (lymphocyte-predominant) cell or 'popcorn' cell. Typically, R–S cells are absent or infrequent. L and H cells are found against a background of mantle zone B cells, T cells, germinal centre cells and follicular dendritic cells. This form often presents as localized disease and is more common in males, and has a tendency to evolve into diffuse large B cell lymphoma (DLBCL), a form of non-Hodgkin's

---

Box 15.2 Reed–Sternberg cells

Reed–Sternberg cells are named after Dorothy Reed Mendenhall of Johns Hopkins School of Medicine and the Austrian pathologist Carl Sternberg who made the first authoritative microscopic descriptions of Hodgkin disease and disproved the prevalent theory that the disease was a form of tuberculosis.

lymphoma (NHL). Formal diagnosis of this form of HD requires immunohistochemical studies to differentiate it from lymphocyte-rich HD or some forms of NHL.

The first four types named above are considered to be variants of classical HD and are treated in the same way. The fifth subtype, nodular lymphocyte-predominant HD has distinct biological characteristics and requires a different treatment approach.

Epidemiology of HD

In the UK, HD accounts for about 1 in 200 cases of all cancers diagnosed, with an annual incidence of around 1600 cases. In Europe, there were just over 17 000 new cases in 2008. HD is the third most commonly diagnosed cancer in people aged 15–29 years, and the sixth most commonly diagnosed cancer in children under 15 years.

There is significant geographic variation in the incidence of HD. The disease is most common in western Asia (from the Mediterranean to north-west India), but is rare in Japan, China and Bangladesh. HD is unusual in having a bimodal age distribution with incidence peaks in young (aged 15–34 years) and older people (aged between 55 and 75 years).

The incidence of HD subtypes varies according to age and socio-economic status. In developing countries, the incidence of the mixed cellularity and lymphocyte-depleted subtypes is higher, whereas the nodular sclerosis subtype is most common in developed countries. In the UK, incidence rates for nodular sclerosis HD peak in young adults. Overall, HD is slightly more common in males than in females.

The most common presenting feature in HD is the presence of painless, asymmetrical lymphadenopathy, which may be accompanied by severe, generalized itching in the absence of a skin rash. In contrast to NHL, which is frequently disseminated at presentation, most cases of HD are restricted to a single anatomical site at presentation. The presence of pyrexia and drenching night sweats are associated with more advanced disease. Examination of the peripheral blood seldom affords any useful diagnostic information in HD. The presence of anaemia, lymphocytopenia or leucoerythroblastosis all suggest advanced disease with bone marrow involvement, but this is uncommon at presentation.

Histological examination of an affected lymph node biopsy in classical HD typically reveals the loss of normal architecture and the presence of a diffuse infiltrate of lymphocytes, histiocytes, eosinophils, plasma cells and neutrophils, which are of normal appearance. Scattered among this infiltrate are variable numbers of R–S cells, the hallmark of HD. R–S cells are typically large, with two or more large, oval nuclei, each of which contains a huge nucleolus that is separated from the thickened nuclear membrane by a clear zone. After many years of controversy over the origin of the R–S cell, it is now universally agreed that they are derived from germinal centre or post-germinal centre B cells. R–S cells have an extraordinary immunophenotype with expression of genes typical of several different haemopoietic cell lines, a reflection of the genetic 'reprogramming' typical of these cells.

In the nodular lymphocyte-predominant variant of HD, the malignant cell is not the R–S cell, but the characteristic lymphocyte-predominant (LP) cell. These cells are derived from late germinal centre B cells at the point of transition to memory B cells. In common with the R–S cells of classical HD, LP cells show a partial loss of the B cell phenotype, but usually this is significantly less severe.

The natural history of untreated HD appears to involve the creeping advance of tumour from a single point of origin in a lymph node, first to contiguous nodes by direct contact, then to adjacent and more distant lymph nodes via the lymphatic circulatory system and, finally, to the spleen where further dissemination to the liver and bone marrow occurs via the blood circulatory system. With modern treatment, more than 80% of cases of early HD and 50% of cases of advanced HD survive for more than 10 years after presentation.

Aetiology of HD

The aetiology of HD is not well characterized, although it seems clear that infection with Epstein–Barr virus (EBV) is implicated. EBV is a highly infectious herpes virus. It occurs worldwide and probably infects up to 95% of humans at some time in their lives. Infection most commonly occurs in infancy or early childhood, when it causes a mild, self-limiting 'influenza-like' illness. Later infection (during adolescence or early adulthood) is also relatively common, when it causes a condition called infectious mononucleosis, or glandular fever.

EBV DNA is identifiable in R–S cells in around 50% of cases of HD in the developed world and in more than 90% of cases in the developing world. EBV positivity is higher in the mixed cellularity (60–70%) than in the nodular sclerosis (15–30%) subtypes. Almost all cases of HD in HIV patients are EBV-positive.

EBV infection is also associated with the development of Burkitt lymphoma in tropical Africa, nasopharyngeal carcinoma in China, certain post-transplant lymphomas and some AIDS-related lymphomas, and is suspected to be involved in several other malignancies. The possible role of EBV in lymphomagenesis is considered in more detail in the section on aetiology of NHL later in this chapter (see *Section 15.2*).

The incidence of HD is increased in people with AIDS or other forms of chronic immunosuppression. HD has also been shown to cluster in families: about 1% of patients have a family history of the disease. The risk of developing HD is higher in same-sex siblings, monozygotic twins or children of people diagnosed with HD. Siblings of an HD patient have a 3–7-fold increased risk of developing HD. The risk is higher in monozygotic twins. These observations suggest either a genetically determined susceptibility or shared environmental exposure.

Presentation and clinical features of HD

Most HD patients present with asymptomatic lymphadenopathy, most commonly above the diaphragm. Affected nodes are described as having a 'rubbery' texture. Patients may also have unexplained weight loss, fever or drenching night sweats. These are known as B symptoms and are associated with more advanced disease. Other specific symptoms may be associated with localized infiltration of tumour. For example, chest pain, cough or other respiratory symptoms may indicate involvement of mediastinal nodes or lungs. Symptoms such as pruritus (itching), urticaria and fatigue are attributable to cytokine release by R–S cells. Splenomegaly, hepatomegaly or both may be present.

Investigation of HD

No single routine laboratory test is diagnostic for HD. Instead, a battery of tests provides information that may aid diagnosis and determination of prognosis. Useful laboratory tests include:

- full blood count with white cell differential to check for cytopenia or anaemia. Most commonly, the FBC is normal at presentation. Where present, anaemia is usually of the chronic disorder type, although it may also reflect bone marrow involvement or haemolysis due to the presence of an autoantibody. If haemolysis is suspected, a Coombs' test should be performed.
- serum lactate dehydrogenase (LDH) is a useful indicator of tumour size. Markedly raised LDH may indicate advanced disease or bulky tumour.
- serum alkaline phosphatase to check for liver or bone involvement. Markedly raised ALP may indicate such involvement.
- an HIV test.

- renal and liver function tests to check for involvement.
- assessment of acute phase reactants (erythrocyte sedimentation rate, C-reactive protein, etc.) as a non-specific indicator of disease.
- immunohistochemistry to demonstrate clonality and phenotype. The classic subtypes of HD are positive for CD15 and CD30 and may be positive for CD20. Nodular lymphocyte-predominant HD is negative for CD15 and CD30 but positive for CD20 and CD45. Other immunohistochemical stains recommended to exclude forms of NHL that may mimic HD include CD3 and anaplastic lymphoma kinase (ALK). These should be negative.
- lymph node biopsy histology (supplemented by immunohistochemistry) is an absolute requirement for diagnosis and subtyping. The most suitable biopsy techniques for HD diagnosis and subtyping are excisional biopsy (removal of an entire lymph node) or incisional biopsy (removal of a section of lymph node). Fine-needle aspiration is seldom used because it does not provide samples suitable for classifying HD subtypes.
- bone marrow biopsy is required in all patients with suspected marrow involvement. Because involvement can be patchy, bilateral biopsies are recommended. Marrow involvement is more common in the elderly and in patients with advanced disease.

Imaging studies such as plain chest X-ray, computed tomography (CT), magnetic resonance imaging (MRI) and [^{18}F]fluorine-deoxyglucose positron emission tomography (FDG-PET) provide useful additional information.

Staging and prognosis of HD

Staging is a formal procedure that identifies and classifies the extent and location of disease and is used to assess prognosis and to inform treatment selection. HD tends to spread in a fairly predictable way, e.g. HD that starts in the lymph nodes in the neck may spread first to the lymph nodes above the collarbones, and then to the lymph nodes under the arms and within the chest. In time, the HD can invade blood vessels and spread to almost any other part of the body, particularly the liver, lungs, bone and bone marrow.

The most commonly used staging system for HD is the Ann Arbor Staging System. This system allocates patients to four stages (designated Stages I–IV) as shown in *Table 15.1*. Following allocation of a stage, certain letters are added to signify additional useful information about the disease.

- The subscript letter B is appended to the stage if the patient has a fever > 38 °C, night sweats or loss of at least 10% of body weight in the six months prior to diagnosis (e.g. Stage II$_B$). These symptoms are commonly referred to as 'B symptoms'. If these symptoms are absent, the letter A is appended (e.g. Stage II$_A$).

Table 15.1 The Ann Arbor Staging System

Stage	Definition
I	Disease is located in a single lymph node region, or a single extranodal organ
II	Disease is present in two distinct locations; both affected areas are on the same side (above or below) of the diaphragm. The affected locations may be two distinct nodal regions or one nodal region and one extranodal organ
III	Disease is present on both sides of the diaphragm and may involve both nodes and extranodal organ(s)
IV	Diffuse or disseminated involvement of one or more extralymphatic organs, including any involvement of the liver, bone marrow, or nodular involvement of the lungs

- If tissues close to, but distinct from the major lymphatic regions are affected, the letter E (for extranodal) is appended to the stage (e.g. Stage III_E). Contiguous involvement of extranodal sites due to direct extension of nodal disease is designated with the E suffix.
- If the spleen is involved, the letter S is appended to the stage (e.g. Stage II_S or II_{ES}). About 30% of new cases have splenic involvement (67% for mixed cellularity HD).
- If bulky disease (defined as a mass > 10 cm in diameter or a mediastinal mass that occupies more than one-third of the chest diameter) is present the letter X is appended to the stage (e.g. Stage III_X).
- Examples of Ann Arbor staging are illustrated in *Figure 15.1*.

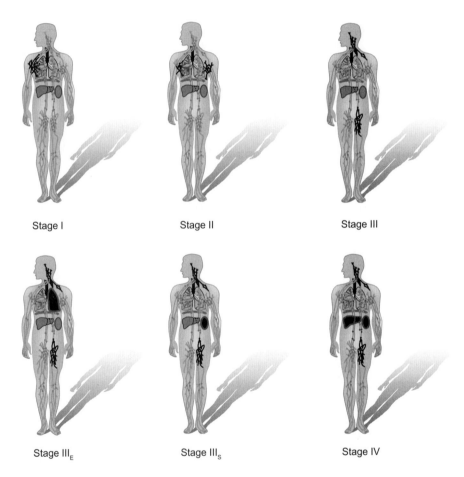

Stage I   Stage II   Stage III

Stage III_E Stage III_S Stage IV

Figure 15.1
Examples of Ann Arbor staging of NHL. From left to right the illustration shows involvement of a single lymph node region (Stage I); involvement of two distinct lymph node regions, both of which are above the diaphragm (Stage II); involvement of two distinct lymph node regions, one above and one below the diaphragm (Stage III); involvement of two distinct lymph node regions, one above and one below the diaphragm and the left lung (an extranodal site; Stage III_E); involvement of two distinct lymph node regions, one above and one below the diaphragm and the spleen (Stage III_S); involvement of two distinct lymph node regions, one above and one below the diaphragm and infiltration of both the liver and spleen (Stage IV_{S+H}).

Determination of the stage of HD should be supplemented by assessment of prognosis. In patients with Stage I or II disease, the following factors are considered to indicate an unfavourable prognosis:

- the presence of bulky disease
- an ESR ≥ 50 mm/hour in an otherwise asymptomatic patient
- more than three sites of disease involvement
- the presence of B symptoms
- the presence of extranodal disease.

In patients with advanced HD (defined as Stage III or IV disease), the International Prognostic Factors Project (IPFP) score can be used to provide prognostic information. The score is based on the presence or absence of seven unfavourable features:

- serum albumin < 4 g/dl
- haemoglobin < 10.5 g/dl
- male sex
- Stage IV disease
- age ≥ 45 years
- total white cell count > $15.0 \times 10^9/l$
- absolute lymphocyte count < $0.6 \times 10^9/l$ or < 8% of the total white cell count.

The presence of each of these features at diagnosis scores one. The impact of IPFP score on disease progression and survival at five years is shown in *Table 15.2*. The major limitation of this scoring method is that it is unable to clearly identify high-risk HD patients who might benefit from more aggressive treatment. Currently, no such prognostic scoring system exists. Analysis of gene expression markers, cytokines and other serum markers may help to identify these patients in the future.

Table 15.2 Impact of IPFP score on treatment outcome for advanced HD

IPFP score	% free from progression	% survival
0	84	89
1	77	90
2	67	81
3	60	78
4	51	61
≥ 5	42	56

Treatment of HD

HD is considered to be a curable disease and the intention of therapy is curative, but this needs to be balanced against the need to minimize long-term toxicities. This is achieved by using a multidrug combination chemotherapy supplemented by radiotherapy. The use of a broad spectrum of agents limits exposure to the toxic effects of any one modality, and provides synergistic cytotoxicity. Treatment of resistant or relapsed disease is more aggressive.

Early stage HD

This group includes patients with classical HD at Stage I$_A$ or II$_A$ without any unfavourable features (bulky disease, raised ESR, more than three sites of involvement, B symptoms or extranodal disease). These patients are typically treated with the ABVD regimen (Adriamycin®, bleomycin, vinblastine, dacarbazine) or the Stanford V regimen (doxorubicin, vinblastine, mustard, bleomycin, vincristine, etoposide, prednisone), followed by involved-field radiotherapy. The selection of site(s) that require radiotherapy can be guided using PET to identify residual disease. This approach achieves five-year survival rates of about 95% and five-year freedom from progression rates of around 90%.

Non lymphocyte-predominant HD typically presents as early stage disease that can be treated with surgical removal of infiltrated nodes and localized radiotherapy. The minority of such cases that transform to DLBCL are treated using standard regimens for that disease.

Early stage HD with unfavourable features

This group is defined as patients with Stage I or II HD with bulky disease, with or without further unfavourable factors. Standard treatment for these patients is as above, but more cycles of chemotherapy are given as tolerated by the patient.

Using these approaches, five-year survival rates are almost as high as those achieved in early stage HD without unfavourable factors, particularly in younger patients.

Advanced and/or high-risk HD

This group is defined as patients with Stage I or II HD with B symptoms or Stage III or IV HD. Standard treatment for these patients is as above, but patients are restaged using PET or CT at completion of treatment and further treatment is given to any patients with residual disease. Once a complete response (defined as disappearance of measurable disease) is achieved, involved field radiotherapy is administered.

An alternative approach is to treat with the BEACOPP regimen (bleomycin, etoposide, Adriamycin®, cyclophosphamide, vincristine, procarbazine, prednisone), followed by involved field radiotherapy.

Using these approaches, 3–5-year freedom from treatment failure rates of about 75% are obtained. A more aggressive regimen, escalated BEACOPP (higher doses of etoposide, Adriamycin*, and cyclophosphamide and the addition of granulocyte colony-stimulating factor (G–CSF) for neutrophil support), has improved 10-year freedom from treatment failure and overall survival rates to more than 80 and 85% respectively.

Relapsed or primary refractory HD

HD that does not respond to initial therapy (primary refractory) or that relapses after an initial response is associated with poor long-term outcome. The treatment of choice for these patients is high-dose myeloablative chemotherapy (e.g. BEAM: BCNU, etoposide, ara-C (also known as cytarabine), melphalan) and rescue with autologous stem cell transplantation. Using this approach, durable remissions can be achieved in around half of patients. For patients ineligible for transplant due to age or co-morbidity, salvage chemotherapy can be offered. Salvage chemotherapy regimens typically include drugs that are complementary to those that failed during induction therapy, e.g. ICE (ifosfamide, carboplatin, etoposide), DHAP (cisplatin, cytarabine, dexamethasone), and ESHAP (etoposide, methylprednisolone, cytarabine, cisplatin) (see also *Box 15.3* for explanation of some drug regimen acronyms).

Experience with allogeneic transplant has been discouraging because of unacceptably high transplant-related mortality. Trials of reduced intensity conditioning (mini-allo) transplants offer the potential for long-term survival with lower transplant-related mortality.

Targeted immunotherapy using monoclonal antibodies directed against the R–S cell antigen CD30 are under evaluation in clinical trials.

Treatment of relapsed HD remains suboptimal and clinical trials of alternative approaches are ongoing.

> **Box 15.3 Alphabet soup and drug regimens**
>
> The acronyms used to describe chemotherapy regimens can be confusing because sometimes the initials of the generic drug name are used and sometimes the initials of the trade names. Sometimes extra letters are introduced to make the acronym pronounceable! The resultant 'alphabet soup' approach can be misleading. For example, the common frontline NHL regimens CVP and CHOP sound as if they are very different. In fact, CHOP is CVP with a single additional drug:
>
> CVP – Cyclophosphamide + Vincristine + Prednisolone
>
> CHOP – Cyclophosphamide + Hydroxydaunorubicin + vincristine (Oncovin®) + Prednisolone
>
> Other confusing examples include the regimens ESHAP, which comprises Etoposide, methylprednisolone (Solumedrol®), High-dose cytosine Arabinoside and cisplatin (Platinol®), DHAP, which comprises Dexamethasone, High-dose cytosine Arabinoside and cisplatin (Platinol®) and EPOCH, which comprises Etoposide, Prednisone, vincristine (Oncovin®), Cyclophosphamide and doxorubicin (Hydroxydaunomycin).

15.2   NON-HODGKIN LYMPHOMAS (NHL)

About 85% of all malignant lymphomas are NHL and about 80% of these are of B lymphoid origin, while almost all of the rest are of T lymphoid origin (rare examples of true histiocytic lymphomas have been described). The diversity of NHL is reflected by the more than 30 different subtypes, which can be broadly divided into two groups based on their clinical behaviour:

- **aggressive NHL** (about 67% of cases) includes subtypes that are fast-growing and typically have acute presentation and rapid progression. These forms of NHL often affect younger adults and are considered potentially curable with current treatment modalities.
- **indolent NHL** (about 33% of cases) includes subtypes that are slower-growing and are considered generally incurable with current treatment approaches. Indolent forms of NHL typically affect older adults.

Indolent NHLs grow relatively slowly and may be asymptomatic at presentation. Many patients may not require treatment, sometimes for months or even years. Typically, indolent NHLs respond well to treatment, with most patients achieving a remission and experiencing a variable period of progression-free survival. However, in most cases, patients go on to experience a pattern of repeated relapses and treatment-induced responses. With each relapse, the disease typically becomes more resistant to treatment and the proportion of remissions obtained falls. For this reason, most indolent NHLs are considered to be incurable. A proportion of indolent NHLs undergo transformation into a more aggressive form, which is likely to be resistant to treatment.

Aggressive NHLs grow more quickly and are much more likely to be symptomatic at presentation than the indolent forms. Most patients with aggressive NHL require treatment straight away. Paradoxically, although these diseases are more aggressive and faster-growing than the indolent forms, this makes them more amenable to cure.

Epidemiology of the NHLs

NHL represents a diverse group of haematological malignancies, but epidemiological evidence on individual subtypes is relatively scant. As a group, the NHLs are the most common haematological malignancy and the fifth most common cancer overall in most of the Western world. In the European Union (EU), there are about 52 000 cases diagnosed each year, with a slight excess incidence in males. For example, in the UK, the male age-standardized incidence rate of 16.2 cases per 100 000 population is higher than the female rate of 11.5. In the EU, around 26 000 people die of NHL each year. Worldwide, the annual death rate is around 172 000.

Because many patients survive with NHL for several years after diagnosis, the disease is easily the most prevalent haematological malignancy, with an estimated five-year prevalence of more than 750 000 affected individuals worldwide.

The incidence of NHL increases with age; rates increase sharply in people over 50 years and around two-thirds (70%) of all cases are diagnosed in people over 60 years. The median age at diagnosis of NHL is 67 years.

While for most malignant conditions incidence has decreased over the past few decades, that of NHL has, until very recently, been steadily rising. During the past few years, however, NHL incidence rates have begun to plateau or even decline, particularly in countries of northern Europe. NHL is significantly more common in patients with AIDS. It is likely that some of the increase in NHL incidence seen during the 1980s was attributable to this cause and that, conversely, one of the reasons for the flattening of the incidence curve is the introduction of highly active antiretroviral therapy (HAART) for AIDS patients. In addition, some of the increase may be attributable to an ageing population. However, none of these phenomena seem able to completely explain the changing incidence of NHL. There remain many other possible contributing factors, which are poorly understood.

There are wide geographic variations in the incidence of NHL and the distribution of subtypes, with the highest rates in North America, Australia, New Zealand and western Europe and the lowest rates in eastern and south central Asia. There are also significant variations in the different types of NHL seen around the world. For example, Burkitt lymphoma is endemic in tropical Africa, but occurs only sporadically elsewhere; T cell lymphomas are much more common in east Asia and the Caribbean and gastric lymphoma is most common in northern Italy.

Aetiological factors

The cause of NHL is not well understood, although our knowledge in this respect has improved dramatically in recent years. It is believed that no single factor is responsible for NHL, but rather multiple factors may interact to promote lymphomagenesis. Significant progress has been made in understanding the pathogenesis of NHL as a multistep transformation process. Three main mechanisms of lymphomagenesis have been described, although these mechanisms may overlap and interact:

- viral-induced survival and genetic instability
- chronic immune stimulation by antigen
- chronic immunosuppression

Viral-induced survival and genetic instability
Oncogenic viruses such as human papillomavirus (HPV), hepatitis B virus (HBV) and EBV are known to be responsible for around 15% of all cancers in humans. These viruses interact with acquired genetic mutations that permit transformed cells to escape the normal regulatory controls over cell growth and death, the defining feature of malignancy. The best understood mechanism of viral lymphomagenesis involves EBV.

Epstein–Barr virus. EBV is a highly infectious herpes virus. It occurs worldwide and probably infects up to 95% of humans at some time. EBV infection is associated with the development of the aggressive malignancies Burkitt lymphoma in tropical Africa and nasopharyngeal carcinoma in China. It has also recently been shown to be implicated in the aetiology of HD, certain post-transplant lymphomas, some AIDS-related lymphomas and is suspected to be involved in several other malignancies.

These multiple disparate outcomes of the same virus puzzled scientists for decades. How can the virus that infects almost all of the world's population, and causes a relatively mild illness in most people, also be responsible for the development of malignant diseases that kill nearly 100 000 people around the world each year?

The answer lies in complex interactions of geography, environment and immune system subversion. Normal B cell differentiation is an immensely wasteful process. Every day, billions of different B cell precursors are produced but the majority of these undergo apoptosis before they reach maturity. The cells that die have been selected for death because they are auto-reactive or they may carry genetic rearrangements that are non-functional or otherwise unstable. EBV specifically infects B cells at several stages of their development, including pro-B, pre-B, immature and mature B cells. Once established within B cells, EBV exerts two important effects:

- it establishes a chronic infection that elicits a polyclonal B cell proliferative response
- it expresses a series of viral proteins that are structurally similar to, or are capable of interacting with, human anti-apoptotic proteins, cytokines and signal transduction molecules. These proteins subvert the normal regulatory mechanisms of cell growth and death, effectively 'immortalizing' infected cells.

These twin effects can allow abnormal B cells that would normally be deleted not only to survive, but also to proliferate, creating multiple clones of abnormal, genetically unstable B cells. As these clones continue to proliferate, they are likely to accumulate new mutations that progressively lead towards malignant transformation.

The region of Africa associated with endemic Burkitt lymphoma coincides with the malarial belt. It is believed that the pattern of repeated parasitic infestations and the chronic immunosuppression that results, further increases the risk of an immortalized (i.e. EBV-infected) B cell surviving and acquiring oncogenic chromosomal abnormalities.

Because of the nature of B cell differentiation, the likelihood that mutations involving immunoglobulin genes will arise is increased. One particular genetic rearrangement, t(8;14), places the gene for the transcription factor c-*MYC* in the immunoglobulin heavy chain locus, leading to markedly increased expression and deregulated cell growth. The t(8;14) translocation is characteristic of Burkitt lymphoma in tropical Africa.

Human T-lymphotropic virus-I. An unusual form of T cell lymphoma, adult T cell leukaemia/lymphoma (ATLL) is found mainly in Japan, the Caribbean and in other pockets around the world and is linked to infection with human T lymphotropic virus-I (HTLV-I). This virus is endemic in the parts of the world where ATLL is most common. For example, up to 20% of the adult population in southern Japan has evidence of HTLV-I infection.

HTLV-I specifically infects mature T cells. A viral protein, TAX, induces T cell proliferation and also inhibits apoptosis by induction of I-κB degradation, which activates the NF-κB pathway. Thus, HTLV-I infection establishes a latent infection that results in a chronic, polyclonal T cell proliferation. Over time, new genetic lesions such as mutations of the *P53* gene, deletion of the tumour-suppressor genes *P15* and *P16*, and alterations in the pattern of DNA methylation develop, leading to malignant transformation.

Other viruses have been implicated in the aetiology of lymphoid malignancy, including HTLV-II, the herpes viruses HHV-6 and HHV-8 and hepatitis C.

Chronic immune stimulation by antigen

There is an emerging body of evidence suggesting that chronic infection with certain bacteria causes persistent inflammation and is strongly linked with gastric mucosa-associated lymphoid tissue (MALT). *Helicobacter pylori* is a Gram-negative rod that causes peptic ulceration and is associated with an increased incidence of gastric carcinoma and MALT lymphoma. Strong evidence for the aetiological role of the infecting organism emerged from the observation that antibiotic treatment for *H. pylori* caused regression of the lymphoma in over two-thirds of patients.

H. pylori infection triggers recruitment of both B and T cells to the gastric mucosa, where the immunoreactive T cells drive continuous polyclonal B cell proliferation. The mechanism of lymphomagenesis appears to involve the accumulation of genetic lesions in the proliferating B cell clone with gradual progression towards malignant transformation. The most common genetic abnormality in gastric MALT lymphoma is t(11;18), which is found in around 30% of cases. Other abnormalities commonly seen include t(1;14) and t(1;2) and trisomy 3.

Other infections associated with specific MALT lymphomas include *Campylobacter jejuni*, which is associated with immunoproliferative small intestinal disease (also called Mediterranean lymphoma), *Borrelia burgdorferi* (which causes Lyme disease) with primary cutaneous B cell lymphoma, and *Chlamydia psittaci* (which causes the respiratory condition psittacosis) with ocular adnexal MALT lymphoma.

Autoimmune conditions involving site-specific inflammation, such as Sjögren syndrome and Hashimoto's thyroidosis, are also associated with an increased risk of NHL.

Chronic immunosuppression

Acquired immunodeficiency syndrome (AIDS) is associated with an excess incidence of lymphoma, commonly with extranodal disease. The most common extranodal sites include meninges, GI tract, bone marrow, liver, and lungs. NHL in AIDS patients is most commonly of B cell origin (especially large B cell and Burkitt or Burkitt-like subtypes). The risk of lymphoma is increased 150–650-fold among HIV-infected patients compared to the general population and is associated with older age, severe immunodeficiency and prolonged HIV infection.

Although the pathogenesis of HIV-NHL is only partly elucidated, possible pathways include viral cofactors such as EBV, HHV-8 (Kaposi sarcoma-associated herpesvirus) and HCV (Hepatitis C virus), chronic antigen stimulation and cytokine dysregulation.

Classification of NHL

Several NHL classification systems have been developed over the years, but none, until recently, had found universal favour. Gall proposed one of the first widely used lymphoma classifications in 1942. This classification was based predominantly on the morphology of the lymphocytes and tumour structures under light microscopy and became the mainstay for diagnosis at this time.

Other early systems proposed in the late 1960s and early 1970s, including the Rappaport, Lukes and Collins, and Lennert (Kiel classification) systems, incorporated subdivisions of NHL based on characteristics such as microscopic appearance and immunological features of malignant cells. For example, the Rappaport system was based on lymphoma cell morphology and tissue histology with classification according to differentiation and diffuse or nodular appearance. In 1982, the International Working Formulation (IWF) was created in an attempt to unify these different systems in a universal system with clinical and prognostic significance. The IWF grouped NHL into 3 main categories:

- **low-grade lymphomas:** slow-growing lymphomas, also referred to as indolent lymphomas
- **intermediate-grade lymphomas:** considered to be moderately aggressive lymphomas
- **high-grade lymphomas:** considered to be more aggressive than those in the other two categories.

The IWF was widely used in clinical practice in the USA, whereas the Kiel classification system was preferred in Europe. The Revised European–American Classification of Lymphoid Neoplasms (REAL) was created in 1994 by the International Lymphomas Study Group and rapidly superseded the IWF. The REAL system was developed for consensus of terminology and was based on the immunological principles used by Lennert and Lukes and Collins. This system recognized new disease entities and was proposed as the international replacement for all previous classification systems.

The new World Health Organization (WHO) classification of lymphomas represents a development of the REAL system and is the current standard classification system.

The WHO classification of NHL

The WHO classification identifies four features: morphology, immunophenotype, genetic and clinical features, and is currently the 'gold standard' for classification of all haematological malignancies. The WHO classification proposes three major groups of lymphoid neoplasms: B cell lymphomas/leukaemias, T/natural killer-cell lymphomas/leukaemias and Hodgkin disease. The WHO classification of the lymphoid neoplasms is summarized in *Table 15.3.*

Table 15.3 The WHO classification of lymphoid neoplasms

Lymphoid neoplasms	Aggressive (A) / Indolent (I)
Precursor lymphoid neoplasms	
B-lymphoblastic leukaemia/lymphoma NOS (B-ALL)	A
B-lymphoblastic leukaemia/lymphoma with recurrent genetic abnormalities (B-ALL)	A
T-lymphoblastic leukaemia/lymphoma (T-ALL)	A
Mature B cell neoplasms	
Chronic lymphocytic leukaemia/small lymphocytic lymphoma (CLL/SLL)	I
B cell prolymphocytic leukaemia (B-PLL)	A
Lymphoplasmacytic lymphoma	I
Waldenström macroglobulinaemia (WM)	I
Splenic marginal zone lymphoma	I
Hairy cell leukaemia (HCL)	I
Extranodal MALT lymphoma	I
Nodal marginal zone lymphoma	I
Follicular lymphoma (FL)	I
Primary cutaneous follicle centre lymphoma	I
Mantle cell lymphoma (MCL)	A
Diffuse large B cell lymphoma (DLBCL)	A
Primary mediastinal large B cell lymphoma	A
Primary effusion lymphoma	A
Burkitt lymphoma	A
Precursor T cell neoplasms	
T cell prolymphocytic leukaemia (T-PLL)	A
T cell large granular lymphocytic leukaemia	I
Aggressive NK cell leukaemia	A
Adult T cell lymphoma/leukaemia (HTLV-1+)	A

Lymphoid neoplasms	Aggressive (A) / Indolent (I)
Extranodal NK/T cell lymphoma, nasal type	A
Enteropathy-associated T cell lymphoma	A
Hepatosplenic T cell lymphoma	A
Subcutaneous panniculitis-like T cell lymphoma	A
Mycosis fungoides	I
Sézary syndrome	I
Anaplastic large cell lymphoma, ALK+	A
Peripheral T cell lymphoma	A
Angioimmunoblastic T cell lymphoma	A
Primary cutaneous T cell lymphoma	A
Some rare forms have been omitted; MM and related disorders are discussed in *Chapter 16*.	

Clinical features of NHL at presentation

The presenting features of NHL patients vary widely according to the stage and subtype of the disease and whether significant extranodal disease is present. Patients with indolent forms such as follicular lymphoma (FL) often present with a painless peripheral lymphadenopathy and may be otherwise symptomless. Symptoms such as fever, drenching night sweats and weight loss (so-called B symptoms) are unusual in such patients. Patients with MALT lymphoma or other extranodal disease may present with mild symptoms traceable to the site of infiltration. For example, abdominal pain, back pain or bloating may suggest GI tract involvement or bulky mesenteric or retroperitoneal lymphadenopathy.

Aggressive lymphomas such as diffuse large B cell lymphoma (DLBCL) can also present as painless lymphadenopathy without other symptoms, but those presenting with advanced disease often have B symptoms or other symptoms associated with extranodal involvement. Primary extranodal disease occurs in up to 20% of cases of DLBCL and frequently presents as an unexplained mass in the GI tract, tonsils, nasopharynx or oropharynx. Less commonly, bone, testis, thyroid, skin, orbit, salivary glands, sinuses, liver, kidney, lung or central nervous system may be involved.

There are few presenting features that are specific for NHL and this can result in delayed or missed diagnosis. It is the grouping of symptoms and signs, coupled with features such as age and exclusion of less sinister diagnoses that usually leads to a referral for specialist investigation and the subsequent diagnosis of NHL being made.

Clinical evaluation of the NHL patient

In cases of suspected NHL, every patient will undergo a physical examination and some routine tests to rule out other, less serious explanations for the presenting signs and symptoms. If these fail to exclude the possibility of a diagnosis of NHL, more extensive investigation will be performed.

History and physical examination

Patient characteristics such as age, symptoms, co-morbidities, general health, etc. are gathered during a thorough study of the patient's medical history. This helps to determine possible risk factors of NHL. Important features of the examination include determination of HIV risk, history of infections, autoimmune disease or immunosuppressive therapy.

Physical examination will include a thorough search for obvious lymphadenopathy, particularly under the chin (parotid, submandibular, submental and sublingual nodes), in the neck and tonsil area (cervical nodes), above the shoulders (supraclavicular nodes), on the elbows (epitrochlear nodes) and in the groin (axillary nodes). If lymphadenopathy is found, the nodes will be examined for their size, texture, erythema and whether they are painful. The sites affected and the number of affected sites will be noted.

The presence of lymphadenopathy in deep nodes that cannot be directly palpated is assessed by looking for secondary signs such as swelling or discomfort. For example, bulky mediastinal lymphadenopathy may be indicated by abdominal discomfort, mild back pain or a sensation of bloating. Enlarged nodes can compress nearby structures so a check for signs of compression of major veins, arteries, nerves, vital organs, and spinal cord will be conducted.

Extranodal disease may also cause suggestive symptoms. For example, gastric lymphoma may present with symptoms similar to an ulcer, i.e. pain and gastric bleeding. In advanced disease, hepatomegaly and/or splenomegaly may be present, so an abdominal examination will be performed.

Close assessment of persistent symptoms such as fever, chills, sweats (often at night), unexplained weight loss and pruritus will add significant information.

A definitive NHL diagnosis requires a lymph node biopsy. The architecture of an entire lymph node can provide valuable information. For example, in FL the follicular architecture of the lymph node is typically maintained, while in diffuse lymphomas it is effaced.

Laboratory and imaging studies

For most suspected cases of NHL, routine blood tests are performed:

- haematology profile including a full blood count, white blood cell differential count and examination of a peripheral blood smear
- clinical chemistry profile, particularly lactate dehydrogenase; alkaline phosphatase, uric acid, creatinine, calcium, and albumin.

Blood tests cannot usually detect lymphoma directly but abnormal blood counts and derangement of blood chemistries can provide some clues to assist in diagnosis.

Immunophenotyping

Immunophenotyping is a technique that uses monoclonal antibodies to identify protein markers present in the cytoplasm, nucleus or surface membrane of cells, thereby identifying the cell type and degree of differentiation. There are two main aims of performing an immunophenotype on biopsy tissue. First, it is important to determine whether any lymphocytes present are polyclonal or monoclonal. The former is likely to indicate an ongoing immune response, whereas the latter is indicative of malignancy. A monoclonal proliferation is characterized by the presence of the same set of cell markers on all of the lymphoid cells present. Once clonality has been established, determination of the pattern of expression of cell markers present is an important way of determining the subtype of lymphoma (see *Table 15.4* and later in this chapter).

Many forms of NHL are accompanied by characteristic chromosomal abnormalities. Although there is no unique abnormality that always clinches a diagnosis, demonstration of the presence of particular cytogenetic abnormalities can augment other diagnostic information. For example, the translocation t(11;14)(q13;q32) is often found in cases of mantle cell lymphoma.

Once diagnosis of NHL is made, imaging studies are performed to determine the stage of the disease. The imaging studies most often employed include the following:

Table 15.4 The International Prognostic Index for NHL

Prognostic factor	Negative prognostic indicator
Ann Arbor stage	Stage ≥ III
Patient age	> 60 years
Lactate dehydrogenase (LDH)	Raised
Performance status	ECOG performance score ≥ 2
Extranodal disease	≥ 2 sites involved

■ Chest X-rays: these are a form of electromagnetic radiation (like light); they are of higher energy, however, and can penetrate the body to form an image on film. Structures that are dense (such as bone) will appear white, air will be black, and other structures will be shades of grey depending on density. Plain X-ray can be used to visualize enlarged lymph nodes in the chest and neck area.

■ Computed tomography (CT) scans are X-ray images taken from multiple angles or planes of a particular area of the body and assembled into a cross-sectional image using a computer. CT is a more accurate method than plain X-ray for detection of lymphoma in chest and neck or abdominal and pelvic areas, but is unable to detect bone involvement.

■ Magnetic resonance imaging (MRI) is a technique that uses magnetic fields instead of X-rays to generate an image. An MRI produces images by exposing the hydrogen nuclei in body tissue to strong, external magnetic fields, causing tiny, harmless movements of atoms in the area of the body being studied that can be detected and converted to a clear and detailed image of the tissue. Numerous variations of MRI have been developed and each has a particular strength in imaging. MRI is very good for detecting involvement of the central nervous system and bone marrow.

■ Positron emission tomography (PET) scans evaluate and produce images of the metabolic activity of cells in different parts of the body using an injected radioactive tracer. As the tracer decomposes in the body, it gives off positron emissions that are sensed by detectors that assemble and record the emissions into a high-resolution two- or three-dimensional image indicating a particular metabolic process in a specific anatomical site. A radioactive chemical called [18F]fluorine-deoxyglucose is an effective tracer because most cells use glucose as an energy source. PET can detect disease in non-enlarged lymph nodes, bone and mesentery. PET can provide more accurate results than CT, for example in detecting hepatic and splenic involvement or distinguishing between fibrosis from active tumour, but can suffer from false positive findings due to infections, sarcoidosis or thymic hyperplasia. Low grade NHL may be detected less well using PET, particularly small tumours.

■ Lymphangiography: this a form of X-ray of the lymphatic system obtained after injection of a radio-opaque contrast medium. It provides additional information on lower parts of the body and can be useful if CT fails to show abnormal lymph nodes but the index of suspicion of NHL remains high. Lymphangiography is not particularly sensitive and may produce a false negative finding: the technique is not commonly used for staging NHL.

Staging and prognosis of NHL

Following diagnosis of NHL, accurate staging evaluation is important for treatment selection and management. The aims of staging cancer patients include:

■ informing treatment selection
■ establishment of an accurate prognosis

- accurate stratification of patients, e.g. for clinical trials
- establishment of criteria that permit rational response assessment.

Development of a clinically useful staging system for NHL has proven difficult, partly because of the heterogeneous nature of the disease. The recommended staging system for NHL is the Ann Arbor Staging System described earlier in this chapter. This system is primarily an anatomical staging system, i.e. it is based on the location and spread of disease, but it also encompasses the presence or absence of systemic symptoms. However, this system takes no account of the grade of the lymphoma and does not subdivide certain clinically distinct forms of the disease. For these reasons, it is recommended for use in conjunction with a clinical scoring system such as the International Prognostic Index (IPI).

The IPI was designed to augment lymphoma staging by taking account of factors known to affect patient prognosis as well as the anatomical site and spread of the disease. The IPI has become the primary clinical scoring system used to predict disease recurrence and overall survival in patients with NHL. IPI is strongly predictive of outcome in aggressive lymphomas such as DLBCL, but is less accurate for indolent lymphomas. Derivation of the IPI for an individual patient requires assessment of the presence or absence of five negative prognostic features present at the time of diagnosis, as shown in *Table 15.4*.

An IPI score is calculated by counting the number of adverse prognostic indicators present at diagnosis (0 to 5). The scoring system is predictive of risk and identifies patients as belonging to one of four distinct outcome groups with a 5-year survival ranging from 26% to 73%, as shown in *Table 15.5*. Survival data are based on outcomes following anthracycline-based combination chemotherapy. Updated versions of the IPI have been proposed for patients under the age of 60 years, and for modern immunochemotherapy treatment regimens. Subtype-specific prognostic indices have also been developed for follicular lymphoma (FLIPI) and mantle cell lymphoma (MIPI). The basic principles of operation of all of these indices are similar to those of the IPI.

A number of molecular aberrations have been shown to impact prognosis for some NHL subtypes. For example, in patients with DLBCL or FL, *BCL-2* overexpression has been associated with poorer survival whereas, in contrast, *BCL-6* expression has been associated with a more favourable outcome. Molecular markers such as these impact on prognosis by interfering with important mechanisms such as apoptosis, cell cycle regulation and angiogenesis.

Table 15.5 Impact of IPI risk group on five-year survival

IPI score	Risk category	Five-year survival
≤ 1	Low	73%
2	Low–intermediate	51%
3	High–intermediate	43%
≥ 4	High	26%

Some important subtypes of NHL

Diffuse large B cell lymphoma

Diffuse large B cell lymphoma (DLBCL) is the most common lymphoid malignancy in adults, accounting for 31% of all adult NHL and with an annual incidence in the USA of more than 25 000 cases. DLBCL is a group of heterogeneous neoplasms with several morphological and immunophenotypic variants. Some cases of DLBCL arise following transformation of an underlying indolent lymphoma, such as FL, small lymphocytic lymphoma (SLL), lymphoplasmacytic lymphoma (WM), splenic marginal zone lymphoma or extranodal marginal zone (MALT) lymphoma.

DLBCL is an aggressive lymphoma and is characterized by a diffuse pattern of malignant cells spread throughout the lymph node with effacement of the normal nodal architecture.

Bone marrow involvement in DLBCL may take two forms:

- in about 10% of cases, large cell lymphoma is present in the marrow
- in about 20% of cases, the bone marrow is infiltrated by aggregates of small atypical lymphoid cells; this can indicate that the DLBCL is in the early stages of transformation from an indolent lymphoma such as FL.

DLBCL cells typically express B cell-associated antigens such as CD19, CD20, CD22 and CD79a as well as CD45 and often surface immunoglobulin (sIg). They may co-express CD5 or CD10.

There is no single characteristic cytogenetic abnormality that defines DLBCL. In 20–30% of cases, *BCL-2*, (e.g. t(14;18)(q32;q21) and/or *BCL-6* (involving 3q27) rearrangements are found. The t(8;14)(q23;q32) characteristic of Burkitt lymphoma has been described and is associated with a particularly aggressive clinical course. Additional cytogenetic abnormalities are common and some cases may have complex karyotypes. Mutations and deletion of the *P53* gene are common in DLBCL but some cases also overexpress the wild-type protein.

Gene expression profiling has identified at least two subtypes of DLBCL called the germinal centre B cell (GCB) and activated B cell (ABC) subtypes. The GCB subtype is associated with a better prognosis and correlates with the presence of t(14;18)(q32;q21), suggesting a transformed follicular cell origin.

DLBCL patients often present with a rapidly growing mass (up to 40% of DLBCL is extranodal with GI tract, bone and CNS all commonly involved). B symptoms are present in about 30% of cases at presentation. Around one-third of cases present with localized (Stage I or II) disease. Bone marrow involvement is seen in about 16% of cases. The prognosis of DLBCL is highly associated with IPI score.

CHOP chemotherapy had been the standard of care for DLBCL since its introduction in the 1970s, but has now been improved by the addition of rituximab (R-CHOP). R-CHOP is associated with improvements in overall survival (OS), and event-free survival (EFS) or progression-free survival (PFS) without increased toxicity, in all patient groups studied (see *Box 15.3*). Current studies are investigating possible improvements in therapy using dose intensification of CHOP or R-CHOP. Radiotherapy may be useful in early stage or bulky disease.

Follicular lymphoma

FL is the second most frequent type of NHL, accounting for around 22% of cases. There are marked geographical differences in the incidence of follicular NHL, although the reasons for this remain unclear.

FL appears in lymph node sections as a variable mixture of centrocytes and centroblasts, with an at least partially follicular pattern. The clinical aggressiveness of the disease increases broadly in line with an increasing proportion of centroblasts. The WHO classification uses the Mann and Berard criteria to divide cases into one of three grades:

- Grade I is characterized by a small-cleaved cell (centrocyte) proliferation
- Grade II is characterized by a mixed proliferation of small-cleaved (centrocyte) and large (centroblast) cells
- Grade III is characterized by the proliferation of large (centroblast) cells.

The bone marrow is frequently involved. Some cases of FL present in an already transformed state, when they may more closely resemble DLBCL.

FL cells are usually sIg+, CD10+, CD5– and CD23–/+. Most cases are BCL-2+, and nuclear BCL-6 is expressed by at least some of the malignant cells. The frequency of Ki-67+ is lower than that seen in reactive follicular hyperplasia.

Immunoglobulin heavy and light chain genes are rearranged, reflecting the germinal centre origin of the cells. The t(14;18)(q32;q21) cytogenetic abnormality is present in up to 90% of cases, which explains the commonly observed BCL-2 overexpression. Abnormalities of BCL-6 expression are seen in 40–50% of cases and appear to be associated with an increased risk of transformation to DLBCL. Most cases of FL have complex karyotypes; t(14;18)(q32;q21) is rarely the sole abnormality.

Gene expression profiling has revealed the presence of two distinct 'signatures' that have prognostic significance. Transformation of FL into DLBCL has also been investigated with gene expression profiling, and the results suggest that there is more than one mechanism underlying FL transformation.

FL affects predominantly older adults, with no gender imbalance. Most patients present with generalized lymphadenopathy and advanced disease. Only a relatively small proportion presents with apparent Stage I disease. There are FL cells in the bone marrow in about half of cases, although it is less common to find them in the peripheral blood. Extranodal disease is rarely seen and is almost never a presenting feature.

The disease is often incurable because, in the majority of patients, it is diagnosed at an advanced stage (Stage III or IV). The gradual histological transformation into a more aggressive type of lymphoma, which is much harder to treat successfully, occurs in about 50% of cases. The current median survival of FL is 8–10 years.

Radiotherapy offers the prospect of cure in FL patients with Stage I or II disease. However, for most FL patients who have advanced disease, treatment is not curative. Many patients are not offered treatment until they become symptomatic (a strategy called 'watch and wait'). Primary treatment typically consists of chemotherapy using an alkylating agent-based regimen such as CHOP or a fludarabine-based regimen; rituximab ± chemotherapy; radioimmunotherapy or stem cell transplantation.

Marginal zone B cell lymphoma

Marginal zone B cell lymphomas (MZL) can be classified according to their location as extranodal marginal zone B cell lymphoma (or MALT lymphomas), nodal marginal zone B cell lymphoma and splenic marginal zone lymphoma. This indolent B cell lymphoma occurs in various extranodal sites, such as the GI tract, lung, salivary gland, thyroid, breast and skin. Extranodal marginal zone B cell lymphoma is characterized by an infiltration of centrocyte-like small B cells occupying the marginal zone and surrounding secondary lymphoid follicles. MALT-type lymphoma accounts for approximately 5–6% of all NHLs, and 50% of gastric lymphomas, with a median age at presentation of 60 years. Translocations t(11;18), t(14;18) and t(1;14) are relatively common in MALT lymphomas. Gastric MALT lymphoma is caused by infection with *H. pylori*, and there is evidence to link non-gastric MALT lymphoma with infection by microbial pathogens. Antibiotic treatment is the standard first-line therapy for gastric MALT lymphoma, and remission can be expected in more than 70% of patients.

Mantle cell lymphoma

Mantle cell lymphoma (MCL) comprises 6% of all cases of NHL. Clinical presentation is typically between 50 and 70 years, with a striking male predominance (male:female about 3:1). Most patients present with advanced disease, with bone marrow and peripheral blood involvement. Extranodal involvement is common and may be the presenting feature.

The majority of MCLs (> 90%) contain a t(11; 14)(q13; q32) translocation resulting in overexpression of cyclin D1, a protein involved in regulation of the cell cycle at the G1–S checkpoint. Additionally, the immunoglobulin heavy chain (IgH) gene is mutated in approximately 25% of cases. MCL displays the worst features of indolent and aggressive lymphomas; it has an aggressive clinical course without a curative option. MCL has the lowest five-year survival rate of any NHL.

Small lymphocytic lymphoma

Small lymphocytic lymphoma (SLL), is an indolent neoplasm characterized by an accumulation of small, mature-appearing lymphocytes in the blood, bone marrow, and lymphoid tissues. B-CLL accounts for 30% of all leukaemias and approximately 6% of all NHL cases, with a median age at diagnosis of 72 years. Incidence rates are nearly double in men than women. SLL is considered to be the same condition as CLL (see *Chapter 12*).

Waldenström macroglobulinaemia

Waldenström macroglobulinaemia (WM) is an indolent lymphoma characterized by the presence of a lymphocytic plasma cell and lymphoplasmacytic infiltrate in the bone marrow and the presence of a serum monoclonal immunoglobulin M (IgM). WM occurs in 1–2% of NHL patients, and has a global incidence of 2.5 million per year. The median age of onset is 63 years. This NHL type nearly always involves the bone marrow, with about one-third of patients presenting with lymphadenopathy, splenomegaly or hepatomegaly. To date, WM remains incurable, with a median survival of 5–10 years.

Clinical management of NHL

The appropriate choice of treatment for a patient with NHL is a key determinant of success and is based on a combination of disease subtype, stage and patient factors such as age and co-morbidity. The types of treatment options currently used for NHL include:

- 'watch and wait'
- radiotherapy
- single agent or combination chemotherapy
- immunotherapy
- radioimmunotherapy
- high-dose chemotherapy followed by stem cell transplantation.

Chemotherapy remains the mainstay treatment, although these days it is often combined with immunotherapy to increase treatment effectiveness. Ongoing patient participation in clinical trials is essential to improve outcomes. Clinical trials can help to determine whether the use of prognostic factors can identify patients with low risk who can receive less intensive treatments, or how to reduce the toxicity and long-term effects of treatment.

Some patients with indolent forms of NHL have no symptoms at presentation and a 'watch and wait' approach may be appropriate. This strategy is based on balancing the risks of treatment against the benefits of treatment to the individual. For patients with early stage indolent disease, it may be appropriate to withhold initial treatment to avoid possible risks and side-effects until the disease progresses or the patient becomes symptomatic. 'Watch and wait' is seldom appropriate for patients with aggressive NHL.

Selection of treatment strategy for NHL patients is dependent on grade and extent of disease. In effect, patients can be grouped into four broad categories:

- indolent with early stage disease
- indolent with late stage disease
- aggressive with early stage disease
- aggressive with late stage disease.

Indolent NHL with early stage disease

About 20% of cases of indolent lymphoma are diagnosed in Stage I or II. The most common approaches here are either localized radiotherapy to affected nodes, which may be curative or induce prolonged remission or a 'watch and wait' approach, which may delay chemotherapy for 2–3 years. Disease progression requires treatment as for late stage disease.

Indolent NHL with late stage disease

With advanced indolent NHL, the primary aim of therapy is to achieve prolonged remission; the disease is not considered curable with current conventional treatments. However, the disease can often be controlled for several years. The natural history of advanced indolent NHL is for treatment to induce a series of remissions with inevitable relapses. Early remissions can last for 2–3 years, but subsequent remissions tend to become progressively shorter. Indolent lymphomas frequently evolve into a more aggressive form such as DLBCL, which is much harder to treat.

Front-line treatment. Asymptomatic patients are commonly observed and treatment withheld until the disease progresses or symptoms develop. With conventional methods, early treatment does not confer a survival advantage. Symptomatic patients require chemotherapy. There are several regimens from which to choose including cyclophosphamide, vincristine and prednisone (CVP); CVP with rituximab (R-CVP); cyclophosphamide, doxorubicin, vincristine and prednisone (CHOP); CHOP with rituximab (R-CHOP); fludarabine (± mitoxantrone); chlorambucil and prednisone; single-agent rituximab; rituximab with fludarabine; radioimmunotherapy with ^{131}I-tositumomab; ibritumomab tiuxetan; and various other combinations.

The choice of treatment varies depending on the type of NHL. Until recently, there was no single regimen that had clearly demonstrated an overall survival advantage over the others in NHL patients. However, the addition of rituximab to combination chemotherapy has been shown in a recent meta-analysis to improve overall survival in previously untreated follicular lymphoma patients.

Maintenance treatment. Maintenance treatment is given to patients in remission, with the intention of gradually increasing tumour cell kill, thereby prolonging remission duration. The role of maintenance therapy in some lymphoproliferative diseases such as acute lymphoblastic leukaemia in children is well established, but it is still the subject of clinical trials in indolent lymphoma. Maintenance with rituximab has been shown to prolong remission in patients with follicular lymphoma. Ibritumomab has been licensed in Europe as a maintenance treatment for follicular lymphoma in remission.

Second-line treatment. At present, relapse is inevitable in indolent NHL patients. There is no universally agreed standard treatment for relapsed indolent NHL because no single approach has been shown to provide substantially superior survival. Treatment selection is based on consideration of the age and co-morbidities of each patient, stage, sites of involvement and treatment history. In later relapses, the emphasis of treatment may shift from tumour reduction towards palliation. Options include:

■ repeated front-line chemotherapy: in patients that responded well to front-line chemo-therapy and enjoyed an extended remission, it might be worthwhile repeating the same regimen. Responses are frequently obtained using this approach but are generally shorter-lived than previously.

■ chemotherapy: in patients who experienced a short remission or toxicity with their front-line regimen, an alternative regimen may be tried as relapse therapy. The range of choices is similar to those available for front-line use.

■ aggressive chemoradiotherapy: some centres are experimenting with the role of aggressive chemotherapy and radiotherapy in relapsed indolent NHL patients. The intention here is to maximize tumour cell kill and thereby provide extended remissions.

■ allogeneic stem cell transplant (alloSCT): this treatment can provide extended remissions, but is only suitable for the youngest and fittest patients and is also limited by the availability of matched donors. The most worthwhile results in alloSCT are obtained in patients in first or second relapse.

■ radioimmunotherapy: targeted against CD20 using ^{90}Y-ibritumomab tiuxetan or ^{131}I-tositumomab. This approach has the advantage of being able to specifically target even small pockets of lymphomatous tissue, with minimal toxicity to surrounding normal tissue.

■ proteasome inhibition using bortezomib: many of the cellular processes that drive malignant transformation and progression are mediated by the proteasome. Inhibition of the proteasome has yielded promising results in relapsed mantle cell lymphoma and follicular lymphoma. Trials in other subtypes are ongoing.

Aggressive NHL with early stage disease

For patients with aggressive lymphoma, the definition of early stage disease is typically limited to Stage I_A, i.e. a single lymph node region involved and absence of B symptoms (fever, night sweats or severe, rapid weight loss). Such patients are often treated with localized radiotherapy or a short course of chemoradiotherapy, with the intention of effecting a cure.

Aggressive NHL with late stage disease

In practice, all stages of aggressive NHL other than I_A are treated as if they were late stage disease. Paradoxically, aggressive lymphomas that are rapidly growing and rapidly fatal without treatment are the forms most amenable to cure. The exception is MCL, which remains an incurable condition. Overall, with current conventional chemotherapy, about 40% of aggressive NHL patients are cured, about 40–50% experience a response but eventually relapse, and the rest are refractory to front-line treatment. This heterogeneity of outcome probably reflects the heterogeneous nature of this group.

Front-line treatment. For aggressive NHL, the goal of treatment is cure. For this reason, aggressive lymphomas are typically treated early and intensively. Most patients are treated with an anthracycline-based regimen such as CHOP, R-CHOP, CVP or hyper-CVAD (cyclophosphamide, vincristine, doxorubicin (Adriamycin®), dexamethasone). A growing concern for clinicians is to identify upfront patients that are more likely to relapse and to consider treating them even more aggressively. Gene expression profiling has begun to offer some insight into the heterogeneity of outcome within particular disease entities and may inform treatment selection.

Maintenance treatment. The role of maintenance therapy in aggressive NHL is to maintain the period of remission, which may increase the number of patients achieving a cure. The role of rituximab-based maintenance therapy is currently under investigation in aggressive NHL.

Second-line treatment. Patients who relapse may be offered high-dose chemotherapy with autologous stem cell transplantation, alloSCT if possible or chemotherapy with one of several platinum-based regimens (ICE: Ifosfamide + Cis-platinum + Etoposide; DHAP: Dexamethasone + High-dose AraC + Cis-platinum; ESHAP: Etoposide + Methylprednisolone + High-dose AraC + Cis-platinum or EPOCH: Etoposide + Vincristine + Doxorubicin + Cyclophosphamide + Prednisone) (see also *Box 15.3* for explanation of some drug regimen acronyms).

SUGGESTED FURTHER READING

Armitage, J.O., Mauch, P.M., Harris, N.L. & Coiffier, B. (eds) (2009) *Non-Hodgkin Lymphomas*. Lippincott Williams and Wilkins.

Craig, F.E. & Foon, K.A. (2008) Flow cytometric immunophenotyping for hematologic neoplasms. *Blood*, **111**: 3941–3967.

Hatton, C., Collins, G. & Sweetenham, J.W. (2008) *Fast Facts: Lymphoma*. Health Press.

Marcus, R., Sweetenham, J.W. & Williams, M.E. (eds) (2007) *Lymphoma: Pathology, Diagnosis and Treatment*. Cambridge University Press.

Swerdlow, S.H., Campo, E., Harris, N.L. *et al.* (eds) (2008). *WHO Classification of Tumours of Haematopoietic and Lymphoid Tissues, volume 2*. WHO Press.

SELF-ASSESSMENT QUESTIONS

1. 'HD is of B cell origin'. True or false?
2. Name the two types of malignant cells in classical forms of HD and in nodular lymphocyte-predominant HD.
3. Is HD more common in Japan or the Mediterranean region?
4. 'Disease is present in two distinct locations; both affected areas are on the same side (above or below) of the diaphragm. The affected locations may be two distinct nodal regions or one nodal region and one extranodal organ'. Which Ann Arbor stage of HD is described here?
5. In the Ann Arbor staging system, what letter is used to denote bulky disease?
6. Name the seven adverse prognostic factors used to define the IPFP score for HD.
7. Are indolent forms of NHL generally considered to be curable or incurable using current standard therapies?
8. Name the five adverse prognostic factors used to define the IPI score for NHL.
9. Which of the following are aggressive forms of NHL?
   a. FL
   b. DLBCL
   c. MZL
   d. SLL

Myeloma and related disorders

Learning objectives
After studying this chapter you should confidently be able to:

■ **Outline the WHO classification system for the immunosecretory disorders**
The WHO system is the standard system for the classification of the haematological malignancies worldwide and takes account of morphology, cytogenetics and immunophenotyping data. However, in some disease states, earlier classification schemes such as the FAB scheme are still used because they describe clinical entities more precisely.

■ **Clearly differentiate between MGUS and multiple myeloma**
MGUS is characterized by an unexplained, symptomless M protein at levels less than those found in multiple myeloma (MM) patients. Patients with MGUS do not have a malignant condition. MM is a B lymphoid malignancy affecting immunoglobulin-producing plasma cells and is the second most common of the haematological malignancies. MM is characterized by higher M protein expression, bone marrow plasmacytosis and clinical impairments known as ROTI.

■ **Demonstrate knowledge of the laboratory investigation of multiple myeloma**
Laboratory investigation of a suspected MM requires demonstration and quantitation of M protein in serum and/or urine and demonstration of bone marrow plasmacytosis. Other laboratory measures such as raised plasma viscosity, leucoerythroblastic blood picture, rouleaux, cytogenetic abnormalities, abnormal renal function tests, etc. provide useful supplementary information.

■ **Demonstrate knowledge of the pathophysiology of multiple myeloma**
MM is associated with a wide spectrum of complications, including osteolytic bone disease and renal impairment. All of the sequelae of MM are attributable to two causes: the uncontrolled growth of a plasma cell tumour that actively modulates the bone marrow microenvironment and the inexorable and pointless synthesis and secretion of large quantities of monoclonal immunoglobulin by the malignant plasma cells.

The immunosecretory disorders are all malignant B cell disorders that are characterized by pointless secretion of a monoclonal immunoglobulin (M protein). This chapter focuses on the most common of the immunosecretory disorders, myeloma. The other members of this group are dealt with in outline only.

The WHO classification of the immunosecretory disorders is outlined in *Table 16.1.*

16.1 MULTIPLE MYELOMA

Multiple myeloma (MM) is a B lymphoid malignancy affecting immunoglobulin-producing plasma cells and is the second most common of the haematological malignancies (see also

Table 16.1 WHO classification of the immunosecretory disorders

Monoclonal gammopathy of undetermined significance (MGUS)
Plasma cell myeloma:
Indolent myeloma
Smouldering myeloma
Osteosclerotic myeloma (POEMS syndrome)
Plasma cell leukaemia
Non-secretory myeloma
Plasmacytomas:
Solitary plasmacytoma of bone
Extramedullary plasmacytoma
Waldenström macroglobulinaemia (immunocytoma / lymphoplasmacytic lymphoma)
Heavy chain disease (HCD):
γ HCD
α HCD
μ HCD
Immunoglobulin deposition diseases:
Systemic light chain disease
Primary amyloidosis

Box 16.1). The disease is currently incurable. In many respects, MM behaves as a solid tumour with a particular predilection for bone marrow. The major clinical features of MM result from:

- the accumulation of malignant plasma cells within the bone marrow and other tissues causing disruption of normal bone marrow function, resulting in anaemia, leucopenia and thrombocytopenia
- destruction of bone caused by localized stimulation of osteoclast function
- synthesis of monoclonal immunoglobulin (M-Protein) by the myeloma cells, which accumulates in the blood and urine, causing increased blood viscosity and renal failure
- impairment of normal immune function, due to reduced normal immunoglobulin synthesis, leucopenia, and the release of inhibitory cytokines by the myeloma cells.

Box 16.1 History of myeloma

Multiple myeloma was first described in 1844 by Samuel Solly, almost a year before the first descriptions of leukaemia by Virchow and Bennett. Solly called the condition *'mollities and fragilitas ossium'*, which means soft and fragile bones. The first patient to be fully described was called Thomas Alexander McBean, and was diagnosed in 1845 by William Macintyre, a physician in Harley Street, London. The unusual urine problem (urinary M protein) he discovered was fully investigated by Henry Bence Jones, who published his findings in 1848. Macintyre published the full details of this case of Bence Jones myeloma in 1850. The term 'multiple myeloma' was coined in 1873 by Rustizky.

Epidemiology and aetiology

Multiple myeloma primarily affects older adults, with the median age at diagnosis being 68–73 years. The incidence rises exponentially with age, tapering off after the age of 84 years, possibly due to under-reporting. Only 1% of cases are diagnosed in people younger than 40 years old. The incidence of MM has been increasing over the past several decades. In the European Union, the incidence of MM is 5.72 per 100 000 people, and about 27 500 new patients develop the disease each year. Currently, around 70 000 people are living with MM in the European Union. The condition is slightly more common in men than women and more common in people of African descent than in Caucasians. The incidence is lower still for those of Chinese heritage. Five-year survival rates of around 28% have not improved significantly since the early 1970s, although this is beginning to change with improvements in autologous stem cell transplantation and the use of novel agents such as the proteasome inhibitor bortezomib and the thalidomide derivative lenalidomide. An estimated 19 000 deaths from MM occur each year in the EU.

Familial clustering and a higher incidence of the disease in people of African heritage suggest a genetic component to MM, with a possible autosomal dominant inheritance pattern. Use of sensitive tests such as fluorescent *in situ* hybridization (FISH) has led to the detection of genetic abnormalities in at least 90% of multiple myeloma patients. Abnormalities of chromosome 13 are found in about 45% of patients.

Environmental factors that have been associated with MM include engine exhaust fumes, solvents (benzene, creosote), other chemicals, and ionizing radiation (in atomic bomb survivors, radiation workers, and patients undergoing radiotherapy for ankylosing spondylitis). In most cases, the evidence of association is relatively weak.

Diagnosis

The clinical presentation of multiple myeloma and related conditions is highly varied, but the main clinical features are related to progressive osteolytic bone destruction (bone pain, pathological fractures, symptoms indicative of spinal cord/nerve root compression and hypercalcaemia), disease infiltration of the bone marrow compromising normal haemopoiesis (normocytic, normochromic anaemia and increased susceptibility to infection and bleeding secondary to leucopenia and thrombocytopenia), and high levels of circulating M protein (which can result in renal insufficiency or failure and persistent blood hyperviscosity). Less frequently, symptoms indicative of amyloidosis, such as nephrotic syndrome and cardiac failure, or evidence of extramedullary plasmacytoma may be present.

The International Working Group on Myeloma (IMWG) recommends that the diagnosis of MM should be based on the level/concentration of serum M-protein, the percentage of bone marrow plasma cells and the presence of myeloma-related organ or tissue impairment (ROTI). The IMWG recognizes asymptomatic and symptomatic MM.

Asymptomatic myeloma

The diagnosis of asymptomatic multiple myeloma is based on the demonstration of M protein (> 30 g/l) in serum or urine and/or the presence of > 10% plasma cells in the bone marrow, but with no evidence of ROTI.

ROTI is defined as any of the following:

- increased serum calcium levels
- renal insufficiency
- anaemia
- bone lesions
- other organ or tissue impairment relatable to myeloma.

About 70% of patients have normocytic, normochromic anaemia at the time of diagnosis, but eventually almost all patients develop this symptom. A raised serum calcium level is found in 15–20% of patients at presentation, and is an important treatable cause of renal insufficiency. The serum creatinine level is 173 mmol/l or more in 20% of patients at diagnosis. Conventional radiographs show abnormalities consisting of lytic lesions, osteoporosis or fractures in up to 80% of patients at diagnosis, with the vertebrae, skull, thoracic cage, pelvis, humeri and femurs most frequently involved. Additional evidence of ROTI includes symptomatic hyperviscosity, primary systemic amyloidosis, or recurrent bacterial infections (> 2 episodes in 12 months).

The evidence of ROTI is frequently not clear-cut, and the diagnosis of transition from asymptomatic to symptomatic myeloma may need multidisciplinary critical assessment (see also *Box 16.2*).

Box 16.2 Myeloma and hyperviscosity

Raised plasma viscosity (hyperviscosity) results from the great increase in plasma protein concentration due to synthesis of the monoclonal immunoglobulin (M protein).

Symptomatic myeloma

Three criteria are required for a diagnosis of symptomatic myeloma:

- the identification of an M protein in serum and/or urine (no specific level is required for a diagnosis, although 60% have a serum M protein > 30 g/l)
- the presence of a clonal proliferation of plasma cells in the bone marrow (95% of patients have > 10% monoclonal plasma cells in the marrow but no diagnostic level is specified) and/or a biopsy-proven plasmacytoma
- evidence of any ROTI.

The differential diagnosis of MM should include monoclonal gammopathy of undetermined significance (MGUS), AL amyloidosis, B cell non-Hodgkin lymphoma (including Waldenström macroglobulinaemia), chronic lymphocytic leukaemia, and connective tissue disorders.

Haematological examination typically reveals rouleaux formation secondary to the increased immunoglobulin concentration and normocytic, normochromic anaemia secondary to depression of erythropoiesis, variable thrombocytopenia and leucopenia (see *Box 16.3*). The high concentration of serum immunoglobulin (which is basic) confers a bluish background staining to the blood film. In a minority of cases, a leucoerythroblastic blood picture with atypical plasma cells in the peripheral blood is strongly suggestive of the diagnosis. The plasma viscosity is raised, occasionally markedly so. Examination of the bone marrow reveals an increased number of atypical plasma cells. Immunofluorescent staining of the myeloma plasma cells confirms that they are all synthesizing a single form of immunoglobulin heavy chain and light chain.

The investigations required to establish a diagnosis of MM are summarized in *Table 16.2*.

Box 16.3 Rouleaux formation

'Rouleaux' describes a condition where the red cells coalesce into long chains which characteristically resemble 'stacks of coins'. Rouleaux formation is triggered by an increase in the concentration of plasma proteins such as immunoglobulins, and is clearly evident on microscopic examination of a blood film.

Staging and prognosis

The staging of multiple myeloma is intended to provide prognostic data and to provide a guideline for treatment. The International Staging System (ISS) is an updated staging system that separates patients into three prognostic groups based on serum levels of β_2-microglobulin and albumin at presentation (*Table 16.3*).

Table 16.2 The investigations required to establish a diagnosis of MM

Screening tests	Diagnostic tests	Prognostic tests	Tests for ROTI	Optional tests
FBC, ESR or plasma viscosity, blood film examination	Bone marrow aspirate ± trephine biopsy	Bone marrow cytogenetics or FISH analysis	FBC (anaemia)	Bone marrow immunohistology or flow cytometry
Serum/plasma electrolytes, urea, creatinine, calcium, albumin and uric acid	Immunofixation of serum and urine	Quantification of monoclonal protein in serum and urine	Serum/plasma urea, creatinine Creatinine clearance (measured or calculated)	Vitamin B$_{12}$ and folate assays*
Electrophoresis of serum and concentrated urine		Serum/plasma calcium, albumin, β$_2$-microglobulin	Serum/plasma calcium, albumin, lactate dehydrogenase, C-reactive protein (CRP)	
Quantification of non-isotypic immunoglobulins			Quantification of non-isotypic immunoglobulins	
X-ray of symptomatic areas	Skeletal survey	Skeletal survey	Skeletal survey	Magnetic resonance imaging (MRI) Computed tomography scan

FBC, full blood count; ESR, erythrocyte sedimentation rate; FISH, fluorescent *in situ* hybridization

*only required in the presence of macrocytosis

Table 16.3 The International Staging System (ISS) for MM

Stage	Features	Median survival (months)
1	β$_2$M < 3.5 mg/l; albumin ≥ 3.5 g/dl	62
2	β$_2$M < 3.5 mg/l and albumin < 3.5 g/dl; or β$_2$M 3.5–5.5 mg/l	44
3	β$_2$M ≥ 5.5 mg/l	29

β$_2$M – serum β$_2$-microglobulin level; albumin – serum albumin level. Age is the only other factor that significantly affects outcome. Survival > 5 years is associated with age < 60 years and survival for < 2 years with age > 60 years. Other correlations include platelet count < 130 x 10^9/l and/or serum LDH above normal. Cytogenetics also influence outcome but chromosome 13 deletion and complex abnormalities do not add to the impact of age, β$_2$M and albumin.

The ISS is a simple way to assess prognosis in newly-diagnosed myeloma patients because it uses universally available laboratory tests. Some groups have suggested that it underestimates the heterogeneity of myeloma and have proposed cytogenetic and proliferation-based risk stratification models. In most cases, these are intended to supplement rather than supplant the ISS.

Pathophysiology of MM

Immunoglobulin structure

Antibodies belong to a family of plasma proteins called the immunoglobulins. The different members of the immunoglobulin family share a similar monomeric structure. The main structure of the immunoglobulin molecule is formed by two identical polypeptide chains which are about 430 amino acids in length and are designated the 'heavy' or H chains. These H chains are linked by a disulphide bridge (as shown in *Figure 16.1*). The remainder of the structure is formed by a pair of identical 'light' or L chains which are about 220 amino acids long: one L chain is bound to each H chain by a disulphide bridge.

There are two different types of L chain, which are designated κ and λ. Each immunoglobulin molecule will include either κ chains or λ chains, never both. There are five different types of H chain, which are designated α, δ, ε, γ and μ. The H chains determine the 'class' to which an immunoglobulin molecule belongs. The five different classes of immunoglobulin are designated IgA, IgD, IgE, IgG and IgM respectively. Each class of immunoglobulin is characterized by different biological, biochemical and physical properties that determine its function.

L chains consist of two major domains, the constant region (C) and the variable region (V). The genes that encode κ chains are located at chromosome 2p11–12. A single gene encodes the κ chain constant region but the synthesis of the variable regions is considerably more complex (see *Box 16.4*). The κ chain variable regions are encoded by two distinct gene segments: a VL segment which codes for the N-terminal 95 amino acid residue segment of the variable region and a JL joining segment which codes for the remaining 13 amino acid residues of the variable region. DNA sequencing has shown that 40 functional V_κ and five J_κ genes exist. The synthesis of a κ light chain involves the random selection of a single V_κ gene and a single J_κ gene. These are then brought into apposition with the Cκ gene by the rearrangement of the germline DNA within the developing B lymphocyte. The rearranged genes are then transcribed into mRNA in the normal manner. This process of rearrangement allows the generation of a huge variety of different κ chains from a relatively small number of genes.

The generation of diversity in λ chains is achieved by a similar means. In this case, the λ chain gene complex is located on chromosome 22q11.2 and consists of four functional C_λ genes, 39 functional V_λ genes and four J_λ genes.

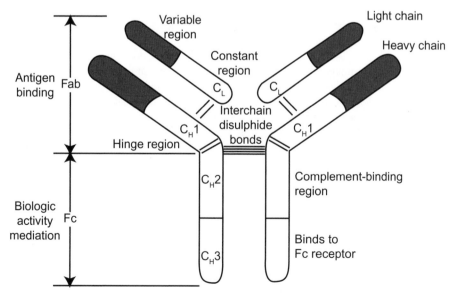

Figure 16.1
Structure of immunoglobulins.

Box 16.4 Somatic hypermutation

Susumu Tonegawa, a Japanese molecular biologist, made the discovery of the genetic mechanisms involved in the generation of antibody diversity, known as somatic hypermutation. In a landmark series of experiments beginning in 1976, he showed that the B cell DNA of embryonic and adult mice differed in sequence and that the genes in the mature cells of the adult mice had moved around, recombined, and deleted to form the diversity of the variable region of antibodies being produced. Tonegawa won the Nobel Prize for Physiology or Medicine in 1987 for this seminal work.

The heavy chain gene complex is located on chromosome 14q32 and consists of 51 functional VH genes, 27 functional DH genes, 6 functional JH genes and genes for each of the heavy chain isotypes (α, δ, ϵ, γ and μ). Although the basic principles for assembly and rearrangement of heavy chains are similar to those for light chains, there are three (designated V, D and J), not two gene segments used in each variable region.

The synthesis of an immunoglobulin heavy chain requires two germ-line DNA rearrangements:

- the first rearrangement results in the selection of one D and one J gene and places them together
- the second rearrangement results in the addition of a V gene to the DJ segment, thereby determining the antigenic specificity of the heavy chain. The resultant VDJ segment is transcribed along with the two C genes that are in close proximity, i.e. the μ and δ genes. Thus, an unstimulated B lymphocyte can express both IgM and IgD immunoglobulins with identical antigenic specificity.

Although the antigenic specificity of the immunoglobulin that a given B lymphocyte can synthesize is irrevocably determined by the particular V, D and J segments that are brought into apposition, the class of immunoglobulin can be changed, a phenomenon known as isotype switching. At the 5′ end of each C gene except the δ gene there is a region of repeating base sequences called a switch region. B lymphocytes are capable of rearranging their DNA by aligning the VDJ segment with the switch region of any of the downstream C genes, resulting in the deletion of the intervening C region DNA and the loss of the ability to synthesize immunoglobulin of those classes.

The biological advantage of the ability to break and recombine the DNA strands in the immunoglobulin light and heavy chain gene complexes is the generation of enormous diversity of antibody production. However, the price that must be paid is that these regions of DNA are highly susceptible to genetic mutation. The immunoglobulin gene loci are heavily implicated in the pathogenesis of a wide range of lymphoid malignancies.

MM is characterized by the synthesis of a monoclonal immunoglobulin by the malignant plasma cells. There are subtypes of myeloma for each immunoglobulin isotype i.e. IgA IgD, IgE, IgG and IgM. Each of these monoclonal immunoglobulins can carry either a κ or a λ light chain, resulting in ten different myeloma subtypes, e.g. IgG κ. In addition, a form of myeloma exists that secretes only light chains, either κ or λ. This is known as Bence Jones myeloma. The frequency of these subtypes is shown in *Table 16.4* (see also *Box 16.5*).

Table 16.4 Distribution of MM subtypes

	IgG		IgA		IgD		IgM		IgE	
	κ	λ	κ	λ	κ	λ	κ	λ	κ	λ
Frequency (%)	35	20	15	11	0.2	1.3	0.1	0.1	8	7

Box 16.5 Myeloma subtypes

Diagnosis of myeloma requires the demonstration of a monoclonal immunoglobulin or immunoglobulin light or heavy chain in serum and, where proteinuria is present, in the urine. Determination of the immunoglobulin subclass and light chain class of the monoclonal protein provides important prognostic information. IgG myeloma is associated with a slower tumour growth rate than the other types of myeloma. However, the rate of synthesis of monoclonal immunoglobulin is highest in this form, so the total serum immunoglobulin concentration also is highest in IgG myeloma. IgA myeloma is associated with hyperviscosity because of the tendency of this form of immunoglobulin to polymerize. IgD myeloma is a particularly malignant form, which is associated with a younger age group and is most common in men. The median survival time for this form of myeloma is about a year. IgE myeloma is extremely rare and is associated with the presentation of plasma cell leukaemia (PCL). This rare disease presents as an acute leukaemia with a circulating plasma cell count greater than 2×10^9/l, anaemia, thrombocytopenia, hepatosplenomegaly, osteolysis and renal failure. The white cell count at presentation frequently exceeds 80×10^9/l of which more than half are atypical plasma cells. Bence Jones (BJ) myeloma occurs when immunoglobulin light chains are synthesized in the absence of heavy chains. This form of myeloma is associated with the most rapid tumour growth. The prognosis is particularly grim for λ chain BJ myeloma.

Cytogenetics

MM is genetically diverse, and most likely results from accumulated mutations that sequentially drive the abnormal plasma cells towards full malignant proliferation. Almost 40% of myeloma patients at diagnosis have an abnormal karyotype and genomic changes are identifiable in around 70% of patients (see *Box 16.6*). Aneuploidy is common, with monosomies being more common than trisomies. Hypodiploidy is found in up to 14% of patients, with monosomies and deletions of chromosomes 6, 13, 16 and 22 being most common. Hyperdiploidy is found in almost one third of patients, including trisomies of chromosomes 3, 5, 7, 9, 11, 15, 19 and 21. Structural abnormalities include deletion and monosomy of chromosome 13, translocations involving chromosome 14q32 and deletions of chromosome 17p13. Cytogenetic abnormalities have a significant influence on disease outcome.

Box 16.6 Cytogenetics and myeloma prognosis

Cytogenetic abnormalities in MM have prognostic significance, presumably because implicated oncogenes affect the biology and behaviour of the disease. In general, patients with t(4;14) or t(14;16) have the worst survival, those with del(17)(p13.1) and/or chromosome 13 anomalies have poor survival and those with t(11;14) have favourable survival.

The pathophysiological significance of some of these mutations has been elucidated. For example, the immunoglobulin genes are among the most heavily transcribed genes in the body. Reciprocal translocations involving the immunoglobulin heavy chain gene locus at 14q32 can involve relocation of a proto-oncogene into this locus, thereby markedly up-regulating its expression. For example, the translocation t(4;14)(p16.3;q32) is present in about 15% of MM patients and leads to up-regulation of at least four oncogenes; fibroblast growth receptor 3 (*FGFR3*), multiple myeloma SET (*MMSET*), an erythropoietin-induced gene *TACC3* and the gene for the cell cycle regulator cyclin D2 (*CCND2*). The result is increased resistance to apoptosis and enhanced proliferation in MM cells that carry this translocation. The translocation t(11;14) (q13;q32) is present in up to 20% of cases of myeloma and results in up-regulation of the cyclin D1 (*CCND1*) and *MYEOV* genes. Several other translocations involving 14q32 are commonly found in MM patients.

Chromosome 17p13 deletion is found in 10% of MM patients and involves the *p53* tumour suppressor gene. *p53* is involved in the regulation of cell proliferation, differentiation and apoptosis, as well as in DNA replication and repair. Dysregulation of *p53* is common in many different cancers and leads to impaired apoptosis and genomic instability, promoting the development of further genetic abnormalities.

Deletions of chromosome 13 usually involve the region 13q14, which includes the retinoblastoma (*RB-1*) gene. The retinoblastoma protein plays an important role in the control of the cell cycle and suppresses the transcription of interleukin (IL)-6, an important growth factor for myeloma cells. Other genes probably contribute to the clinical importance of the 13q deletion.

MM and the marrow microenvironment

Myeloma cells actively modulate their bone marrow microenvironment in such a way as to potentiate their growth and survival. Myeloma cells express multiple adhesion molecules including ICAM-1, the fibronectin receptor VLA-4, the lymphocyte homing receptor CD44 and the neural cell adhesion molecule N-CAM. Bone marrow stromal cells express the adhesion molecule VCAM-1. Binding of myeloma cells to bone marrow stromal cells stimulates a storm of cytokine synthesis and secretion:

- interleukin-6 is secreted by both the stromal cells and the myeloma cells. This cytokine is an important growth and survival factor for myeloma cells.
- several osteoclast-activating factors, such as IL-1β, IL-6, and TNFβ are secreted by stromal cells. These induce differentiation and maturation of the bone-resorbing cells (osteoclasts), and are major contributors to the bone disease that characterizes multiple myeloma.
- syndecan-1 (CD138) also stimulates osteoclastic activity and leads to release from the bone matrix of several cytokines, such as TGFβ, IL-6, bFGF and IGF. These cytokines directly or indirectly stimulate MM cell growth and secretion of parathyroid-hormone-related protein, thereby creating a vicious circle, with MM cells stimulating bone resorption, and bone resorption leading to increased MM cell growth.
- increased expression by stromal cells of proangiogenic factors such as VEGF, bFGF and IL-8. Neovascularization of the bone marrow is an important determinant of the progression of MM.
- increased expression of the anti-apoptotic proteins bcl-2 and bcl-xL, which increases drug resistance of the MM cells and promotes accumulation of genetic mutations, an important facet of MM progression.

The complexity of these multiple interactions is only beginning to be unravelled, but it is already clear that MM cells actively manipulate their bone marrow microenvironment in many different ways that support their growth and survival and promote disease progression. The multiple interactions between MM cells and the microenvironment are depicted in *Figure 16.2*.

Myeloma bone disease

Bone is continuously being remodelled. Bone marrow osteoclasts resorb bone and osteoblasts are charged with its replacement. In health, these competing processes are tightly regulated so that the changing demands of the body are met. For example, during childhood the demand for bone growth and repair of bone is met by favouring osteoblast activity over osteoclast activity and during much of adulthood, the requirement for growth is minimal so resorption and replacement are held in balance.

In MM patients, the balance between osteoclast and osteoblast activity is disturbed by:

- increased expression of cytokines such as IL-6, IL-3, VEGF, TNFα and MIP-1α, that exert direct or indirect osteoclastogenic activity
- expression of potent osteoclast activating factors such as IL-1β, HGF and osteopontin

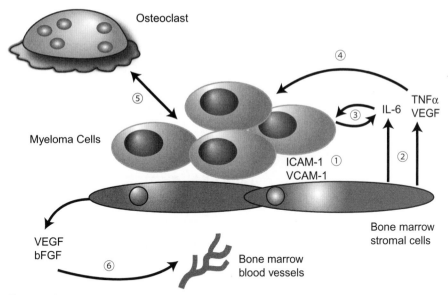

Figure 16.2
Interaction of MM cells with the bone marrow microenvironment. (1) MM cells bind to bone marrow stromal cells via adhesion molecules including ICAM-1 and VCAM-1 (2) adhesion of MM cells to each other and to stromal cells stimulates cytokine secretion, including IL-6, TNFα and VEGF (3) IL-6 is a potent growth factor for MM cells and can act in both paracrine and autocrine fashions (4) and (5) the action of various cytokines on MM cells stimulates secretion of many factors that promote osteoclastogenesis and potentiate osteoclast function (6) VEGF and bFGF stimulate neovascularization, an important component of MM disease progression.

■ inhibition of osteoblast differentiation via bone morphogenic protein-2, the Wnt signalling inhibitor Dikkopf-1 (DKK-1) and IL-3
■ dysregulation of the RANK-RANKL-OPG pathway, the primary regulator of bone remodelling and maintenance of the stable equilibrium necessary for bone strength and repair (see also *Box 16.7*).

Box 16.7 Myeloma and bone remodelling

Activation of the transcription factor NFκB by binding of the receptor activator of NFκB (RANK) on the surface of myeloid progenitors to its ligand (RANKL) is a key requirement for osteoclast differentiation and production. RANKL is normally expressed by bone marrow stromal cells, which also produce osteoprotegerin (OPG), a soluble inhibitor of RANK–RANKL interaction. In health, this pathway is the primary regulator of bone remodelling and maintains the stable equilibrium necessary for bone strength and repair. Myeloma cells disrupt this equilibrium by up-regulating RANKL expression, down-regulating OPG synthesis and secretion and sequestering circulating OPG by binding to surface syndecan-1. Myeloma cells also express RANKL and so can directly affect osteoclast differentiation.

The consequent imbalance in bone remodelling leads to osteopenia and the development of osteolytic lesions. More than 80% of myeloma patients have concomitant osteopenia, which can be the most distressing complication of this disease.

The mechanisms involved in myeloma bone disease are illustrated in *Figure 16.3*.

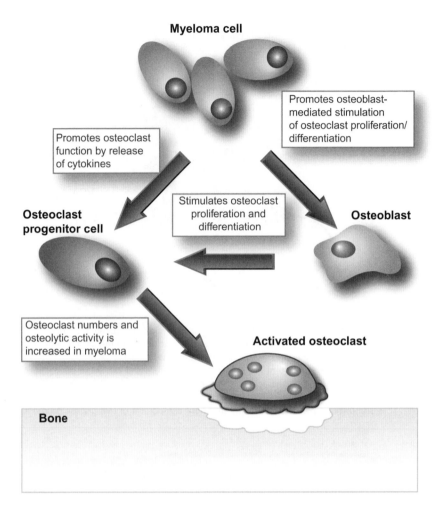

Figure 16.3
Mechanism of myeloma bone disease.

Myeloma renal disease

Impairment of renal function is a common complication in myeloma. Up to one third of patients will have some degree of renal impairment at diagnosis, and about 50% will develop this complication at some point during the course of the disease. The renal impairment is sufficiently severe to warrant haemodialysis in 2–3% of cases. Renal impairment is associated with a high tumour load, and with optimal modern treatment of the renal impairment, it is this that explains the poor prognosis seen in such patients.

The two main causes of renal impairment in myeloma are:

- deposition of light chains (Bence Jones protein) in the renal tubules, which results in loss of nephron function and progressive renal impairment. This results in the formation of casts and is known as 'myeloma kidney'. There is also a direct nephrotoxic effect of light chains. Effective treatment of the myeloma with reduction in light chain concentration can induce some degree of recovery of renal function.

■ hypercalcaemia, caused by bone destruction causes hypercalciuria and dehydration and so contributes to renal failure. Hypercalcaemia is present at diagnosis in 15–30% of patients and 30–40% of patients will have hypercalcaemia at some point in their disease. Patients who develop hypercalcaemia usually have a large tumour burden. Calcium deposits in the kidneys may also cause inflammatory damage to the kidney (interstitial nephritis).

More rarely, deposition of light chains in the glomeruli can cause renal impairment. This is called light-chain nephropathy. Other factors causing or contributing to renal impairment include nephrotoxic drugs, infection, amyloidosis and dehydration. Non-steroidal anti-inflammatory drugs often contribute to renal failure in myeloma patients and should be avoided. Bisphosphonate therapy may have an adverse effect on renal function, and close monitoring of renal function is recommended if these drugs are used.

Treatment strategies

At diagnosis, symptomatic multiple myeloma is heterogeneous and the course and response to treatment are affected by many disease and patient variables, including disease stage and prognostic factors, patient age, performance status, and renal function. Median survival of patients with newly diagnosed multiple myeloma is 6–12 months in the absence of treatment and 2–4 years with standard chemotherapy.

The preferred front-line treatment is autologous haemopoietic stem cell transplantation, but this is available for only a minority of patients due to age or comorbidity. The conventional induction therapy for stem cell transplantation is vincristine, adriamycin and dexamethasone (VAD), but this is beginning to be supplanted by novel combination therapies including thalidomide, lenalidomide and bortezomib.

Conventional chemotherapy for *de novo* myeloma patients unsuitable for transplant involves melphalan or cyclophosphamide with prednisone. Responses (defined as ≥ 50% reduction in M protein) in up to 50% of patients are commonly obtained with these regimens, but complete responses (100% reduction in M protein) are rare. Newer combinations that add thalidomide or bortezomib to this combination appear to increase both the response rate and the proportion of high quality responses and may, in the near future, become the new standard.

Although responses to therapy are common, repeated relapses are inevitable. Treatment, therefore, is centred on a sequence of therapies aimed at achieving durable responses and treatment of relapsed disease with subsequent courses of treatment, assuming increasing refractoriness to therapy with each relapse (*Figure 16.4*).

Eventually, all patients have disease relapse that is refractory to further therapy. Patients with relapsed/refractory multiple myeloma have a median survival of only 6 to 9 months, and treatment at this stage is mainly palliative, to reduce disease-related symptoms (see also *Box 16.8*).

Box 16.8 Myeloma and the microenvironment

Improved understanding of the ways in which MM cells modulate their microenvironment has led to identification of novel targets for therapy and the introduction of new treatments. The first major improvement in drug treatment of MM for more than 20 years came with the use of thalidomide in patients with advanced disease. The rationale for this was that thalidomide has antiangiogenic properties and that neoangiogenesis is important to MM disease progression. The successful use of thalidomide led to the development of a less toxic but equally effective analogue called lenalidomide. The fact that the transcription factor NF-κB is central to the expression of the multiple cytokines and other factors that modulate MM cell and osteoclast biology led to the development of bortezomib, an entirely unique agent that acts by reversibly inhibiting the proteasome and modulating NF-κB activation. These drugs are beginning to transform MM therapy and have all been found to exert several other anti-myeloma effects at the molecular level.

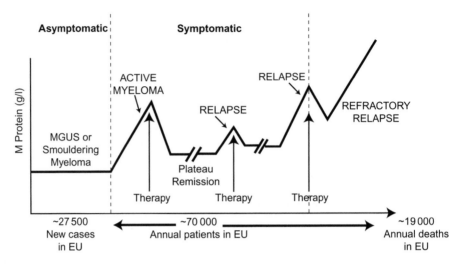

Figure 16.4
Schematic representation of the course of MM.

Supportive care is an important facet of myeloma treatment and requires the use of blood and platelet transfusion or recombinant haemopoietic growth factors to address cytopenia, bisphosphonates for secondary prevention of bony complications, including hypercalcaemia, pathological fracture, and spinal cord compression and analgesia.

16.2 VARIANTS OF MYELOMA

Indolent myeloma

A diagnosis of indolent myeloma can be made in a patient with:

- fewer than three osteolytic lesions, without compression fractures
- M protein levels IgG ≤ 7 g/dl, IgA ≤ 5 g/dl
- no symptoms or associated disease features
- performance status > 70%
- haemoglobin > 10 g/dl
- serum calcium normal
- serum creatinine < 2 mg/dl
- no infections.

Smouldering myeloma

Smouldering myeloma is the same as indolent myeloma apart from having 10–30% plasma cells in the bone marrow and an absence of bone disease.

Osteosclerotic myeloma (POEMS syndrome)

POEMS is a very rare plasma cell disorder that is characterized by the presence of:

- Polyneuropathy (sensorimotor demyelination)

■ Organomegaly (hepatosplenomegaly)
■ Endocrinopathy (diabetes, gynaecomastia, testicular atrophy, impotence)
■ Monoclonal gammopathy
■ Skin changes (hyperpigmentation, hypertrichosis).

POEMS accounts for around 1% of the plasma cell malignancies and differs from myeloma in that there are fewer than 5% plasma cells in the bone marrow and that renal failure and severe bone disease are rare. The nature of the relationship between POEMS syndrome and MM is not well understood. This disorder has also been called osteosclerotic myeloma, Crow–Fukase syndrome, PEP syndrome (**p**lasma cell dyscrasia, **e**ndocrinopathy, **p**olyneuropathy), and Takatsuki syndrome.

Plasma cell leukaemia

Plasma cell leukaemia accounts for about 2% of plasma cell malignancies and can be divided into primary and secondary forms. Primary PCL is diagnosed without evidence of pre-existing myeloma, whereas secondary PCL clearly evolves as a terminal complication of MM, most commonly Bence Jones or IgD subtypes. The disease is characterized by $> 2 \times 10^9/l$ or 20% plasma cells in the peripheral blood and an aggressive course with short survival. Most of the clinical features of MM are also seen in PCL, although osteolytic lesions and bone pain are less frequent and lymphadenopathy and organomegaly are more frequent. Renal failure is particularly common.

Non-secretory myeloma

This variant presents diagnostic challenges because patients with non-secretory myeloma have no detectable M protein in either their serum or urine. About 3% of symptomatic MM patients are non-secretory. Confirmation of the diagnosis relies on identification of the clonality of the plasma cells using immunoperoxidase or immunofluorescence. Renal impairment is less common than in patients with secretory multiple myeloma. The treatment and outcomes for non-secretory myeloma are the same as for secretory MM.

16.3 MONOCLONAL GAMMOPATHY OF UNDETERMINED SIGNIFICANCE

Monoclonal gammopathy of undetermined significance (MGUS) is characterized as the presence of an unexplained, symptomless M protein at levels less than that found in MM patients (see *Box 16.9*). The level of M protein may remain stable for several years. MGUS is identifiable in about 3% of people aged > 70 years and in 1% of people older than 50 years.

Patients with MGUS do not have a malignant condition, but should be monitored periodically because about 25–30% eventually progress to MM or a related disorder. Progression can occur

---

Box 16.9 MGUS

MGUS has been called many different things over the years, including essential hyperglobulinaemia, benign, idiopathic, asymptomatic, non-myelomatous, discrete, cryptogenic, lanthanic and rudimentary monoclonal gammopathy, dysimmunoglobulinaemia, asymptomatic paraimmunoglobulinaemia and idiopathic paraproteinaemia. The term unattributed or unassociated monoclonal gammopathy MG(u) has been suggested, but has yet to gain acceptance.

after up to three decades of stable MGUS. The criteria recommended by the International Myeloma Working Group for the diagnosis of MGUS are:

- serum M protein < 30 g/l
- clonal plasma cells in bone marrow < 10% (if done)
- low level of plasma cell infiltration in a trephine biopsy (if done)
- no evidence of other B cell proliferative disorders
- no evidence of ROTI.

16.4   SOLITARY PLASMACYTOMA OF BONE

A plasmacytoma is a discrete, usually solitary mass of malignant plasma cells. They can occur in bone or in one of several extramedullary sites.

Solitary plasmacytoma of bone occurs in 3–5% of patients with plasma cell malignancy. It is twice as common in men than in women and the median age at diagnosis is about 55 years. The most common symptom at presentation is pain at the site of the skeletal lesion, and may be the result of pathological fracture. Plasmacytoma of bone can present as a palpable mass where the tumour has broken through the bone into surrounding tissue. The site of a solitary plasmacytoma of bone is more common in the axial skeleton and in the thoracic vertebrae.

For a diagnosis of solitary plasmacytoma of bone, skeletal survey must reveal no other myelomatous lesions, anaemia, hypercalcaemia or renal impairment. If these are present, a diagnosis of asymptomatic or smouldering myeloma should be made. A minor M protein may be present in serum or urine. Treatment involves localized radiotherapy of the affected area. Progression to MM occurs in around 50% of patients, usually within four years or so.

16.5   EXTRAMEDULLARY PLASMACYTOMA

Plasmacytomas can occur in extramedullary sites such as the upper respiratory tract, gastrointestinal tract, central nervous system, urinary bladder, thyroid, breasts, testes, parotid gland or lymph nodes. Diagnosis relies on finding a plasma cell tumour in an extramedullary site in the absence of signs of MM on bone marrow, blood urine and radiological examination. Treatment consists of localized radiotherapy of the affected area and may be curative. Progression to symptomatic MM occurs in about 15% of patients.

16.6   WALDENSTRÖM MACROGLOBULINAEMIA

Waldenström macroglobulinaemia (WM) is an uncommon B lymphoid malignant disorder, which is characterized by hyperviscosity secondary to the excessive secretion of a monoclonal IgM immunoglobulin by the malignant clone (see also *Box 16.10*). Prior to the publication of the

---

Box 16.10 History of WM

Waldenström macroglobulinaemia was first described by Jan G. Waldenström (1906–1996) in 1944 in two patients with bleeding from the nose and mouth, anaemia, hypofibrinogenaemia, swollen lymph nodes, malignant plasma cells in the bone marrow, and increased blood viscosity due to increased levels of a class of heavy proteins called macroglobulins.

WHO classification, WM was thought to be related to MM because of the presence of monoclonal gammopathy and infiltration of the bone marrow and other organs by plasmacytoid lymphocytes. It is now classified as a lymphoplasmacytic lymphoma, a subcategory of the indolent (low-grade) non-Hodgkin lymphomas. The median age of presentation of WM is 60–65 years.

WM is an indolent disease which typically presents with variable combinations of weight loss, hepatosplenomegaly, lymphadenopathy, peripheral neuropathy and a bruising or bleeding tendency, following a long history of vague malaise, weakness and weight loss. Because of the large size and chemical properties of IgM the most common cause of morbidity is hyperviscosity syndrome, which causes blurring or loss of vision, headache and (rarely) stroke or coma.

Haematological examination reveals marked rouleaux and normocytic, normochromic anaemia. The total white cell count may be normal or depressed but relative lymphocytosis is common. The platelet count is normal at presentation in 50% of cases. However, neutropenia and thrombocytopenia often become more troublesome as the disease advances. Attempts to aspirate bone marrow frequently fail due to hypercellularity and the extremely high viscosity of the marrow blood. The malignant cells are pleomorphic: some resemble lymphocytes whereas others clearly resemble plasma cells; most, however, have an intermediate appearance and are described as being lymphoplasmacytoid.

Treatment of WM is usually reserved for symptomatic patients and includes the monoclonal antibody rituximab, sometimes in combination with chemotherapy such as chlorambucil, cyclophosphamide or vincristine, with or without concurrent corticosteroids. Autologous stem cell transplantation may be offered to younger patients. Symptomatic relief from hyperviscosity syndrome can be achieved using plasmapheresis, but does not address the underlying disease.

Median survival is about five years from time of diagnosis. Transformation to MM can occur, but this is a rare event.

16.7 HEAVY CHAIN DISEASES

The heavy chain diseases (HCD) are rare B cell proliferative disorders characterized by the uncontrolled synthesis and secretion of abnormal, often structurally incomplete, immunoglobulin heavy chains in serum, urine, or both. HCD is classified according to the immunoglobulin heavy chain type, i.e. α, γ and μ HCD. Up to a third of patients have an associated autoimmune disorder.

Patients usually present with evidence of systemic disease, such as weight loss, fever, anaemia, and recurrent infection. Splenomegaly usually is present. Hepatomegaly and peripheral lymphadenopathy are common findings. Patients may have osteolytic lesions and pathological fractures. Renal impairment is uncommon.

There is no specific treatment for HCD. Symptomatic patients may be offered treatment similar to MM or CLL. Where remissions are obtained, they are usually short-lived. Overall, the prognosis is poor, but there is wide variation. Some patients remain asymptomatic for several months, while in others the disease progresses rapidly, with survival of only a few months.

16.8 IMMUNOGLOBULIN DEPOSITION DISEASES

Systemic light chain disease

Light chain disease (LCD) is characterized by deposition of monoclonal, amorphous immunoglobulin light chains in the kidney, liver, heart, small intestine, spleen, skin, nervous system and bone marrow. In the majority of cases, the monoclonal light chain is identified as a κ chain and a κ M protein is present in serum and/or urine.

The most common morbidity associated with LCD is renal failure, but hepatic failure, congestive heart failure, peripheral neuropathy and skin lesions secondary to the deposition of light chains can all occur. Some cases of LCD transform to lymphoma, multiple myeloma or Waldenström macroglobulinaemia.

Primary amyloidosis

Amyloidosis is an umbrella term given to a group of diverse diseases characterized by the deposition and accumulation in the tissues of aggregates of an abnormal form of a variety of different proteins. These aggregates are called amyloid. Accumulation of amyloid in the tissues ultimately leads to widespread organ dysfunction and failure.

There are several different forms of amyloidosis, including:

- **AL amyloidosis**, which used to be called primary amyloidosis, is caused by a low-grade plasma cell disorder. The abnormal plasma cells secrete unstable monoclonal immunoglobulin light chains that form insoluble aggregates (amyloid). **AH amyloidosis** is a variant of AL amyloidosis in which the precursor protein is immunoglobulin heavy chain.
- **AA amyloidosis** used to be called secondary amyloidosis because it occurs following chronic inflammatory disorders such as tuberculosis or rheumatoid arthritis, chronic infections and occasionally malignant disease.
- **Aβ amyloidosis** is caused by accumulation of the transmembrane glycoprotein amyloid beta precursor protein (AβPP). This form of amyloidosis is seen in Alzheimer's disease and certain other degenerative brain disorders.
- **PrP amyloidosis**, where the precursor is a misfolded prion protein. This form of amyloidosis can follow an infection (e.g. kuru, transmissable spongiform encephalopathy) or may be inherited (Creutzfeldt–Jakob disease, Gerstmann–Sträussler–Scheinker syndrome, fatal familial insomnia). The infectious animal diseases scrapie and bovine spongiform encephalopathy are related to the human forms.
- **Familial or hereditary amyloidosis**, in which amyloid formation is caused by the presence of mutated genes that synthesize abnormal proteins e.g. transthyretin, fibrinogen Aα and apoprotein A-1.

Diseases other than AL amyloidosis are outside the scope of this book.

Most cases of AL amyloidosis have a low-grade plasma cell disorder with minimal infiltration of the bone marrow. In many ways, the plasma cell component is similar to monoclonal gammopathy of undetermined significance (MGUS). Monoclonal immunoglobulin light chains can be measured in the blood of about 95% of patients with AL amyloidosis. Chromosomal abnormalities that frequently occur in MGUS and myeloma such as 13q14 deletion and 14q translocations are also found in AL amyloidosis patients.

About 20% of AL amyloidosis patients at diagnosis have a more obvious plasma cell proliferation and also satisfy the criteria for a diagnosis of myeloma. In addition, about 20% of myeloma patients are also diagnosed as having AL amyloidosis, either at the time of their myeloma diagnosis or later in the course of their disease. It is rare, however, for AL amyloidosis patients with a subtle plasma cell disorder to progress to overt myeloma. This may be because of the short median survival time from diagnosis of AL amyloidosis, but may also reflect a real biological distinction between the disease entities. The prognosis for myeloma patients with coincident AL amyloidosis is significantly poorer than for uncomplicated myeloma, with an average survival after diagnosis of 1–2 years.

Epidemiology

AL amyloidosis is a rare condition with an estimated prevalence rate of about 1 in 91 000 people. In common with other plasma cell disorders, the frequency of AL amyloidosis increases with age: the median age at presentation is 65 years, with only 10% of patients aged below 50 years. About 60–65% of cases are male. There are no known racial predispositions and risk factors for developing AL amyloidosis have not been identified.

The prognosis for patients with AL amyloidosis is poor, with progressive organ failure and death usually occurring within 1–2 years following diagnosis.

Clinical features and diagnosis

AL amyloidosis is a multiple system disorder that can affect almost any organ except the brain. The wide variety of non-specific clinical features that result often delays diagnosis. A high proportion of newly diagnosed patients report a recent history of fatigue, fluid retention and weight loss. Most patients are diagnosed only after symptoms specific to a particular organ are present. Thus, a variable history of investigation and treatment for renal, cardiac, hepatic or neurological symptoms is common before referral to a haematologist is made following suspicion of amyloidosis. Significant physical findings in AL amyloidosis include tongue enlargement, periorbital purpura (the raccoon eye sign), and periarticular amyloid infiltration (the shoulder pad sign). When present, these are specific for amyloidosis but can easily be overlooked and only occur in about 15% of patients.

Although almost any organ of the body may be involved, usually one or two are predominantly affected in an individual patient. Commonly, patients will be described as having amyloidosis of a particular organ, for example, cardiac amyloidosis or renal amyloidosis. This is potentially misleading because it reflects only the organ most affected and does not imply that other organs are not affected. Neither does it mean that these are in any way different to AL amyloidosis.

The most common clinical manifestations of AL amyloidosis at diagnosis include:

- **renal involvement.** About one third of AL amyloidosis patients have dominant renal amyloid at diagnosis.
- **gastrointestinal and hepatic involvement.** Amyloid involvement of the GI tract or liver can occur simultaneously or separately. GI tract involvement may be focal or diffuse and symptoms relate to the location, size and extent of AL amyloid deposits. Up to 25% of AL amyloidosis patients have hepatic involvement, with hepatomegaly and increased serum alkaline phosphatase concentration.
- **cardiac involvement.** About 20% of AL amyloidosis patients have dominant symptomatic cardiac amyloid at diagnosis.
- **nerve involvement.** Peripheral and autonomic neuropathy is seen in 15% of AL amyloidosis patients.

AL amyloidosis is considered an incurable disease and has a relatively poor long-term prognosis with a median survival of 12–24 months; 51% of patients survive for one year; 16% of patients for five years and less than 5% of patients for 10 years. The main determinants of prognosis are the extent and location of amyloid deposition and the degree of organ impairment at diagnosis. For example, the median survival of patients with dominant cardiac involvement is only six months and for hepatic failure 21 months.

Principles of treatment

There is no drug available at present that specifically targets AL amyloid deposits. The major principles of treatment then, are to treat the underlying plasma cell disorder to minimize further amyloid deposition and to support the function of damaged organs. Most of the treatment options are those that have proved useful in the treatment of myeloma. Successful reduction of the plasma cell clone can lead to stabilization or even partial regression of amyloid deposits. However, this process is slow and it can take up to 12 months after the end of chemotherapy for patients to experience a significant improvement in their health. Because of this, most physicians aim for rapid suppression of the underlying disorder. Existing organ damage frequently hampers this aim by reducing the ability of the patient to tolerate aggressive treatment. Treatment is often tailored along the way according to rapidity and depth of response and adverse events. Optimal management of AL amyloidosis requires a multi-speciality approach adapted to the specific requirements of each patient.

SUGGESTED FURTHER READING

Alexander, D.D., Mink, P.J., Adami, H., *et al.* (2007) Multiple myeloma: A review of the epidemiologic literature. *Int. J. Cancer,* **120 (S12):** 40–61.

Comenzo, R.L. (2006) Amyloidosis. *Curr. Treat. Options Oncol.* 7: 225–236.

Dimopoulos, M.A. & Anagnostopoulos, A. (2005) Waldenström's macroglobulinemia. *Best Pract. Res. Clin. Haematol.* **18:** 747–765.

Kyle, R.A. & Rajkumar, S.V. (2005) Monoclonal gammopathy of undetermined significance. *Clin. Lymphoma Myeloma,* **6:** 102–114.

Malpas, J.S., Bergsagel, D.E., Kyle, R.A. & Anderson, K.C. (2004) *Myeloma: Biology and Management,* 3rd edn. W.B. Saunders, Oxford.

Rajkumar, S.V., Dispenzieri, A. & Kyle, R.A. (2006) Monoclonal gammopathy of undetermined significance, Waldenström's macroglobulinemia, AL amyloidosis, and related plasma cell disorders: diagnosis and treatment. *Mayo Clin. Proc.* **81:** 693–703.

Smith, A., Wisloff, F. & Samson, D. (2006) Guidelines on the diagnosis and management of multiple myeloma 2005. *Br. J. Haematol.* **132:** 410–451.

SELF-ASSESSMENT QUESTIONS

1. Is multiple myeloma a B cell, T cell or NK cell disorder?
2. What is ROTI in the context of myeloma?
3. What are the three criteria required for a diagnosis of symptomatic multiple myeloma?
4. A newly diagnosed MM patient has a serum β_2M of 2.1 mg/l and a serum albumin of 2.8 g/dl. What is their ISS stage?
5. Name the five classes of immunoglobulin.
6. What is the most common subtype of multiple myeloma?
7. Which of the following are adhesion molecules?
   a. ICAM-1
   b. IL-6
   c. CD44
   d. IL-8
   e. VEGF
8. Complete the sentence:
   Osteo _____ resorb bone while osteo _____ replace bone.
9. What is the alternative name for free monoclonal immunoglobulin light chains secreted in myeloma?
10. What is the difference in laboratory test results between indolent myeloma and smouldering myeloma?
11. Is MGUS a malignant disease?

Bone marrow failure

Learning objectives
After studying this chapter you should confidently be able to:

■ **Define the scope and nature of bone marrow failure**
Bone marrow failure encompasses all forms of peripheral blood cytopenias that are caused by a failure of haemopoiesis: it is not restricted to red cell cytopenias. Disorders such as the myelodysplastic syndromes, which are characterized by bone marrow hypercellularity and ineffective haemopoiesis, or hypersplenism where cytopenia is secondary to peripheral blood cell destruction, are specifically excluded by this definition.

■ **Compare and contrast the pathophysiology of selected inherited and acquired bone marrow failure states**
Almost one third of childhood cases of bone marrow failure are inherited and most of these can be classified as Fanconi anaemia or Diamond–Blackfan syndrome. These conditions are genetically diverse. Other inherited bone marrow failure states are relatively rare. Acquired aplastic anaemia is an immune mediated condition.

■ **Review the pathogenesis and pathophysiology of PNH**
Paroxysmal nocturnal haemoglobinuria (PNH) is an acquired clonal haemopoietic stem cell disorder characterized by haemolysis, bone marrow failure and a thrombotic tendency. PNH is caused by somatic mutations in the *PIGA* gene (Xp22.1), encoding a protein involved in the biosynthesis of the glycosylphosphatidylinositol (GPI) anchor, leading to a deficiency of all GPI-anchored cell membrane proteins. Treatment is primarily symptomatic, but allogeneic stem cell transplantation may offer a cure.

■ **Outline the available treatment strategies for aplastic anaemia**
Supportive care is an important component of the treatment of aplastic anaemia, but only allogeneic haemopoietic stem cell transplantation offers the prospect of cure. Non-transplant candidates are offered immunosuppressive treatment to control the disease.

Bone marrow failure includes both inherited and acquired conditions and is characterized by damage or defect of haemopoietic stem cells or the bone marrow microenvironment that results in some degree of hypoplasia affecting one or more cell lines (see also *Box 17.1*). Disorders such as the myelodysplastic syndromes, which are characterized by bone marrow hypercellularity and ineffective haemopoiesis, or hypersplenism where cytopenia is secondary to peripheral blood cell destruction are specifically excluded by this definition.

Bone marrow failure is a relatively rare condition with an overall incidence in Western Europe of about 1 per 200 000. The incidence of bone marrow failure is estimated to be around three times higher than this in Japan and the Far East, and also is greater in certain underdeveloped countries where it more commonly affects children. The condition can present at any age, but is seen most commonly in young adults aged 15–25 years and in patients aged over 60 years.

> **Box 17.1 Definitions of anaemia**
>
> Anaemia is often used in the sense of a reduced number of red blood cells e.g. iron deficiency anaemia. However, the term is derived from the Ancient Greek *an* (none) and *haima* (blood), so its original meaning relates to a reduction in any or all of the blood cells. It is in this wider sense that the term hypoplastic anaemias is used. Thus, the hypoplastic anaemias are a group of haematological disorders characterized by bone marrow failure and include thrombocytopenias, leucopenias and pancytopenias as well as anaemias (in the narrower sense).

17.1 CLASSIFICATION OF THE BONE MARROW FAILURES

There is no universally agreed classification scheme for the different forms of bone marrow failure. In this book they are classified according to three criteria:

- whether they are inherited or acquired disorders
- the haemopoietic cell line(s) affected
- aetiology.

17.2 THE INHERITED BONE MARROW FAILURES

Fanconi anaemia

Almost one third of childhood cases of bone marrow failure are inherited and most of these can be classified as Fanconi anaemia. A range of congenital abnormalities are present including patchy brown skin pigmentation, stunting of growth, microcephaly, renal and skeletal malformations and, classically, absence or underdevelopment of both thumbs (see *Box 17.2*).

> **Box 17.2 Microcephaly**
>
> Microcephaly is a medical term that means an abnormally small head in relation to the rest of the body.

Fanconi anaemia is inherited as an autosomal recessive disorder and is caused by mutations in one of 11 different genes, designated *FANCA* (16q24.3), *FANCB* (Xp22.31), *FANCC* (9q22.3), *FANCD1* (13q12.3), *FANCD2* (3p25.3), *FANCE* (6p21.3), *FANCF* (11p15), *FANCG* (9p13), *FANCL* (2p16.1), *FANCI* (unknown locus), and *FANCJ* (unknown locus; see *Box 17.3*). There is no *FANCH* gene. Affected individuals are homozygous or doubly heterozygous for mutations in these genes. The protein products of these genes appear to function to protect against genotoxic stress at least in part by forming complexes with each other and they also play a role in cell survival pathways.

> **Box 17.3 *FANCD1* and *BRCA2***
>
> The *FANCD1* gene is also known as *BRCA2* (Breast Cancer Type 2 susceptibility gene). The encoded protein is involved in the repair of chromosomal damage and it also plays a critical role in embryonic development. Mutated forms of this gene cannot repair DNA effectively, allowing mutations in other genes to accumulate. Mutations of the *FANCD1* / *BRCA2* gene cause an increased risk for breast cancer. Fanconi anaemia results from homozygosity for abnormalities of this gene.

Mutations of the *FANCA* gene are the most common in patients with Fanconi anaemia, accounting for almost two-thirds of cases. The spectrum of *FANCA* mutations is very wide and includes nonsense, mis-sense, and splicing mutations as well as microdeletions, microinsertions and duplications.

The most common presenting features for Fanconi anaemia are bleeding secondary to thrombocytopenia and a request for investigation of short stature. Typically, thrombocytopenia develops first as an isolated abnormality, followed some months or even years later by the development of anaemia. Neutropenia is usually a relatively late manifestation of the disease. Bone marrow examination reveals hypocellularity with a reduction in the number of CFU-GEMM, CFU-GM and BFU-E and extensive fatty replacement of haemopoietic tissue. Dysplastic features are usually minimal and reflect the stress imposed on the dwindling haemopoietic tissue in trying to maintain circulating blood cell counts.

More than 10% of Fanconi anaemia cases progress to acute leukaemia or develop a tumour of the gastrointestinal tract or skin (see also *Box 17.4*). Allogeneic stem cell transplantation is a successful form of treatment for hypoplastic anaemia but does not correct the other congenital abnormalities or the tendency to develop non-haemopoietic malignancy. In the absence of a suitable bone marrow donor, administration of high dose anabolic steroids produces a temporary recovery in peripheral blood cell counts but at the cost of development of male secondary sexual characteristics in both boys and girls, liver damage and bouts of uncontrolled hyperactivity and aggression.

Box 17.4 Fanconi anaemia and chromosome fragility

Standard cytogenetic preparations of bone marrow from cases of Fanconi anaemia typically show some increase in the number of chromosomal breakages and complex rearrangements present. However, pretreatment of the bone marrow samples with cyclophosphamide or mitomycin C increases the incidence of these abnormalities markedly. Using this technique, Fanconi homozygotes are readily and reliably detectable. The cells of Fanconi heterozygotes may also show an increase in the number of chromosomal aberrations but cannot be separated from normal cells with absolute certainty.

Pearson syndrome

Pearson syndrome is a rare, refractory macrocytic sideroblastic anaemia with pancytopenia, defective oxidative phosphorylation, exocrine pancreatic insufficiency, and variable hepatic, renal and endocrine failure. It is caused by mutations of mitochondrial DNA. Death often occurs in infancy or early childhood due to infection or metabolic crisis. Treatment is largely symptomatic; stem cell transplantation might cure the haematological abnormality, but not the other organ dysfunction.

Diamond–Blackfan syndrome

Diamond–Blackfan syndrome typically presents in the first two years of life as a severe anaemia and reticulocytopenia in the presence of normal white cell and platelet counts. Bone marrow examination reveals either a complete absence of erythropoietic precursors or a maturation arrest in erythropoiesis. Almost half of affected individuals also have congenital abnormalities, including craniofacial malformations, thumb or upper limb abnormalities, cardiac defects, urogenital malformations, and cleft palate. Diamond–Blackfan syndrome may be confused with Fanconi anaemia, although cytogenetic abnormalities are absent.

Diamond–Blackfan syndrome is genetically heterogeneous. About 20–25% of affected individuals have a mutation in the RPS19 gene on chromosome 19q13.2, which encodes a protein involved in both ribosome construction and other extra-ribosomal functions. A second genetic link has been demonstrated in some families that maps to chromosome 8p23.3–8p22. The nature of this gene remains to be determined. There is evidence for further genetic heterogeneity.

The treatment of choice for Diamond–Blackfan syndrome is allogeneic stem cell transplantation but if this option is not available most cases respond well to high dose corticosteroids or cyclosporine. The success of corticosteroid therapy in inducing prompt and sustainable remission of the anaemia suggests an immune-mediated pathogenesis.

The congenital dyserythropoietic anaemias

The congenital dyserythropoietic anaemias (CDAs) are a group of rare inherited disorders of unknown cause that are characterized by a variable degree of anaemia, reticulocytopenia, marked ineffective erythropoiesis and erythroblast multinuclearity. Three types of CDA are recognized.

- **Type I CDA** is associated with mild to moderate macrocytic anaemia, megaloblastoid bone marrow appearances and an autosomal recessive mode of inheritance. The hallmark of this form of CDA is the presence in the bone marrow of up to 3% binucleated erythroblasts with intranuclear chromatin bridges. Dysmorphic features may be present. The causative gene has been identified as *CDAN1*, but the function of the transcribed protein is unknown.

- **Type II CDA** is the most common form of CDA and is characterized by a mild to severe normocytic anaemia, the presence of up to 50% multinucleated erythroblasts in the bone marrow, enhanced expression of Ii antigens on red cells and an autosomal recessive mode of inheritance. Mature peripheral blood red cells in this disorder are highly susceptible to lysis in acidified serum. The gene for CDA type II has been mapped to chromosome 20q11.2, but has not been definitively identified. CDA type II is also known by the descriptive title hereditary erythroblast multinuclearity with positive acidified serum test (HEMPAS; see *Box 17.5*).

- **Type III CDA** is the rarest form of CDA and is associated with a mild macrocytic anaemia, the presence of highly multinucleate erythroblasts in the bone marrow and an autosomal dominant mode of inheritance. The abnormal erythroblasts may contain up to 12 nuclei and are sometimes known as gigantoblasts. The gene for CDA type III has been mapped to chromosome region 15q21–q25, but has not been definitively identified.

Several other types of CDA have been described, but these are all extremely rare.

Box 17.5 Ham's test – part 1

In Ham's acidified serum test, the patient's red cells are incubated for 1 hour at 37 °C with a selection of ABO compatible acidified sera and the samples are examined for the presence of haemolysis. A 'positive' result (i.e. haemolysis) is obtained in cases of paroxysmal nocturnal haemoglobinuria (PNH) and HEMPAS (see also *Box 17.9*).

Inherited neutropenias

Cyclic neutropenia

Cyclic neutropenia is a rare congenital disorder, which is characterized by recurrent neutropenia with oral ulceration, pharyngitis with lymphadenopathy and, in severe cases, pneumonia. The neutrophil count in affected individuals follows a regular cyclic pattern with bouts of neutropenia occurring at about three-weekly intervals and lasting for about four days. A sharp fall in the numbers of CFU-GM present in the bone marrow and an arrest of granulopoietic activity occurs about one week before the neutropenic phase. These changes remit spontaneously after a few days and the neutrophil count climbs back into the lower reaches of normality for about 2–3 weeks before the cycle repeats itself.

Cyclic neutropenia is typically an autosomal dominant abnormality due to mutations in *ELA2*, the neutrophil elastase gene. Usually, cyclic neutropenia is relatively benign, requiring only antimicrobial therapy to treat the minor infections that occur during the neutropenic phase of the cycle.

Kostmann infantile genetic agranulocytosis (Kostmann syndrome)

Infantile agranulocytosis is a rare, autosomal trait characterized by profound neutropenia despite the presence of normal numbers of CFU-GM in the bone marrow that are capable of terminal differentiation in culture and a severe susceptibility to infection. Most affected infants die from overwhelming infection within the first year of life, but some respond to treatment with recombinant human G-CSF. Kostmann syndrome is genetically diverse; several gene mutations have been identified in different families including autosomal dominant mutations in *ELA2*, the neutrophil elastase gene, autosomal recessive mutations in the *HAX1* gene, which encodes a protein associated with the actin cytoskeleton and *GFI1*, a zinc-finger transcriptional repressor gene that is involved in haemopoietic stem cell function and lineage commitment.

Familial benign neutropenia

Familial benign neutropenia is a rare condition that is inherited in an autosomal dominant fashion and is characterized by chronic mild neutropenia with a compensatory increase in the cell count of the other leucocytes and a relatively mild clinical course. Bone marrow examination typically reveals mild granulocytic hypoplasia but normal erythropoietic and thrombopoietic activity.

Reticular dysgenesis

Reticular dysgenesis is a rare condition of unknown aetiology, which is characterized by a selective and complete absence of leucopoiesis. Affected infants lack any identifiable granulocyte, monocyte or lymphocyte precursors in the bone marrow and lymphoid organs, and so are extremely immunosuppressed. Erythropoiesis and thrombopoiesis appear to be normal. Allogeneic stem cell transplantation is the only effective treatment for this condition.

Shwachman–Diamond syndrome

This disorder has an autosomal recessive inheritance and presents as a moderate to severe neutropenia in infancy. Affected infants have recurrent infections, diarrhoea, and difficulty in feeding. Dwarfism, chondrodysplasia, and pancreatic exocrine insufficiency may also be present. Most cases of Shwachman–Diamond syndrome are caused by mutations in the *SBDS* gene, which is involved in ribosome synthesis and RNA processing reactions. The most effective treatment is recombinant human G-CSF.

Cartilage–hair hypoplasia

Cartilage–hair hypoplasia is an autosomal recessive condition and is due to mutations in the *RMRP* gene, which encodes the RNA component of the ribonuclease mitochondrial RNA processing complex. The condition is seen most often in Amish and Finnish families and it presents as a moderate to severe neutropenia, defective cell-mediated immunity, macrocytic anaemia, gastrointestinal disease, and dwarfism. Affected individuals appear to be predisposed to the development of lymphoma. The treatment is allogeneic stem cell transplantation.

Dyskeratosis congenita (Zinsser–Cole–Engman syndrome)

This condition presents with mental retardation, pancytopenia, and defective cell-mediated immunity and is haematologically similar to Fanconi anaemia. Typically, congenital abnormalities such as alopecia, abnormal sweating, telangiectasia and mental retardation are joined by the development of progressive hypoplastic anaemia in early adulthood. Dyskeratosis congenita is usually X-linked recessive, although autosomal dominant and autosomal recessive forms also exist. The X-linked recessive form of the disorder has been linked to mutations in the *DKC1* gene, which encodes dyskerin, a nucleolar protein associated with ribonucleoprotein particles. The autosomal dominant form of dyskeratosis congenita is associated with mutations in the *TERC* gene, which encodes the RNA component of telomerase. Patients with this disorder have shorter telomeres than normal. The treatment is recombinant human G-CSF, GM-CSF and allogeneic stem cell transplantation.

Barth syndrome

Barth syndrome is an X-linked recessive disorder presenting in infancy as cardiomyopathy, skeletal myopathy, recurrent infections, dwarfism, and moderate to severe neutropenia.

Chédiak–Higashi syndrome

Chédiak–Higashi syndrome is an autosomal recessive disorder with recurrent infections, learning difficulties, bleeding disorders and numerous other phenotypic abnormalities. The neutropenia is moderate to severe, and the treatment is allogeneic stem cell transplantation.

Congenital amegakaryocytic thrombocytopenia

Amegakaryocytic thrombocytopenia is a rare condition which is inherited as an autosomal recessive disorder and is characterized by a severe thrombocytopenia secondary to deficiency of megakaryocyte production, platelet dysfunction and, usually, absence of the bones of the lower arms. The condition is also known as the thrombocytopenia with absent radii (TAR) syndrome. Haemorrhage is a major cause of mortality in the first year of life. This condition is due to mutations in the c-*MPL* gene, which encodes the thrombopoietin receptor.

Familial platelet disorder

Familial platelet disorder is a rare autosomal dominant disorder caused by mutations in the RUNX1 gene at 21q22. Affected individuals have mild to moderate thrombocytopenia with platelets of normal size. There is also a functional abnormality, resulting in bleeding problems more severe than expected from the platelet count. Patients with FPD are much more likely to develop haematological malignancies including acute myeloid leukaemia (AML) and myelodysplastic syndrome (MDS; see *Chapter 13*), often in early middle age. Leukaemia development appears to require acquisition of secondary genetic mutations.

17.3 ACQUIRED BONE MARROW FAILURE

Acquired bone marrow failure is more commonly known as aplastic or hypoplastic anaemia. The term aplastic anaemia is sometimes used interchangeably with bone marrow failure but, in this book, we reserve the term for acquired bone marrow failure, usually of immune aetiology (see *Box 17.6*).

Box 17.6 Aplastic anaemia

Paul Ehrlich made the first description of a case of aplastic anaemia in 1888 in a pregnant young woman who died following an acute illness with severe anaemia, bleeding, fever, and a markedly hypocellular bone marrow. However, the term aplastic anaemia was not coined until six years later by Anatole Chauffard. The first successful allogeneic bone marrow transplantation was performed in 1972 in a patient with aplastic anaemia.

Aplastic anaemia and chemical or physical agents

A wide range of chemical, physical and infectious agents are capable of inducing bone marrow hypoplasia. Historically, great emphasis has been placed on the causative role of chemicals such as benzene or drugs such as chloramphenicol. This led to the search for a causative agent in all cases of acquired aplastic anaemia, and the failure to find any resulted in most cases being defined as idiopathic aplastic anaemia. More recently, the emphasis on causative factors has altered such that most cases of acquired aplastic anaemia are considered to have an immune pathophysiology and cases that are clearly attributable to chemical, physical or infectious insult are considered to be a distinct minority.

Broadly, the various agents associated with aplastic anaemia can be divided into two types:

- those agents that always induce hypoplasia in all of those exposed and in whom the degree of hypoplasia induced is proportional to the degree of exposure
- those agents that are innocuous to most people but which induce hypoplasia in a minority of susceptible individuals. This is the larger group, and includes a huge number of widely used drugs.

Ionizing radiation

Exposure to ionizing radiation such as X-rays, γ-rays, α-particles and β-particles inflicts serious damage to cellular DNA, involving the introduction of strand breaks, base deletions and the promotion of inappropriate base pairing. The degree of damage inflicted is typically proportional to the dose of radiation received, although actively cycling cells are much more radiosensitive than those in G_0. Because of this, the most radiosensitive tissues are the haemopoietic stem cells, gut mucosal cells and germ cells. A dose of 7 Gy or more of penetrating ionizing radiation such as X-rays completely ablates the bone marrow and other rapidly dividing tissue and, in the absence of stem cell transplantation, is uniformly fatal. With lesser doses, the effect of the radiation is dose-related. Exposure to a single, short-lived dose of ionizing radiation may inflict serious damage to the bone marrow and mucosae leading to severe gastrointestinal disturbances, haemorrhage secondary to thrombocytopenia and infectious complications secondary to neutropenia, commonly resulting in death. However, given supportive care to maintain life, such individuals may recover following repopulation of the bone marrow by haemopoietic stem cells, which were in G_0 at the time of exposure.

Chronic or repeated exposure to ionizing radiation is associated with the development of profound aplastic anaemia because, as resting haemopoietic stem cells are spurred into the cell cycle to replace damaged stem cells, they too are subject to the damaging effects of the radiation. This relentlessly destructive cycle eventually leads to severe depletion of the haemopoietic stem cell pool. Ionizing radiation is also associated with an increased incidence of haematological malignancies secondary to sublethal stem cell damage.

Cytotoxic chemotherapy

Cytotoxic drugs are extremely toxic substances that are used deliberately to kill malignant cells. However, they are not selective for malignant cells; both normal and malignant cells are poisoned by these agents. The degree of hypoplasia that results is dose-related. Long experience with the therapeutic use of cytotoxic drugs has enabled the selection of dose regimens that induce temporary bone marrow hypoplasia so that recovery of normal haemopoietic tissue occurs quickly after withdrawal of the drug. Occasionally, prolonged use of alkylating agents such as busulphan can lead to prolonged hypoplasia from which recovery is slow or incomplete. Certain forms of cytotoxic chemotherapy (e.g. alkylating agents and epipodophyllotoxins) are also associated with an increased incidence of secondary haemopoietic malignancy.

Benzene

Chronic exposure to benzene has long been associated with the induction of aplastic anaemia, myelodysplasia and acute myeloid leukaemia. Benzene is widely used as an organic solvent, as a cleaning agent and is added to petrol as an anti-knocking agent. Most recorded cases had been exposed to high concentrations of benzene over many years, usually at their place of work. In modern epidemiological studies, benzene-associated aplastic anaemia is rare. This may be due to improved industrial practices or may raise a question over the accuracy of diagnosis in earlier case reports.

Idiosyncratic responses

Many widely used drugs have been reported to induce aplastic anaemia in a tiny percentage of those taking them. The best-known example is the antibacterial agent chloramphenicol, which has been used with safety for decades. At the doses that are in everyday use, chloramphenicol therapy is not associated with clinically significant myelotoxicity. However, about 1 in 20 000 of the population appears to be exquisitely sensitive to this drug: even the tiny amount present in eye drops has been reported to be sufficient to cause profound and refractory aplastic anaemia, which may result in death. Many other widely used drugs have been implicated in idiosyncratic induction of aplastic anaemia, including nonsteroidal analgesics such as indomethacin, ibuprofen and diclofenac, penicillamine, gold and sulfonamide antibiotics. Some such cases are thought to result from genetically determined deficiency in drug detoxification mechanisms, but others appear to be immune-mediated. Unfortunately, withdrawal of the drug does not usually bring about reversal of the aplasia. Such cases are treated in the same way as immune-mediated aplastic anaemia.

Infection

Many infections are, to some degree, myelosuppressive. Chronic haemolytic states such as sickle cell disease and hereditary spherocytosis are occasionally complicated by a sudden arrest of erythropoietic activity. These so-called aplastic crises are thought to result from the myelosuppressive effects of infection on an already severely stressed bone marrow. The most common infective trigger is parvovirus B19, which specifically infects erythroid precursors. In the absence of chronic haemolysis, parvovirus B19 causes a flu-like illness, which is variously known as fifth disease, erythema infectiosum or, more colourfully, slapped cheek disease. Other infectious agents implicated in causing transient aplasia are Epstein–Barr virus and hepatitis viruses.

Immune-mediated aplastic anaemia

The evidence for an immune mechanism underlying acquired aplastic anaemia includes the following observations:

- early attempts to treat aplastic anaemia with allogeneic bone marrow transplantation often resulted in a failure to engraft, but sometimes triggered recovery of normal host haemopoiesis. This was thought to be the result of the immunosuppressive effects of the transplant conditioning regimen.

- the majority of syngeneic (i.e. identical twin) bone marrow transplants conducted without conditioning failed, suggesting that immunosuppression caused by conditioning was an important prerequisite for the return of normal haemopoiesis.
- *in vitro* cell culture experiments showed that lymphocyte-depletion of marrow from aplastic anaemia patients improved cell growth and addition of lymphocytes from aplastic anaemia patients inhibited the growth of normal marrow cells.
- early experimental attempts to treat aplastic anaemia with antithymocyte globulin and cyclosporine were often at least partially successful.

These and many other observations have led to the settled view that acquired aplastic anaemia is caused by autoimmune activation of cytotoxic T lymphocytes with secretion of interferon-γ and tumour necrosis factor-α. These cytokines promote apoptosis of CD34-positive haemopoietic progenitor cells. The mechanism of immune activation is still unknown, but there is some evidence for a genetic basis. There is also some evidence for a humoral autoimmune component in at least some cases of aplastic anaemia. Autoantibodies directed against kinectin or diazepam-binding inhibitor-related protein-1 (DRS-1) can be demonstrated in almost half of patients, suggesting that these proteins may serve as autoantigens and so elicit immune attack against haemopoietic stem cells.

Aplastic anaemia is associated with the presence of clonal haemopoiesis indicative of other acquired clonal stem cell disorders, mainly paroxysmal nocturnal haemoglobinuria (PNH; see later) and myelodysplastic syndrome (MDS; see *Chapter 13*). A minority of cases of aplastic anaemia evolve into PNH or MDS, and the rate of evolution appears to be increased by immunosuppressive therapy. Up to two thirds of cases of aplastic anaemia have minor clones of PNH present, but these do not generally result in clinically significant haemolysis.

Classification of aplastic anaemia

The clinical severity of aplastic anaemia varies widely. In general, the severity of symptoms and the risk of death correlate inversely with the severity of peripheral blood cytopenias. Clinically, there are three recognized categories of severity:

- *severe aplastic anaemia* is defined as a hypocellular bone marrow (< 25% cellularity) with any two peripheral blood cytopenias (absolute neutrophil count < 0.5×10^9/l, platelet count < 20×10^9/l, reticulocyte count < 0.06×10^{12}/l).
- *very severe aplastic anaemia* is defined using the same criteria as severe aplastic anaemia, except that the definition of neutropenia is < 0.2×10^9/l.
- *non-severe aplastic anaemia* is defined as a hypocellular bone marrow (< 25% cellularity), but the peripheral blood cell counts do not meet the criteria for severe aplastic anaemia.

The development of aplastic anaemia can be acute, or there may be a history of slowly declining peripheral blood counts. The presenting symptoms relate to the severity of the cytopenia(s) and are generally predictable (pallor, lassitude and exercise intolerance secondary to anaemia; frequent and recurrent bacterial and fungal infections secondary to neutropenia and a tendency to bruise easily secondary to thrombocytopenia). Lymphadenopathy and splenomegaly are typically absent. Without immunosuppressive therapy, severe or very severe aplastic anaemia is fatal in the majority of cases, most often as a result of overwhelming infection. Non-severe aplastic anaemia is significantly less clinically severe, and may only require supportive therapy.

Diagnosis of aplastic anaemia

Diagnosis and clinical classification of aplastic anaemia requires a full blood count with differential count and reticulocyte count to establish the presence and severity of cytopenia(s) and demonstration of hypocellularity on a bone marrow aspirate and biopsy. Examination of a bone marrow biopsy is important because pockets of normal haemopoiesis may be present and an aspirate may erroneously appear to be only mildly hypocellular.

To differentiate aplastic anaemia from PNH, flow cytometry for the demonstration of GPI-AP deficient cells is required (see later), and the rare hypoplastic MDS variant can be excluded by demonstration of a normal karyotype. In younger patients, the possibility of inherited aplastic anaemia should be considered and a family history taken. Fanconi anaemia can be excluded by the lack of morphological stigmata and a negative test for chromosomal fragility.

On the other hand, the presence of increased myeloblasts and obvious dysplastic features may indicate hypoplastic MDS, particularly in older patients.

Treatment of aplastic anaemia

Supportive care is an important component of the treatment of aplastic anaemia and includes blood transfusion to correct anaemia and antibiotics, both as treatment for established infections and as prophylaxis to minimize future infections. Blood for transfusion should be irradiated to prevent graft versus host disease and cytomegalovirus negative.

Patients with non-severe aplastic anaemia who are not symptomatic may require no treatment, but should be monitored for an increase in the severity of disease over time. Occasionally, non-severe aplastic anaemia remits spontaneously. Symptomatic patients may be supported by judicious use of blood products and antibiotics. Treatment with cyclosporine ± antithymocyte globulin or with daclizumab (an anti IL-2 monoclonal antibody) may help to control the condition.

Patients with severe aplastic anaemia should, wherever possible, be offered allogeneic haemopoietic stem cell transplantation. The prospect of cure is markedly increased and the treatment-associated mortality risk significantly reduced when an HLA-matched sibling donor is used, particularly in younger patients. In patients that are not candidates for stem cell transplantation, immunosuppression with the combination of cyclosporine and antithymocyte globulin can induce remissions in more than two thirds of cases. However, immunosuppression does not offer the prospect of cure and many patients experience only partial remission or relapse following a period of disease remission. Relapsed patients may respond to a second course of immunosuppressive therapy, or may be offered allogeneic stem cell transplantation.

Transient erythroblastopenia of childhood

Transient erythroblastopenia of childhood (TEC) is an anaemia that gradually develops in early childhood. The cause of this condition is unknown, although several viral and immunological mechanisms have been proposed. As the name suggests, patients with TEC recover completely with no sequelae.

Acquired pure red cell aplasia

Acquired pure red cell aplasia (PRCA) is most commonly attributable to an infectious cause as described above. However, a hitherto unknown form of PRCA, caused by antibodies directed against erythropoietin, has recently been characterized. This condition has only been described in patients with chronic kidney disease being treated with recombinant human erythropoietin and is manifest as a loss of effect of the exogenous erythropoietin, with consequent severe anaemia. EPO-associated PRCA has been reported as a rare, sporadic event since 1998, and has been seen with all forms of recombinant erythropoietin when administered subcutaneously. An increase in the number of cases in 2001–2002 associated with one particular product, epoetin alfa, was attributed to the extraction of adjuvants from the rubber plunger of the syringe in which the product is supplied. A change to Teflon®-coated syringe plungers appears to have resolved this problem.

Paroxysmal nocturnal haemoglobinuria

Paroxysmal nocturnal haemoglobinuria (PNH) is an acquired clonal haemopoietic stem cell disorder characterized by haemolysis, bone marrow failure and a thrombotic tendency (see *Box 17.7*). PNH can occur at any age but is most commonly seen in young to middle aged adults. Men and women are affected equally, but there do appear to be differences in frequency and clinical manifestations in different races. Clinically, PNH is highly diverse and may evade accurate diagnosis for several months or even years. Clinical manifestations include:

- variable episodic haemolysis due to an increased susceptibility to complement
- a thrombotic tendency, often affecting the hepatic, abdominal, cerebral, and subdermal veins
- variable bone marrow failure that can range from minimal changes in the peripheral blood through to severe pancytopenia.

Box 17.7 PNH and sleep

The name paroxysmal nocturnal haemoglobinuria reflects the finding in early cases of an episodic (paroxysmal) intravascular haemolysis that resulted in the passage of free haemoglobin into the urine (haemoglobinuria). The nocturnal part of the name derives from the finding that the haemoglobinuria is most noticeable in the early morning urine. It used to be thought that this was caused by the development of acidosis during sleep, which triggered complement-mediated haemolysis. This is now known to be incorrect. Haemolysis occurs throughout the day, but appears more obvious in the concentrated early morning urine.

The presentation of PNH is highly variable; only about a quarter of cases present with acute haemoglobinuria. The remainder present with non-specific (and frequently episodic) symptoms of anaemia, jaundice, haemorrhage, aplasia or thrombosis and may also have non-haematological symptoms such as abdominal pain, bloating, back pain, headaches, oesophageal spasms, erectile dysfunction, renal impairment and fatigue. Typically, although the features of PNH vary widely between individuals, the clinical course in a single individual is generally stable. The course of the disease in most people is one of some degree of chronic haemolysis, punctuated by haemolytic crises that last for several days. Common triggers of such crises include vaccination, surgery, antibiotic treatment and infections. Median survival from diagnosis of PNH is about 10 years, with the cause of death most frequently being thrombosis or complications due to pancytopenia.

Clinically, PNH is divided into three types:

- *Classical PNH* with clear evidence of intravascular haemolysis but no obvious bone marrow failure. These cases often show marrow erythroid hyperplasia with normal morphology and no cytogenetic abnormalities.
- *PNH in the setting of another specified bone marrow disorder*, in which evidence of haemolysis is associated with a current or antecedent bone marrow disorder such as myelodysplastic syndrome, myelofibrosis or aplastic anaemia.
- *Subclinical PNH (PNH-sc)*, where there is no clinical or laboratory evidence of PNH, but GPI-AP-deficient cells (see below for explanation) can be identified in the peripheral blood. PNH-sc is identified most commonly in association with aplastic anaemia or myelodysplastic syndrome.

Molecular pathogenesis of PNH

PNH is caused by an acquired mutation of the PIGA gene located at Xp22.1. This gene encodes a protein called phosphatidylinositol glycan class A (PIG-A) that is involved in the synthesis of the GPI anchor, a membrane protein required for attachment of multiple proteins to the cell membrane. Two GPI-anchored proteins (GPI-AP) are important in the pathogenesis of PNH, the complement regulatory proteins CD55 (decay accelerating factor, DAF) and CD59 (membrane inhibitor of reactive lysis, MIRL). More than 100 different PIGA mutations have been identified, making molecular diagnosis of PNH impractical. The PIG-A mutation arises in a haemopoietic stem cell. The mutant stem cells appear to have a growth advantage over normal stem cells, and so form an expanded clone of GPI-AP deficient blood cells. Because these cells lack CD55 and CD59, they are more sensitive to lysis by complement (see *Box 17.8*).

Box 17.8 Ham's test – part 2

Until relatively recently, the standard tests for PNH were to screen for haemolysis using the sucrose lysis test in which fresh, pooled normal serum is mixed with a low ionic strength sucrose solution and incubated with patient red cells at 37 °C for 30 minutes. These low ionic strength conditions promote complement-mediated haemolysis. Following incubation, if there is obvious haemolysis present, PNH remains a possible diagnosis so a Ham's test should be performed.

In the Ham's test, patient red cells are incubated with acidified serum (pH 6.5–7.0). The acid conditions activate the alternate pathway of complement, triggering haemolysis of PNH red cells. The test is conducted using both patient serum and normal serum. Haemolysis in both the patient serum and normal serum tests is indicative of PNH. Haemolysis in normal serum but not patient serum or sucrose lysis is indicative of HEMPAS. Severe hereditary spherocytosis can also give positive results in both patient and normal serum. To exclude this possibility, the test can be repeated using heat-inactivated serum when HS samples will still show haemolysis but PNH samples, because of the absence of complement, will be negative.

One of the most remarkable characteristics of PNH is that it exists as a genotypic and phenotypic mosaic, with normal stem cells coexisting with clone(s) of GPI-AP-deficient stem cells. In many cases, multiple different clones (each with a distinct PIG-A mutation) of GPI-AP-deficient stem cells are present.

The genotypic mosaicism is manifest phenotypically as the presence in the peripheral blood of a mixture of red cells and granulocytes with different degrees of sensitivity to complement-mediated lysis. Phenotypically, cells are categorized as:

- PNH I cells, which have normal or nearly normal sensitivity to complement
- PNH II cells, which are about 3–5 times more sensitive than normal
- PNH III cells, which are up to 25 times more sensitive than normal.

An individual with PNH most often has a mixed population of PNH I and PNH III cells in their peripheral blood, but mixtures of PNH I, II and III or PNH I and II have also been reported. The proportions of the different types of cells vary widely between individuals and this partly explains the inter-individual variability in haemolysis.

Pathophysiology of PNH

Intravascular haemolysis releases haemoglobin into the plasma, where it is rapidly complexed by an abundant plasma protein called haptoglobin. Formation of these haemoglobin:haptoglobin complexes serves as a salvage mechanism because it slows clearance of haemoglobin and facilitates uptake by the reticuloendothelial system where it is broken down and its components reutilized. However, if haemolysis is severe, the released haemoglobin can saturate the available haptoglobin, which results in free circulating plasma haemoglobin.

Free circulating haemoglobin is excreted via the kidney, resulting in haemoglobinuria, and also deposited in various body tissues, primarily the kidneys. In severe, chronic intravascular haemolysis this can lead to a degree of renal failure.

The free circulating haemoglobin plays an important part in the pathophysiology of PNH because it binds irreversibly with nitric oxide (NO), thereby depleting NO peripheral blood levels. Nitric oxide functions as a regulator of smooth muscle tone and depletion is associated with contraction of smooth muscle. This is manifest as constriction of blood vessels, bowel constriction and pulmonary hypertension, explaining some of the symptoms of PNH including abdominal pain, bloating, back pain, headaches, oesophageal spasms, erectile dysfunction and fatigue.

PNH is associated with thrombophilia with an increased incidence of venous thromboembolism, commonly affecting the cerebral, hepatic, portal, mesenteric, splenic and renal veins. The underlying pathophysiology is incompletely understood, but a temporal relationship with haemolytic crises has been suggested. A deficiency of CD59 and urokinase plasminogen activator receptor on platelets, coupled with increased plasma-soluble urokinase plasminogen activator receptor may contribute.

Some degree of bone marrow failure is present in all PNH patients, which can vary from peripheral blood pancytopenia with a hypoplastic bone marrow through to near normal. PNH patients have a risk of up to 20% of developing aplastic anaemia. Similarly, a minority of cases of PNH will have evolved from aplastic anaemia.

Diagnosis of PNH

Diagnosis of PNH requires the demonstration of GPI-AP deficiency in red cells and granulocytes using flow cytometry. Absence or reduced expression of both CD59 and CD55 on red cells and granulocytes is diagnostic of PNH. A more sensitive reagent for flow cytometric diagnosis of PNH is a fluorescent-conjugated and inactive form of the bacterial toxin aerolysin. This toxin, derived from *Aeromonas hydrophila*, binds specifically to the GPI anchor and is capable of demonstrating the presence of very small PNH clones. There appears to be a link between the size of the PNH clone and thrombotic risk.

Where flow cytometry is unavailable, PNH can be diagnosed using a combination of the sucrose lysis, Ham's and osmotic fragility tests (see *Box 17.8*).

Treatment of PNH

The treatment of PNH is primarily symptomatic: blood transfusion or recombinant erythropoietin to combat anaemia and anticoagulant prophylaxis to minimize the risk of thrombosis. A monoclonal antibody that targets the C5 complement component reduces the severity of intravascular haemolysis. However, none of these treatments offer the prospect of cure. Only allogeneic stem cell transplantation can cure PNH, but the transplant-related morbidity and mortality risk are too high for all but the most severe cases of PNH.

SUGGESTED FURTHER READING

Bacigalupo, A. & Passweg, J. (2009) Diagnosis and treatment of acquired aplastic anemia. *Hematol. Oncol. Clin. North Am.* **23:** 159–170.

Dokal, I. & Vulliamy, T. (2008) Inherited aplastic anaemias/bone marrow failure syndromes. *Blood Rev.* **22:** 141–153.

Ganapathi, K.A. & Shimamura, A. (2008) Ribosomal dysfunction and inherited marrow failure. *Br. J. Haematol.* **141:** 376–387.

Gluckman, E. & Wagner, J.E. (2008) Hematopoietic stem cell transplantation in childhood inherited bone marrow failure syndrome. *Bone Marrow Transplant,* **41:** 127–132.

Green, A.M. & Kupfer, G.M. (2009) Fanconi anemia. *Hematol. Oncol. Clin. North Am.* **23:** 193–214.

Guinan, E.C. (2009) Acquired aplastic anemia in childhood. *Hematol. Oncol. Clin. North Am.* **23:** 171–191.

Kirwan, M. & Dokal, I. (2009) Dyskeratosis congenita, stem cells and telomeres. *Biochim. Biophys. Acta,* **1792:** 371–379.

Lipton, J.M. & Ellis, S.R. (2009) Diamond–Blackfan anemia: diagnosis, treatment, and molecular pathogenesis. *Hematol. Oncol. Clin. North Am.* **23:** 261–282.

Myers, K.C. & Davies, S.M. (2009) Hematopoietic stem cell transplantation for bone marrow failure syndromes in children. *Biol. Blood Marrow Transplant,* **15:** 279–292.

Young, N.S. *et al.* (2008) Aplastic anemia. *Curr. Opin. Hematol.* **15:** 162–168.

SELF-ASSESSMENT QUESTIONS

1. Name the most common gene affected in Fanconi anaemia.
2. Diamond–Blackfan syndrome is manifest as reduced production of which cell type?
3. Which form of CDA is associated with a positive Ham's test?
4. Name the gene that is mutated in most cases of cyclic neutropenia.
5. Name the gene that is mutated in most cases of congenital amegakaryocytic thrombocytopenia.
6. Name the virus responsible for fifth disease that can be associated with a transient arrest of erythropoiesis.
7. What are the criteria for a diagnosis of severe aplastic anaemia?
8. If PNH is a genetic disorder, why is it not heritable?
9. What gene is implicated in the aetiology of PNH?
10. Outline the role of aerolysin in PNH diagnosis.

Overview of haemostasis

Learning objectives
After studying this chapter you should confidently be able to:

■ **Name the five main systems involved in haemostasis**
The haemostatic mechanism is the product of complex interactions of five distinct systems: the vascular system, blood platelets, the coagulation cascade, physiological inhibitors of coagulation and the fibrinolytic system. Events that disturb the balance between these opposing forces promote either haemorrhage or clot formation.

■ **Outline the contribution of the vascular system to haemostasis**
Constriction of the injured blood vessel is an early means of minimizing blood loss. Vascular endothelial cells play an important role in haemostasis as they are the major source of many factors that regulate haemostasis. When a blood vessel is injured, this regulatory system is locally interrupted and exposed sub-endothelial layers provide a surface for activation of platelets and the coagulation system.

■ **Discuss the role of platelets in haemostasis**
Adequate numbers of normally functioning platelets are essential for haemostasis. The primary role of blood platelets is to rapidly form a primary haemostatic plug that creates a temporary physical barrier to blood loss following vascular injury. This plug is relatively fragile and needs reinforcement and stabilization for larger wounds. In addition to their role in forming a haemostatic plug, platelets play an important role in blood coagulation by providing a surface for localized clot formation.

■ **Review the importance of the coagulation cascade as a biological amplification system**
The blood coagulation system consolidates and stabilizes the primary haemostatic plug via fibrin formation. From a physiological standpoint, arrest of bleeding requires an emergency response that rapidly generates a large amount of fibrin. This is achieved *in vivo* in a two-step process that allows massive amplification of an initially small biological signal.

■ **Highlight the pivotal role of vitamin K-dependent factors in haemostasis**
Coagulation factors II, VII, IX, X as well as proteins C and S are dependent on vitamin K for their normal function. These factors are synthesized in an inactive form that cannot bind calcium ions. This ability is conferred by a post-translational modification that requires the presence of vitamin K.

■ **Highlight the concept of balance and mutual interdependence of the various systems involved in haemostasis**
Optimal haemostasis is not a single biological pathway, but the product of the complex interactions of five distinct systems. A fault in any of these systems can predispose to either a bleeding or a thrombotic tendency.

One of the most important survival mechanisms in higher animals is the ability to minimize blood loss following injury. Set against this requirement is the necessity to maintain blood in a fluid state in the absence of injury. Thus, in health, a dynamic equilibrium exists between mechanisms that tend to promote clot formation and those that tend to oppose clot formation. Haemostasis may be defined as those mechanisms that maintain the flowing blood in a fluid state and confined to the circulatory system. The haemostatic mechanism is not a single biological pathway, but the product of the complex interactions of five distinct systems:

- the vascular system
- blood platelets
- the coagulation cascade
- physiological inhibitors of coagulation
- the fibrinolytic system.

Events that disturb the balance between these opposing forces promote either haemorrhage or clot formation (see also *Box 18.1*). This chapter presents an overview of the processes involved in maintaining the haemostatic balance.

Box 18.1 Key dates for haemostasis

1686	First separation of blood clot fibres from cells and serum
1731	Observation that clots stem blood loss
1803	Recognition of sex-linking in haemophilia
1819	First observation of the procoagulant effect of tissues (tissue factor)
1845	Recognition that fibrin formed from plasma fibrinogen
1882	Description of platelet function by Bizzozero
1905	Morawitz four-factor theory of blood coagulation
1926	Description of von Willebrand's disease (vWD)
1935	Development of one stage prothrombin time by Quick
1935	Description of the anti-haemorrhagic properties of vitamin K
1944	Recognition that Christmas disease is distinct from haemophilia
1947	Description of serum inhibitor to tissue thromboplastin
1947	Discovery of factor V by Owren
1949	Discovery of factor VII
1952	Discovery of factor IX (Christmas Factor) by Biggs and MacFarlane
1953	Discovery of factor XI
1955	Discovery of factor XII (Hageman Factor)
1956	Discovery of factor X (Stuart–Prower Factor)
1961	Discovery of factor XIII
1964	Waterfall (cascade) hypothesis of coagulation proposed by Davie and Ratnoff in the USA and by MacFarlane in the UK
1971	Use of ristocetin to diagnose vWD
1977	Purification of tissue factor
1982–present	Development of monoclonal antibody and molecular techniques lead to improved understanding of haemostasis
1987	Pathways of blood coagulation revised to take account of central roles of tissue factor and tissue factor pathway inhibitor (TFPI)
1990–present	Increased understanding of the molecular basis of haemostasis and its disorders, and the rise of molecular diagnostics

18.1   THE VASCULAR SYSTEM

Blood vessel walls are composed of three distinct, concentric layers as shown in *Figure 18.1*.

- The intima forms the inner layer and consists of a thin monolayer of flat vascular endothelial cells. Vascular endothelial cells are actively anti-thrombotic and contain Weibel–Palade bodies, the storage site for von Willebrand factor (vWF). The vascular endothelium is mounted upon an internal elastic membrane, which is largely composed of collagen fibres.
- The media forms the central layer and is the most variable component of the blood vessel wall. In elastic arteries, such as the aorta, the media is composed of elastic fibres arranged in concentric, circumferential layers to absorb the huge changes in pressure as the heart beats. In muscular arteries, the media is composed of smooth muscle cells that permit rhythmic contraction and relaxation of the artery, which helps to maintain blood pressure. In arterioles and veins, the media is thin and is primarily involved in regulating perfusion (arterioles) and vascular volume (veins).
- The adventitia forms the exterior coat and is composed of collagen with a scattering of smooth muscle cells. The border between the media and the adventitia may be marked by a collection of elastic fibres, which form the external elastic lamina.

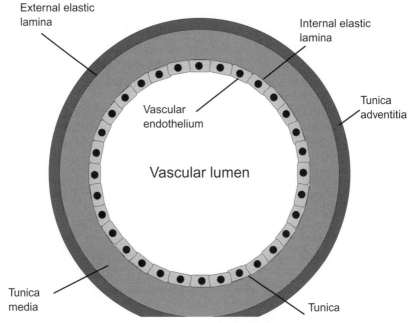

Figure 18.1
General structure of a muscular blood vessel.

Contribution of the vascular system to haemostasis

Constriction of the injured blood vessel is an early means of minimizing blood loss. Vasoconstriction is mediated by substances such as adrenaline, ADP, kinins and thromboxanes. Many of these vasoactive substances are derived from blood platelets.

The metabolic activities of vascular endothelial cells play an important role in haemostasis. These cells are the major source of vWF, thrombomodulin and tissue factor pathway inhibitor

(TFPI). The contribution of these substances to haemostasis is discussed later in this chapter. vWF also is synthesized by megakaryocytes. Endothelial cells also exert inhibitory effects on haemostasis via synthesis of prostacyclin (PGI$_2$) and nitric oxide (NO), potent vasodilators and inhibitors of platelet function.

When the integrity of the vascular endothelial layer is breached, the exposed sub-endothelial layers provide a surface for platelet activation and aggregation as well as activation of the coagulation system. More importantly, the adventitial cells express tissue factor, which is now thought to be the primary activator of blood coagulation. The localized breach of the endothelium is a major factor in localizing clot formation to the site of injury, since the surrounding intact endothelium retains its inhibitory activity.

18.2 BLOOD PLATELETS

Platelets are formed from the cytoplasm of bone marrow megakaryocytes and are the smallest of the blood cells. The normal platelet count lies between 150 and 400 × 10^9/l. Non-activated platelets are disc-shaped, anucleate cells with a relatively complex internal structure reflecting the specific haemostatic functions of the platelet. The ultrastructure of the blood platelet is depicted in *Figure 18.2*.

Of particular importance are the surface glycoproteins and the three types of intracellular granule, the α granules, the lysosomes and the dense granules. The surface glycoproteins are required for the processes of platelet adhesion, aggregation and also, in concert with platelet surface phospholipids exposed during platelet activation, provide a surface on which coagulation factor activation is facilitated. Abnormalities of one or more glycoproteins often lead to a bleeding disorder, as summarized in *Table 18.1*.

The α granules contain the platelet glycoprotein thrombospondin as well as fibrinogen, fibronectin, platelet factor 4 (heparin antagonist, PF4), von Willebrand factor (vWF), β-thromboglobulin (β-TG), platelet-derived growth factor (PDGF) and coagulation factor V and

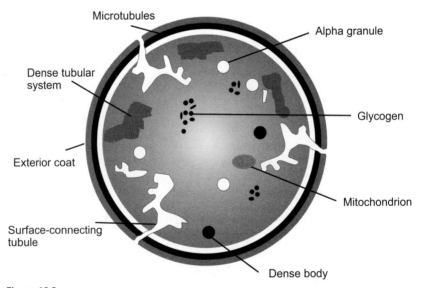

Figure 18.2
Platelet ultrastructure.

Table 18.1 Platelet granule constituents, surface glycoproteins and their most important biological functions

Glycoprotein	Function	
GPIIb–IIIa	Most abundant platelet glycoprotein. Receptor for fibrinogen, vWF and fibronectin. Mediates platelet aggregation. Congenital absence causes Glanzmann's thrombasthenia.	
GPIb–IX–V	Principal receptor for sub-endothelial-bound vWF. Congenital abnormalities include Bernard–Soulier syndrome and pseudo von Willebrand's disease.	
GPIa–IIa	Collagen receptor. Mediates platelet adhesion to sub-endothelium.	
GPVI	Collagen receptor. Mediates platelet adhesion to sub-endothelium.	
Granule	**Compound**	**Function**
α granule	Platelet factor 4 (heparin antagonist)	Neutralizes heparin effect
	β thromboglobulin	Promotes fibroblast chemotaxis
	Platelet derived growth factor	Mitogen for fibroblasts and smooth muscle cells, chemotaxin for neutrophils
	von Willebrand factor	Adhesion molecule, carrier for VIII
	Thrombospondin	Promotes platelet–platelet interaction
	Fibronectin	Adhesion of platelets and fibroblasts
	Fibrinogen	Promotes adhesion and coagulation
	Factor V	Promotes coagulation
Dense granules	ADP	Aggregation of platelets
	ATP	Source of ADP
	Serotonin	Vasoconstriction
	Calcium	Coagulation, platelet function
Lysosome	Hydrolytic enzymes	May participate in clot breakdown

fibrinogen. The dense granules, so called because of their appearance on electron microscopy, contain ADP, ATP, calcium ions and serotonin (5-hydroxytryptamine, 5-HT). The contents of both the α and dense granules are released, via a system of surface-connecting tubules, during platelet activation. These granular contents have a variety of important biological activities as shown in *Table 18.1*.

Both platelets and vascular endothelial cells metabolize arachidonic acid (see *Figure 18.3*). This polyunsaturated fatty acid is mainly present bound to membrane phospholipids, but can be released by the enzyme phospholipase A_2 in activated platelets. The newly liberated arachidonic acid is converted to thromboxane A_2 (TXA_2) by the actions of the enzymes cyclo-oxygenase (COX) and thromboxane synthetase. TXA_2 is a powerful inducer of platelet aggregation, but has a very short half-life (around 30 seconds). Arachidonic acid metabolism within vascular endothelium results in the generation of prostacyclin (PGI_2), which is a potent inhibitor of platelet aggregation.

Platelet function

The primary role of blood platelets is to rapidly form a plug that creates a temporary physical barrier to blood loss following vascular injury. There are four phases of platelet function:

- adhesion to a surface
- shape change

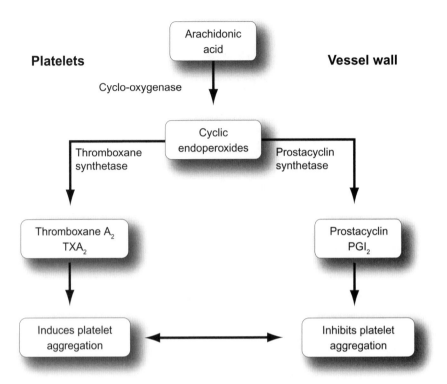

Figure 18.3
Arachidonic acid metabolism in vascular endothelium and platelets.

- ■ release of granule contents
- ■ aggregation.

Adhesion

Blood platelets are activated by contact with a variety of physiological and non-physiological substances, including sub-endothelial tissue, foreign or charged surfaces, ADP, thrombin, TXA_2 and bacterial endotoxin. *In vivo,* damage to the vessel wall causes exposure of sub-endothelial fibres and results in the rapid adherence of circulating platelets to the surface of the wound. Normally, sufficient platelets would be present to completely cover the damaged area. The importance of platelet adhesion *in vivo* is illustrated by the relatively easy bruising and enhanced capillary fragility seen in patients with thrombocytopenia (see also *Box 18.2*).

The mechanisms that govern platelet adhesion differ according to the local blood flow conditions. In areas of high shear such as in arterioles, the platelets do not adhere directly to exposed sub-endothelium. Instead, vWF adheres to the sub-endothelial matrix and platelets

---

Box 18.2 Aspirin and platelet function

The most commonly prescribed antiplatelet drug is aspirin (acetylsalicylic acid), which acts by acetylating the platelet enzyme cyclo-oxygenase, thereby irreversibly inhibiting TXA_2 production. Daily low-dose aspirin therapy is used as an effective prophylactic measure for coronary heart disease.

then bind to the vWF via the GPIb–IX–V surface glycoprotein. This initial attachment facilitates tighter binding of the platelet via GPIIb–IIIa, GPVI and other adhesion molecules. In areas of low shear, the platelets bind directly to sub-endothelial collagen via the surface glycoprotein GPIa–IIa.

Adhesion of platelets via their glycoprotein receptors initiates an internal signalling cascade that leads to functional activation, shape change and release of granule contents.

Shape change

Platelet adhesion is usually accompanied by a transformation in platelet shape from the normal discoid form to one of irregular outline with numerous cytoplasmic projections, the echinocytic configuration (see also *Box 18.3*). This change in shape increases the surface area of the cell and so facilitates surface adhesion interactions. In the early stages of platelet activation the shape changes are reversible, but with increased and continued stimulation the change becomes irreversible and is associated with centralization of the cytoplasmic granules and with degranulation and release of granule contents.

Box 18.3 Echinocytic platelets and spiny sea urchins

Spiculated blood cells are called echinocytes because of their supposed resemblance to the spiny sea urchin *Echinus esculenta*.

Release of granule contents

Platelet degranulation (the release reaction) occurs as a result of the fusion of the cytoplasmic granules with the surface-connected tubular system. The contents of the α and dense granules are thus made available at the platelet surface where they trigger further localized platelet adhesion and aggregation. In particular, release of ADP and TXA_2 results in amplification of platelet activation.

Aggregation

Platelet activation prompts the binding of plasma fibrinogen to specific platelet receptors (GPIIb/IIIa) and the formation of inter-platelet 'bridges'. A variety of compounds are capable of inducing platelet aggregation, including adrenaline, ADP, collagen, thrombin, arachidonic acid and TXA_2. *In vivo*, the ADP released from activated platelets and damaged red cells at sites of injury stimulates the activation of adjacent platelets, which undergo the release reaction and subsequently join the growing aggregate. This self-propagating activation rapidly results in the formation of a primary haemostatic plug, which physically blocks the breach in the vessel wall, thereby staunching blood loss.

The primary haemostatic plug may be sufficient to prevent further blood loss from minor wounds, but it is relatively fragile and needs reinforcement and stabilization for larger wounds. The consolidation of the primary haemostatic plug is brought about by the enzymatic conversion of fibrinogen to fibrin and the subsequent stabilization of the resultant fibrin molecules by blood coagulation factor XIII. Platelets are capable of providing many of the components of the coagulation system in a concentrated form at the local level.

The role of platelets in blood coagulation

In addition to their role in forming a haemostatic plug, platelets play an important role in blood coagulation. Aggregation results in exposure of a previously hidden platelet membrane phospholipid, sometimes called platelet factor 3. This provides a surface for the assembly of three enzyme complexes (the intrinsic and extrinsic tenase complexes and the prothrombinase complex) during the coagulation cascade. The physiological importance of the requirement for platelet phospholipid for coagulation is that it helps to localize clot formation to the area of vascular damage. This limitation is in addition to that provided by intact endothelium. Widespread dissemination of coagulation is a life-threatening condition.

18.3 THE BLOOD COAGULATION SYSTEM

The blood coagulation system is composed of a series of functionally specific plasma proteins (coagulation factors) that interact in a highly ordered and predetermined sequence with the sole object of converting the soluble protein fibrinogen to an insoluble network of fibrin which consolidates and stabilizes the primary haemostatic plug. The coagulation factors are, by convention, referred to by an internationally agreed system of Roman numerals. These numbers are related to the order of discovery of the individual coagulation factors, not the order in which they take part in the coagulation process. Each coagulation factor also has one or more synonyms as shown in *Table 18.2* (see also *Box 18.4*). The coagulation factors are synthesized primarily in the liver, although vWF is produced by endothelial cells and megakaryocytes. Platelets also contain coagulation factors V, XIII, vWF and fibrinogen.

Table 18.2 Nomenclature of the coagulation factors

Coagulation factor	Most commonly used synonym	Activity
I (not normally used)	Fibrinogen	Substrate
II	Prothrombin	Serine protease
III (not used)	Tissue factor (thromboplastin)	Receptor/cofactor
IV (not used)	Calcium ions	Cofactor
V	Labile factor	Cofactor
VI	Originally used to describe activated V (V_a). No longer used	
VII	Stable factor	Serine protease
VIII	Anti-haemophilic factor	Cofactor
IX	Christmas factor	Serine protease
X	Stuart–Prower factor	Serine protease
XI	Plasma thromboplastin antecedent (not normally used)	Serine protease
XII	Hageman factor	Serine protease
XIII	Fibrin stabilizing factor	Transglutaminase
None assigned	Prekallikrein	Serine protease
None assigned	High molecular weight kininogen	Cofactor

Box 18.4 Naming coagulation factors

Many of the alternative names for coagulation factors are derived from the name of the original patient whose deficiency led to their identification. For example, factor X was originally named Stuart–Prower Factor because deficiency states were first identified in a Ms Audrey Prower and a Mr Rufus Stuart in 1956 and 1957 respectively.

There are two types of coagulation factor:

- zymogens, which are inactive plasma proteins (proenzymes), and which, after cleavage by a specific enzyme, are transformed into active enzymes. Coagulation factors that fall into this category include factors II, X, XI, XII and XIII. Most of the coagulation enzymes are serine proteases, i.e. the active site of the proteolytic enzyme contains a serine residue. Factor XIII is a transglutaminase.
- cofactors, which act as accelerators or catalysts for other enzymatic reactions. Factors V and VIII and tissue factor fall into this category.

Two coagulation factors, fibrinogen and factor VII, cannot strictly be classified as either zymogens or cofactors. Fibrinogen is converted to fibrin, which has no enzymatic properties and about 2% of factor VII normally circulates as an active enzyme, although binding to tissue factor potentiates its activity. By convention, activated coagulation factors are denoted by the suffix $_a$, e.g. VII$_a$ is the activated form of factor VII.

The role of vitamin K in blood coagulation

Coagulation factors II, VII, IX and X as well as the natural anticoagulant proteins C and S are dependent on vitamin K for their normal function. These factors are synthesized in an inactive form that cannot bind calcium ions. This ability is conferred by a post-translational modification, which involves γ-carboxylation of glutamic acid residues. Vitamin K *in vivo* continuously cycles between three forms: vitamin K quinone, vitamin K hydroquinone and vitamin K epoxide. The γ-carboxylation reaction is coupled to the conversion of vitamin K hydroquinone to the epoxide form. Thus, in vitamin K deficiency, γ-carboxylation fails and non-carboxylated forms of factors II, VII, IX, X and proteins C and S are released into the circulation (see also *Box 18.5*). Although they are immunologically identical to the normal proteins, these **p**roteins **i**nduced by **v**itamin **K** absence or **a**ntagonism (PIVKA) cannot bind calcium ions, and thus cannot bind to phospholipid surfaces. Because of this, they are activated much more slowly than their normal counterparts, giving rise to the anticoagulant effect, seen, for example, following oral anticoagulant therapy. PIVKA can, however, be activated *in vitro* with the venom of certain snakes such as *Echis carinatus* and this property can form the basis for their laboratory measurement.

Box 18.5 Discovery of warfarin

During the winter of 1921–22, herds of Canadian cattle suffered an epidemic of a haemorrhagic disease. Frank Schofield, a local vet, showed that the disease was caused by feeding the cattle on mouldy silage made from sweet clover. Several years later a vet from North Dakota showed that the disease was secondary to prothrombin deficiency. During a subsequent outbreak in the USA, Wisconsin chemist Karl Link and others identified the agent responsible as bis-hydroxycoumarin (dicoumarol). This substance, under the name of warfarin, is widely used as a rat poison and oral anticoagulant for the treatment of thrombo-embolic disease. Warfarin acts by inhibiting the vitamin K-dependent carboxylation of factors II, VII, IX and X and proteins C and S, without which they are inactive. The name warfarin derives from a combination of the initials of the Wisconsin Alumni Research Foundation (WARF) and the last letters of the chemical name coumarin.

Blood coagulation *in vivo*

From a physiological standpoint, if a wound is sufficiently severe that a platelet plug is insufficient to arrest bleeding, then an emergency response is required that very rapidly generates a large amount of fibrin to strengthen and stabilize the plug. This is achieved *in vivo* in a two-step process that allows massive (around a million-fold) amplification of an initially small biological signal.

The initiation phase

In the first phase of coagulation, known as initiation, circulating activated factor VII (VII$_a$) binds to tissue factor exposed at the site of the injury (see also *Box 18.6* and *Box 18.7*). Tissue factor is expressed on sub-endothelial fibroblasts, injured (but not undamaged) vascular endothelium and activated monocytes. The resulting complex (which is known as the extrinsic tenase complex) activates a small amount of factors IX and X as shown in *Figure 18.4*. The resulting factor X$_a$ can only activate a small amount of prothrombin to form thrombin because its cofactor, factor V$_a$, is not yet available. This small amount of thrombin is insufficient to generate significant amounts of fibrin. Instead, it activates the cofactors V and VIII, and stimulates further platelet activation.

The extrinsic tenase is rapidly inactivated by the formation of a complex with factor X$_a$ and tissue factor pathway inhibitor (TFPI). The initiation phase of coagulation is responsible for the rapid generation of thrombin sufficient to cause localized platelet aggregation and activation of the critical cofactors V and VIII. Rapid inactivation of the extrinsic tenase complex means that continued coagulation requires ongoing generation of factor X$_a$ through the actions of factors VIII$_a$ and IX$_a$, thereby explaining the clinical importance of these coagulation factors.

Box 18.6 The puzzling contact factors

In 1955 a railway worker named John Hageman required surgery for a peptic ulcer, but laboratory tests showed that his blood clotting time was prolonged. Further investigation revealed that he was deficient in a hitherto unknown plasma protein that was involved in contact activation of coagulation. This protein was named Hageman factor. Ten years later, several members of the Fletcher family were shown to have similarly prolonged clotting times and to be deficient in another plasma protein involved in contact activation. This factor was subsequently called Fletcher factor. A further 10 years passed before a Mr Fitzgerald, being treated for gunshot wounds, was shown to have a defect of contact activation and to be deficient in a plasma protein which became known as Fitzgerald factor. All three cases, separated by 20 years, have one important facet in common: gross prolongation of laboratory clotting times but an absence of any bleeding tendency (see also *Box 18.7*). This apparent anomaly cannot be explained by classical blood coagulation theory. Hageman factor is now known as factor XII, Fletcher factor as prekallikrein and Fitzgerald factor as high molecular weight kininogen.

Box 18.7 The contact factor puzzle is solved!

The *in vitro* tests of coagulation such as the activated partial thromboplastin time (APTT) involve a somewhat different mechanism of initiation called contact activation. In this system, factors XII and XI, prekallikrein and high molecular weight kininogen are critical initiation factors. For many years, it was believed that contact activation was also important *in vivo*, but this could not explain the fact that patients with severe deficiency of factors XII or XI do not have a significant bleeding tendency. It was the discovery of TFPI that forced a revision of the accepted mechanisms of blood coagulation *in vivo* and led to the development of the concepts of initiation and amplification detailed in the main text.

The amplification phase

In the amplification phase of coagulation, the formation of two enzyme complexes is responsible for a massive amplification in the amount of thrombin generated and results in rapid and extensive clot formation.

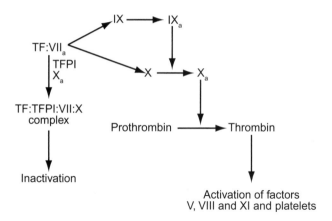

Figure 18.4
Initiation of coagulation *in vivo*. This phase of coagulation is self-limiting and does not generate significant quantities of fibrin. It can be thought of as a preparation for the amplification phase.

In the first step of the amplification phase, factors IX_a and VIII_a that have formed during initiation bind, via calcium ions, to exposed platelet phospholipid on the surface of the haemostatic plug. Binding in this way brings the coagulation factors together in the correct spatial orientation and creates a complex known as the intrinsic tenase complex. Formation of the intrinsic tenase complex prompts a rapid generation of factor X_a. This rapid, localized increase in factor X_a concentration prompts the formation of a second enzyme complex, consisting of factor X_a, calcium ions, platelet phospholipid and factor V_a generated during initiation. This complex, known as the prothrombinase complex, cleaves prothrombin to form the enzyme thrombin. Factors V_a and VIII_a are acting as accelerators, increasing the rate of formation of factor X_a and thrombin.

Thrombin has multiple enzymatic activities, including direct activation of factors V, VIII and XI. By this means, the generation of thrombin produces more of the accelerating cofactors V_a and VIII_a, which produces more thrombin, resulting in an explosive increase in the rate of coagulation.

The primary function of thrombin is the conversion of fibrinogen to fibrin. This is achieved by the cleavage and release of two small peptides from the Aα and Bβ chains of fibrinogen, called fibrinopeptides A and B. This process reduces the overall negative charge of the molecule and allows the spontaneous linear polymerization of the resultant fibrin monomers. At this stage, however, the fibrin clot is held together by hydrophobic and electrostatic bonds alone and is relatively unstable. The final stage of blood coagulation is the stabilization of the fibrin clot by the formation of crosslinks between adjacent linear fibrin molecules. This process is conducted by the transglutaminase, factor XIII_a. This enzyme is produced by the action of thrombin on factor XIII.

The amplification phase of blood coagulation *in vivo* is depicted in *Figure 18.5*.

Blood coagulation *in vitro*

The classical blood coagulation pathway was developed to explain *in vitro* observations made using the standard screening tests, the activated partial thromboplastin time (APTT) and the prothrombin time (PT). This led to the development of two distinct pathways of coagulation, the intrinsic pathway and the extrinsic pathway that converged into a final common pathway

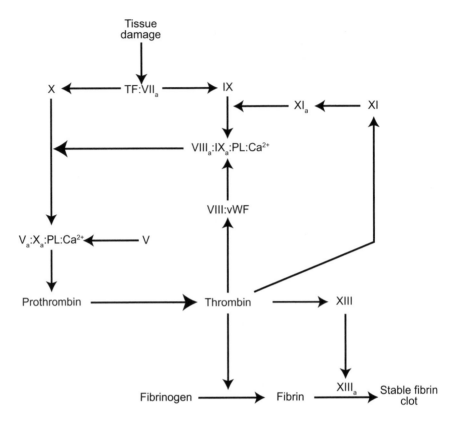

Figure 18.5
The amplification phase of blood coagulation *in vivo*.

as shown in *Figure 18.6*. It is now known that these pathways reflect forms of activation of coagulation that occur *in vitro* but not *in vivo*, and that separate pathways do not exist *in vivo*. The classical concept of blood coagulation has been exceptionally important as a means of understanding the results of laboratory screening tests of coagulation.

The intrinsic pathway
Intrinsic blood coagulation is initiated by contact of the flowing blood with a negatively charged surface such as glass or kaolin. Such exposure causes activation of factor XII, which then converts factor XI to XI$_a$. The factor XI for this reaction is also bound to the activating surface. Factor XI$_a$ activates factor IX, which then forms the tenase complex with factors VIII and X, calcium ions and platelet membrane phospholipid. From this point onwards, the pathway is similar to the *in vivo* pathway, it is only the mechanism of activation that differs (see also *Box 18.8*).

Box 18.8 Conservation of the coagulation mechanism

The coagulation mechanism is highly conserved in mammals. Indeed, any blood coagulation factor from one mammal is capable of activating its target factor from any other mammal. This degree of conservation implies a high level of efficiency.

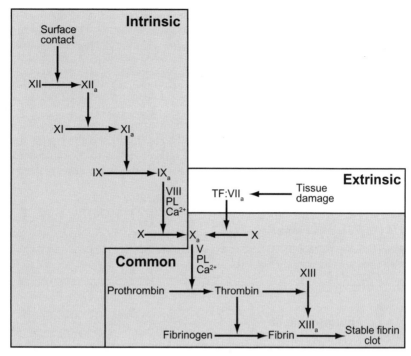

Figure 18.6
The three pathways that constitute the classical blood coagulation pathway.

The extrinsic pathway

In the presence of calcium ions, tissue factor (TF) forms a complex with both factor VII (TF:VII) and factor VII_a (TF:VII_a). The formation of these complexes results in the rapid activation of complexed VII and the enormous potentiation of the action of VII_a, i.e. the activation of factors IX and X. Following factor X activation, coagulation proceeds as described above (see also *Box 18.9*).

Box 18.9 Serine proteases and horseshoe crabs

The only known non-mammalian animal that uses serine proteases as the basis for its blood coagulation system is the horseshoe crab (*Limulus polyphemus*).

The classical concept of blood coagulation has been exceptionally important as a means of understanding the results of laboratory screening tests of coagulation. However, it is now clear that separate coagulation pathways do not exist *in vivo* and that tissue factor is the major physiological activator of blood coagulation.

18.4 INHIBITORS OF BLOOD COAGULATION

The blood coagulation system is a multifactorial biological pathway consisting of zymogens and accelerators. Because of the natural amplification of the enzyme products of the coagulation cascade, there is always a danger that the process may run out of control. A variety of inhibitory mechanisms exist which act to limit coagulation to the site of injury. The major inhibitors of the blood coagulation pathway are tissue factor pathway inhibitor, antithrombin, heparin cofactor II and activated protein C.

Tissue factor pathway inhibitor

Tissue factor pathway inhibitor is synthesized by endothelial cells and circulates in plasma bound to low density lipoproteins (see also *Box 18.10*). It is also present in platelets and bound to heparan sulphate at the endothelial surface. TFPI is the first inhibitor to act and inhibits coagulation by binding to factor X_a and the TF:VII$_a$ complex, thereby inhibiting their proteolytic activity.

Box 18.10 TFPI – what's in a name?

Tissue factor pathway inhibitor (TFPI) is also referred to in older literature as extrinsic pathway inhibitor (EPI) and lipoprotein-associated coagulation inhibitor (LACI).

Antithrombin III

Antithrombin III is a single chain glycoprotein of molecular weight 61 000 that is synthesized in the liver and endothelium and is the main physiological inhibitor of activated coagulation serine proteases. It acts by forming a complex with thrombin and other serine proteases in which both components are inactivated. Complex formation is greatly accelerated (about 2000-fold) by the presence of the anticoagulant heparin.

Heparin cofactor II

Heparin cofactor II is a single chain glycoprotein of molecular weight 65 000, which is synthesized in the liver. It complexes with thrombin in a 1:1 stoichiometric ratio, thereby inactivating the protease. In contrast to antithrombin, heparin cofactor II is specific for thrombin, having no inhibitory activity against the other serine proteases. The activity of heparin cofactor II is amplified 1000-fold by the presence of heparin.

The protein C pathway

Protein C is a vitamin K-dependent protein that plays a dual role in haemostasis by inhibiting blood coagulation and stimulating fibrinolysis (see also *Box 18.11*). Protein C is activated by thrombin in the presence of a cofactor called thrombomodulin. Activated protein C inhibits the coagulation cascade by inactivating factor VIII$_a$ and factor V$_a$, thereby reducing the rate of thrombin generation.

Box 18.11 Naming proteins C and S

Protein C derives its name from the chromatographic separation of the vitamin K-dependent factors from plasma. Using this method, 4 peaks are obtained, and these are labelled A, B, C and D. Protein C is the major constituent of the third peak. Protein S is named after the city of its discovery, Seattle.

Thrombomodulin has a molecular weight of 68 000 and is present in tight association with vascular endothelium. It forms complexes with thrombin in a 1:1 stoichiometric ratio. Complexed thrombin activates protein C several thousand times faster than free thrombin, but does not clot fibrinogen, activate factors V and VIII or aggregate platelets. Thrombomodulin-bound thrombin can still be inhibited by antithrombin.

Protein S is a single chain glycoprotein of molecular weight 69 000, which is synthesized in the liver and endothelium. It is a vitamin K-dependent protein but is not a serine protease. Activated protein C complexes with protein S and calcium ions on platelets and at the endothelial surface, greatly amplifying the inhibitory activity of complexed protein C.

18.5   THE FIBRINOLYTIC SYSTEM

The major function of the fibrinolytic system is the degradation and dissolution of formed fibrin within the circulation. This is achieved by the rapid and localized formation of a powerful proteolytic enzyme called plasmin. As shown in *Figure 18.7*, the fibrinolytic system has four main components:

- plasminogen activators
- plasminogen
- plasmin
- fibrinolytic inhibitors.

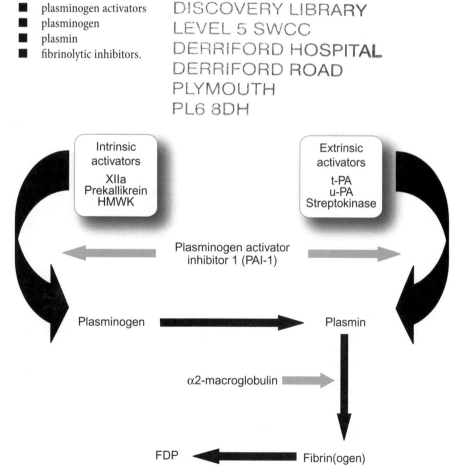

Figure 18.7
The fibrinolytic system.

Plasminogen activators

Plasminogen activation may occur via an intrinsic pathway, possibly mediated by components of contact activation, or via an extrinsic mechanism involving activators released from the blood vessel wall. Plasminogen activators are present in many different human and animal tissues and secretions. This form is known as tissue-type plasminogen activator (t-PA). The other major activator is found predominantly in urine and is known as urokinase-type plasminogen activator (u-PA) (see also *Box 18.12*).

Box 18.12 Exogenous activators of fibrinolysis

In addition to the physiological activators of fibrinolysis, a number of exogenous activators exist. For example, streptokinase is derived from β haemolytic streptococci and has been used as a therapeutic agent for the treatment of established thrombi for many years. However, streptokinase therapy is difficult to control and complicated by the antigenicity of bacterial products. It is likely to be superseded by genetically engineered tissue plasminogen activator, although currently this is extremely expensive.

Tissue plasminogen activator has a molecular weight of 70 000 and is synthesized and stored by vascular endothelial cells, ready for release into the bloodstream when required. It functions as a serine protease in the conversion of plasminogen to plasmin, a process greatly accelerated by the presence of fibrin.

Urokinase (u-PA), a trypsin-like protease, is synthesized in the kidney and is found mainly in urine. It converts plasminogen directly to plasmin in a reaction that does not require the presence of fibrin.

Plasminogen and plasmin

Plasminogen is a single-chain glycoprotein with a molecular weight of about 92 000. The molecule contains five homologous triple loop structures known as kringles, which mediate binding to fibrin and fibrinogen. Both plasminogen and plasmin have a very strong affinity for fibrinogen and fibrin. This means that a fibrin clot will also contain plasminogen activator and plasminogen bound up within it. Thus, activation of plasminogen to form plasmin is localized to the site of clot formation and digestion occurs from the inside of the clot outwards.

Inhibitors of fibrinolysis

As with the coagulation system, uninhibited proteolytic activity is potentially dangerous, and the fibrinolytic pathway is similarly equipped with inhibitory mechanisms. The major physiological inhibitor of plasmin is α_2-antiplasmin; enzyme activity that exceeds the capacity of this inhibitor is neutralized by the high molecular weight plasma protein α_2-macroglobulin or histidine-rich glycoprotein. Inhibition of fibrinolysis is also mediated by inhibition of plasminogen activators via plasminogen activator inhibitor 1 (PAI-1) and plasminogen activator inhibitor 2 (PAI-2).

18.6 TESTS OF HAEMOSTASIS

The first steps in investigation of haemostasis involve clinical examination, history taking and the judicious use of screening tests to narrow the focus of the investigation to the system or systems involved.

Tests of vascular function

There are no specific, reproducible tests of vascular function. Instead, the vascular bleeding disorders are diagnosed by the demonstration of a pattern of bleeding typical of a platelet or vascular disorder, coupled with demonstration of normal platelet number and function. A thorough history and physical examination can help to provide clues as to the diagnosis.

Although not absolute, the pattern of bleeding can help to distinguish between vascular or platelet abnormalities and disorders of blood coagulation as shown in *Table 18.3*. In general, clinical manifestations of bleeding in vascular-platelet disorders occur immediately after trauma, which may often be minimal. These manifestations include petechiae, purpura and mucous membrane bleeding such as epistaxis, gingival bleeding or menorrhagia.

Table 18.3 Patterns of bleeding in disorders of haemostasis

Clinical finding	Vascular-platelet disorders	Coagulation disorders
Mucous membrane bleeding	Common	Unusual
Manifestation after trauma	Immediate after minor trauma	Delayed, sometimes restarting after cessation of primary bleeding (episodic bleeding)
Petechiae	Common	Rare
Haematomas & haemarthroses	Rare	Common, particularly in severe inherited disorders
Superficial bleeding	Common and often prolonged	Commonly normal or minimally prolonged
Gender	No difference	Predominantly male

Tests of platelet number and function

Haemostatic disorders related to platelets can be caused by either thrombocytopenia or decreased function. As in most areas of haematological investigation, a full blood count is essential and examination of a blood film provides useful additional information in many cases. Together, these tests will identify thrombocytopenia and may provide clues about the underlying cause. Platelet morphology can also help to suggest a diagnosis, e.g. giant platelets are often present in Bernard–Soulier syndrome.

The simplest test of platelet function is the bleeding time. This test involves making one or more cuts in the forearm under standardized conditions and timing how long it takes for bleeding to cease. Although this is a relatively crude and non-specific test, it is useful as a first screen for the presence of some platelet disorder.

More specific tests of platelet function include: platelet aggregation studies, measurement of platelet glycoproteins, vWF assay and tests that try to mimic *in vivo* conditions, such as the PFA-100 analyser. Interpretation of platelet function tests is complex and requires both expertise and experience.

Tests of coagulation

The first step in the investigation of coagulation is a coagulation screen, which consists of four tests that together cover most of the likely abnormalities. The tests included in a coagulation screen are the prothrombin time (PT), activated partial thromboplastin time (APTT), thrombin time (TT) and fibrinogen assay. The PT measures the function of the coagulation factors involved in the extrinsic pathway, the APTT measures the intrinsic pathway, the TT measures the conversion of fibrinogen to fibrin by thrombin and the fibrinogen assay measures the concentration of fibrinogen in the plasma. Although these pathways do not exist *in vivo*, abnormalities in one or more of these tests provide strong clues as to the type of coagulation abnormality that may be present (see *Table 18.4*).

If an abnormality is found on a coagulation screen, second-line testing such as specific factor assays may be required, to identify the specific abnormality. The clinical examination and history will help to guide selection of these tests. For example, clinical history may help to differentiate between a likely inherited or acquired disorder. This aspect of investigation is described in the next chapter.

The only coagulation factor not included in the coagulation screen is factor XIII. Those with a deficiency of this factor present with an unusual pattern of bleeding, scarring and poor healing, caused by the formation of unstable clots. Factor XIII deficiency can only be diagnosed using specific factor assays or by molecular methods.

Table 18.4 Interpretation of coagulation screening tests

Test result	Possible disorders
PT prolonged, other tests normal	Factor VII deficiency
	Liver disease
	Vitamin K deficiency
	Warfarin therapy
APTT prolonged, other tests normal	Heparin therapy
	Factor VIII deficiency or inhibitor
	von Willebrand
	Factor IX deficiency or inhibitor
	Contact factor deficiency (XI, XII, PK or HMWK) or inhibitor*
	Lupus anticoagulant
Both PT and APTT prolonged	High-dose heparin therapy
	Warfarin overdose
	Severe vitamin K deficiency
	Moderate-to-severe liver disease
	Common pathway deficiency or inhibitor
	Disseminated intravascular coagulation (DIC)
	Fibrinogen disorder
Prolonged TT	Heparin therapy
	Afibrinogenaemia
	Hypofibrinogenaemia
	Dysfibrinogenaemia

* Prolongation of APTT may be severe in contact factor deficiency but this does not relate to likelihood of bleeding abnormality

SUGGESTED FURTHER READING

Blomback, M. & Antovic, J. (eds.) (2009) *Essential Guide to Blood Coagulation*. Wiley-Blackwell, Oxford.

Kemball-Cook, G., *et al.* (2005) Normal haemostasis. In: *Postgraduate Haematology* (Hoffbrand, A.V., Catovsky, D. & Tuddenham, E.G.D., eds), pp. 783–807. Blackwell Publishing, Oxford.

Nancy, K., *et al.* (2009) Physiology of hemostasis: with relevance to current and future laboratory testing. *Clinics Lab. Med.* **29:** 159–174.

Valerie, L.N. (2009) Prothrombin time and partial thromboplastin time assay considerations. *Clinics Lab. Med.* **29:** 253–263.

Watson, S.P. & Harrison, P. (2005) The vascular function of platelets. In: *Postgraduate Haematology* (Hoffbrand, A.V., Catovsky, D. & Tuddenham, E.G.D., eds), pp. 808–824. Blackwell Publishing, Oxford.

SELF-ASSESSMENT QUESTIONS

1. Name the five main systems involved in haemostasis.
2. Name the three concentric layers in the structure of blood vessels.
3. Which of the following substances are synthesized by vascular endothelial cells?
   a. vWF
   b. PGI_2
   c. thrombomodulin
   d. TFPI
   e. all of the above
4. Which of the following substances are stored in platelet α granules?
   a. ADP
   b. thrombospondin
   c. fibrinogen
   d. serotonin
   e. platelet factor 4 (PF4)
   f. von Willebrand factor (vWF)
   g. β-thromboglobulin (β-TG)
   h. coagulation factor V
5. Name the principal platelet membrane glycoprotein receptor for sub-endothelial-bound vWF.
6. Name the platelet enzyme acetylated by aspirin.
7. Which of the following coagulation factors are vitamin K-dependent?
   a. V
   b. VII
   c. VIII
   d. II
   e. fibrinogen
8. Which coagulation factor acts as a transglutaminase?
9. Name the main physiological inhibitor of activated coagulation serine proteases.
10. Name three components of the protein C inhibitory pathway.
11. What property of plasminogen helps to localize fibrinolysis to the site of clot formation?

Bleeding disorders

Learning objectives
After studying this chapter you should confidently be able to:

- **List selected examples of inherited bleeding disorders associated with defects of primary haemostasis**
  Among the inherited vasculopathies associated with bleeding are hereditary haemorrhagic telangiectasia and Ehlers–Danlos syndrome. Inherited platelet disorders can be quantitative (i.e. resulting in thrombocytopenia) or qualitative (i.e. resulting in disordered platelet function). Among the inherited thrombocytopenias are the rare conditions congenital amegakaryocytic thrombocytopenia and thrombocytopenia with absent radii. Thrombocytopenia is an important component of disease in the inherited conditions May–Hegglin anomaly and Wiskott–Aldrich syndrome. The most important inherited thrombocytopathies include Bernard–Soulier disease, pseudo von Willebrand's disease, Glanzmann's thrombasthenia and the platelet storage pool diseases.

- **Compare and contrast the pathophysiology of Bernard–Soulier disease, von Willebrand's disease and haemophilia**
  Von Willebrand's disease is the most common inherited haemorrhagic disorder and is inherited as an autosomal dominant condition, affecting both males and females. It is characterized by deficiency of vWF with abnormalities in the assembly and processing of vWF multimers. Factor VIII is reduced in vWD, but this is a secondary phenomenon due to loss of the protective function of vWF for factor VIII. Bleeding in most cases is mucous membrane-related. Haemophilia is an X-linked recessive disorder (i.e. affecting males) and is the second most common inherited bleeding disorder. It is characterized by deficiency of factor VIII. Circulating vWF levels are usually normal or raised. Bleeding is primarily into muscles and joints. Bernard–Soulier disease is a rare, autosomal recessive trait and is characterized by deficiency of the GPIb:GPIX:GPV vWF platelet membrane receptor. The pattern of bleeding is similar to vWD, but the circulating vWF and factor VIII levels are normal.

- **Outline the genetic basis of haemophilia and the approach to screening for carrier detection**
  The gene that encodes factor VIII is located on the tip of the q arm of the X chromosome (Xq28). Haemophilia results from mutations of this gene and so is inherited as an X-linked recessive disorder. The gene is highly susceptible to mutation; more than 350 different mutations have been identified, many of which are unique to an individual family. Up to 95% of haemophilia patients have identifiable mutations of the factor VIII gene, enabling accurate gene tracking through families. Carrier detection involves family studies, serial measurement of factor VIII and vWF and screening for common mutations. This approach can identify mutations in up to 97% of carriers of severe forms of haemophilia.

- **Discuss the pathogenesis and pathophysiology of disseminated intravascular coagulation**
  DIC is characterized by the widespread activation of all of the haemostatic mechanisms. Although the early result of DIC is thrombosis, the most

obvious feature in most cases is haemorrhage secondary to the consumption of coagulation factors and platelets. The most common triggers of DIC are infection, malignancy and obstetric complications. Systemic thrombin generation triggers activation of the coagulation cascade and platelets, resulting in the deposition of microthrombi throughout the body and leading to widespread occlusion of the microcirculation. The resulting ischaemic tissue damage propagates haemostatic activation. Widespread activation of platelets and coagulation rapidly and progressively lead to thrombocytopenia, a drop in the circulating levels of coagulation factors and progressive depletion of circulating antithrombin III, secondary to reticuloendothelial clearance of thrombin–antithrombin complexes. Fibrin deposition and local endothelial injury trigger secondary fibrinolysis, resulting in plasmin generation and digestion of fibrin(ogen), factors V and VIII, and a range of other plasma proteins. Fibrin(ogen) degradation products interfere with fibrin polymerization and platelet function. To cap it all, widespread activation of the complement and kinin systems leads to an increase in vascular permeability, hypotension and shock. These secondary events in the pathogenesis of DIC explain the apparently paradoxical thrombohaemorrhagic state that typifies this condition.

■ **List the circumstances in which acquired bleeding disorders may arise**
Acquired bleeding disorders are much more common than inherited disorders. They are commonly associated with infection, malignancy, liver disease and obstetric complications. The acquired purpuras are a group of haemostatic disorders manifest as mucous membrane bleeding and include Henoch–Schönlein purpura, immune thrombocytopenic purpura, heparin-induced thrombocytopenia, thrombotic thrombocytopenic purpura and toxin-induced thrombocytopathy.

Optimal haemostasis requires the interaction of numerous components of the blood vessel wall, platelets, coagulation system and the fibrinolytic system. Defects affecting any of these mechanisms can cause either a bleeding or a thrombotic disorder, which may be hereditary or acquired. This chapter focuses on the inherited and acquired bleeding disorders.

19.1 INHERITED BLEEDING DISORDERS

Haemostasis requires a dynamic equilibrium between clot-promoting and clot-preventing activities. A haemorrhagic diathesis results from any alteration in the haemostatic balance, which either impairs clot-promoting activities or potentiates clot-inhibiting or dissolution activities. A variety of such defects exist including:

■ structural defects of the vascular system, resulting in easy disruption
■ quantitative (thrombocytopenia) or qualitative (thrombocytopathy) defects of platelets, resulting in impaired platelet plug formation
■ deficiency or dysfunction of coagulation factors (coagulopathy), resulting in impaired clot formation
■ deficiency or dysfunction of fibrinolytic inhibitors, resulting in hyperfibrinolysis

Inherited structural defects of the vascular system

Hereditary haemorrhagic telangiectasia
Hereditary haemorrhagic telangiectasia (HHT) is inherited as an autosomal dominant condition and is characterized by malformed, thin-walled capillaries, known as telangiectases, which are

> **Box 19.1 Osler–Rendu–Weber syndrome**
>
> HHT is also known as Osler–Rendu–Weber syndrome. The French physician Rendu was the first to differentiate HHT from haemophilia. In 1876, he described a 52-year-old man with repeated nose bleeds, multiple haemangiomatous spots on the skin of his face, lips, tongue and palate and also on his trunk. Rendu also noted that the man's mother had experienced similar problems.
>
> It was not until 1901 that Dr William Bart Osler of Johns Hopkins hospital wrote the first comprehensive description of the disease, emphasizing the familial nature of the condition. Six years later, Dr Frederick Parkes Weber added significantly to earlier descriptions in a seminal *Lancet* article. The contributions of these three men to the modern understanding of HHT are recognized in the triple eponym that is sometimes used.

highly susceptible to rupture (see *Box 19.1*). Telangiectases are most obvious on the tongue, lips and nose but they occur throughout the body. Clinically, HHT presents as recurrent nosebleeds (epistaxes) and gastrointestinal blood loss. Enlargement and coalescence of telangiectases leads to bleeding in the lungs or brain, which may be life threatening. No treatment is available for HHT other than correction of the recurrent anaemia and cautery of troublesome bleeding points. The genetic basis of HHT is extraordinarily diverse; more than 500 different mutations have been identified as causing this condition. Most of these mutations have been found in the endoglin (*CD105*) gene on chromosome 9q34.1, leading to type 1 HHT, or in the activin A receptor type II-like 1 gene (*ACVRL1*) gene on chromosome 12q11–14, leading to type 2 HHT. Both endoglin and ACVRL1 are involved in transforming growth factor-β (TGFβ) binding on blood vessel endothelium.

Ehlers–Danlos syndrome

Ehlers–Danlos syndrome (EDS) is the name given to a group of collagen disorders characterized by extreme elasticity and fragility of the skin, hypermobility of the joints and a haemorrhagic tendency (see *Box 19.2*). In the most serious variant, EDS type IV, there is a quantitative or qualitative deficiency of type III collagen, the form that predominates in blood vessels. Such a deficiency leads to a tendency for spontaneous rupture of bowel or large arteries, which may be life threatening. This form is linked to mutation of the *COL3A1* gene on chromosome 2q31. There is no treatment for this condition.

> **Box 19.2 Ehlers–Danlos syndrome**
>
> There are indications throughout history of families with unusual symptoms that correspond with Ehlers–Danlos syndrome, but the first clear clinical description of this syndrome in western Europe was made by Dr Edvard Ehlers at a clinical meeting of the Paris Society of Syphilology and Dermatology in 1899. Nine years later, another case was presented to the same society by Dr Henri-Alexandre Danlos.
>
> In 1936, Dr Frederick Parkes Weber (of Osler–Rendu–Weber fame, see *Box 19.1*) suggested that the condition should be named Ehlers–Danlos syndrome.
>
> Interestingly, Edvard Ehlers was not the first physician to diagnose this condition. That achievement belongs to a Russian physician, Dr Chernogubov who presented two cases to the Moscow Dermatological and Venereologic Society in 1892. This presentation was not known of in western Europe, so the condition was named after Ehlers and Danlos. However, in Russia, the condition is known as Chernogubov syndrome.

Inherited defects of platelets

A deficiency of platelet activity may be caused by severe thrombocytopenia or defective platelet function. The clinical manifestations of congenital platelet disorders all follow a similar pattern: easy bruising, petechial rash, mucous membrane bleeding (epistaxis, gastrointestinal bleeding, menorrhagia) or excessive bleeding following minor trauma. The severity of these symptoms varies from a severe, life-long haemorrhagic diathesis to a much milder condition.

Inherited thrombocytopenias

Inherited conditions that cause failure of thrombopoiesis and so lead to thrombocytopenia are rare. The best-described inherited thrombocytopenias include congenital amegakaryocytic thrombocytopenia, thrombocytopenia with absent radii, May–Hegglin anomaly and Wiskott–Aldrich syndrome.

Congenital amegakaryocytic thrombocytopenia

Congenital amegakaryocytic thrombocytopenia (CAMT) is a rare inherited disease characterized by a severe thrombocytopenia with markedly reduced megakaryocytes in the bone marrow. Typically, isolated thrombocytopenia is present at birth but pancytopenia often develops in later childhood. The condition is caused by various mutations in the thrombopoietin receptor gene *c-MPL* at 1p34. This means that platelets and megakaryocytes do not respond to circulating thrombopoietin so thrombopoiesis is severely retarded. The only cure for CAMT is stem cell transplantation.

Thrombocytopenia with absent radii

Thrombocytopenia-absent radii (TAR) syndrome is a rare condition in which thrombocytopenia is associated with a reduction of the number of megakaryocytes in the bone marrow and absence of both radii, causing deformity of the lower arms. Multiple other anatomical abnormalities may be present. TAR syndrome was first described in 1951 and is most often described as an autosomal recessive condition. The mutations that cause TAR have not been identified but studies have shown that a 200 kb microdeletion at 1q21.1 is present in all cases. This microdeletion appears to be required but is not sufficient to cause the condition; another as yet unidentified mutation is also required. Death from haemorrhage is most common in the early months of life. Platelet counts tend to rise after this time and may even normalize.

May–Hegglin anomaly

May–Hegglin anomaly (MHA) is a rare autosomal dominant disorder caused by mutation of the non-muscle myosin heavy chain-9 gene (*MYH9*) at 22q11.2, leading to macrothrombocytopenia secondary to defective megakaryocyte maturation and fragmentation (see *Box 19.3*). MHA is characterized by variable thrombocytopenia with giant platelets containing few granules and the presence of large basophilic, cytoplasmic inclusion bodies (resembling Döhle bodies), consisting

---

Box 19.3 May–Hegglin anomaly

The earliest description of what later came to be known as May–Hegglin anomaly was made by Dr May in 1909 in an asymptomatic young girl with leucocytic inclusion bodies distinguishable on a blood smear. In 1945, Dr Hegglin described a man and his 2 sons who were also healthy but who had thrombocytopenia with giant platelets, and the same leucocytic inclusions observed by Dr May. The work of these two physicians was later recognized when the condition they described became known as May–Hegglin anomaly (MHA).

of precipitated myosin heavy chains in the neutrophils, eosinophils, basophils and monocytes. The condition is often asymptomatic but may be associated with purpura, easy bruising and mucous membrane bleeding, but this is seldom severe. Both neutrophil and platelet function is normal in MHA.

Wiskott–Aldrich syndrome

Wiskott-Aldrich syndrome (WAS) is an X-linked condition with variable expression (see *Box 19.4*). Symptoms commonly include eczema, thrombocytopenia with small platelets and immunodeficiency. There is an increased risk of autoimmune disease and haematological malignancy. The condition is caused by a mutation in the gene for Wiskott–Aldrich syndrome protein (WASp) at Xp11.23–11.22. The exact function of WASp is unknown, but it appears to be involved in the pathways that govern actin filament assembly and cell movement. Most affected boys die in childhood from infection, bleeding or haematological malignancy. Stem cell transplantation offers the only prospect of cure.

Box 19.4 Wiskott–Aldrich syndrome

Wiskott–Aldrich syndrome is named after the German paediatrician Dr Alfred Wiskott and the US paediatrician Robert Anderson Aldrich who described the condition independently.

Inherited thrombocytopathies

Bernard–Soulier disease

Bernard–Soulier disease (BSD) is a rare, autosomal recessive trait, which is characterized by the presence of giant platelets, variable thrombocytopenia, impairment of vWF-mediated platelet adhesion, prolonged bleeding time and a bleeding tendency of variable severity (see *Box 19.5*). BSD platelets are deficient in the GPIb:GPIX:GPV membrane glycoprotein complex, which is the receptor for von Willebrand factor and is required for optimal platelet activation and function. BSD is caused by mutations in the genes that encode GPIbα at 17pter–p12 (type A BSD), GPIbβ at 3q21 (type B BSD) or GPIX at 22q11.2 (type C BSD). Mutations in the GPV gene at 3q29 have not been implicated in BSD.

There is no specific curative treatment for BSD. Supportive therapy includes red cell transfusions to combat anaemia, hormonal control of ovulation to minimize heavy menstruation and platelet transfusions when required.

Box 19.5 Bernard–Soulier disease

The first case of Bernard–Soulier disease was reported in 1948 by two French physicians, Jean Bernard and Jean-Pierre Soulier, in a 5-month-old child with recurrent haemorrhagic problems.

Pseudo von Willebrand's disease

Pseudo von Willebrand's disease (platelet-type vWD) is inherited as an autosomal dominant condition and is characterized by mild thrombocytopenia, moderately reduced plasma vWF concentration and a prolonged bleeding time. Pseudo vWD is caused by mutation of the GPIb gene at 17pter–p12, resulting in enhanced binding of plasma vWF. Careful laboratory testing is required to distinguish between pseudo von Willebrand's disease, true von Willebrand's disease and Bernard–Soulier disease.

Glanzmann's thrombasthenia

Glanzmann's thrombasthenia (GT) is inherited as an autosomal recessive trait and is characterized by a normal platelet count and morphology, impairment or absence of clot retraction and near absence of platelet aggregation (see *Box 19.6*). The disorder is caused by a profound deficiency or defect of the platelet membrane glycoprotein complex (GPIIb:GPIIIa) that mediates platelet aggregation responses by functioning as a surface receptor for fibrinogen and vWF. GT is caused by mutation in the gene for GPIIb at 17q21–32 or the GPIIIa gene at the same locus. In type I GT, platelets show a complete absence of the GPIIb–IIIa complex, deficiency of fibrinogen and severely impaired or absent clot retraction. In type II GT, GPIIb–IIIa complex expression is reduced, platelet fibrinogen is detectable and clot retraction is moderately impaired.

Although Glanzmann's thrombasthenia is a very uncommon disorder, it is one of the most frequently encountered inherited qualitative platelet defects.

Box 19.6 Glanzmann's thrombasthenia

Glanzmann's thrombasthenia is named after Eduard Glanzmann, the Swiss paediatrician who first described the condition. The condition is also (less commonly) known as Glanzmann–Nägeli syndrome, Nägeli syndrome II and Révol's syndrome, recognizing the early descriptions of other physicians.

Storage pool disease

Storage pool disease is a relatively mild autosomal dominant platelet disorder and is caused by a deficiency of platelet dense granules (δ-SPD) or α granules (α-SPD) or, rarely, both (see *Box 19.7*). This causes a deficiency of the important substances stored in these granules and consequent impairment of functional responses.

Box 19.7 Grey platelet syndrome

α-SPD is also known as grey platelet syndrome because, when stained with Romanowsky dyes and viewed by light microscopy, the absence of α granulation in the platelets results in a uniform grey appearance.

Inherited coagulopathies

The inherited coagulopathies are rare, with an overall incidence of about 0.02%, but disorders such as haemophilia are both scientifically and clinically important, and have even been politically and historically important (see *Box 19.8*). Much of our current knowledge of the physiology of coagulation has been derived by studying the pathophysiology of cases of isolated coagulation factor deficiency. The two most commonly encountered inherited coagulopathies are associated with an abnormality or deficiency of the factor VIII:vWF complex. Coagulation factor VIII and vWF normally circulate in plasma as a non-covalently bound complex. Formation of this complex is essential for the survival of factor VIII in plasma. Von Willebrand's disease (vWD) is caused by a deficiency or defect of vWF, while haemophilia is caused by a deficiency or defect of factor VIII.

Von Willebrand's disease

Von Willebrand's disease is the most common inherited haemorrhagic disorder with a worldwide distribution and a particularly high incidence in the Scandinavian countries (see *Box 19.9*). The prevalence of vWD in the general population has been estimated to be about 1%, but it is possible that this is an underestimate since very mild cases may never be detected.

Box 19.8 The royal disease

Haemophilia (deficiency of factor VIII) played a significant role in European political history during much of the 19th and early 20th centuries. The Queen of the United Kingdom at this time was Queen Victoria. With her husband, Prince Albert of Saxe-Coburg-Gotha, Victoria had four sons and five daughters, who went on to marry into other Royal families in Europe and, in turn, went on to have 20 grandsons (two of whom were stillborn) and 22 granddaughters. The importance of these facts lies in the knowledge that Victoria was a haemophilia carrier. It is clear that Queen Victoria passed the affected gene to two of her daughters, Princess Alice and Princess Beatrice and to her son Prince Leopold. A third daughter, Princess Helena, may or may not have been a carrier. Two of Queen Victoria's other sons died in infancy and haemophilia may or may not have been implicated.

Victoria's affected children went on to marry and to pass haemophilia into the royal families of Spain, Germany and Russia. The disease continued to take its toll on these families, with several affected princes dying young and several carrier princesses passing on the affected gene.

Perhaps the greatest impact of what became known as the 'royal disease' came when Princess Alix of Hesse and by Rhine, the daughter of Princess Alice, married Tsar Nicholas II of Russia, and passed it on to her only son: Tsarevitch Alexei. The chronic illness of the Tsarevitch and the increasingly desperate attempts of his mother to find support and solace led her to the mystic healer Grigori Yefimovich Rasputin. Many historians credit the malign influence of Rasputin on the Tsarina as a major contributor to the fall of the Romanov Empire and the success of the Russian Revolution.

Haemophilia now appears to be extinct in the royal families of Europe.

Box 19.9 Von Willebrand's disease

Von Willebrand's disease was first described by the Finnish physician Erik Adolf von Willebrand in 1926 as an apparently inherited haemorrhagic condition in several members of a Finnish family from the Åland Islands in the Gulf of Bothnia. This new condition was readily distinguished from haemophilia by the presence of a prolonged bleeding time test. Von Willebrand suspected that the condition, which he named **pseudohaemophilia** but which later came to bear his name, was a disorder of platelet function. The true nature of von Willebrand's disease has only recently been identified.

---

vWD is a heterogeneous disorder with several subtypes recognized, based on differences in the assembly and processing of vWF multimers (see *Table 19.1*). The vWF gene is located at 12p13.3. Broadly, vWD types 1 and 3 represent a quantitative deficiency of a functionally normal vWF while type 2 variants represent the presence of a qualitatively abnormal vWF. Type 2 vWD is divided into types 2A, 2B, 2M and 2N. Type 1 is the most common form of vWD, accounting for more than 70% of cases. The most common type 2 variant is type 2A, which accounts for about 15% of cases. Type 3 vWD is a severe, life-long haemorrhagic disorder that is clinically similar to severe haemophilia apart from the added complication of platelet dysfunction secondary to deficiency of vWF. Types 2C and 3 vWD are inherited as an autosomal recessive trait, whereas all other types are inherited in an incompletely dominant fashion.

Pathophysiology of vWD. vWF has two functions: it mediates platelet adhesion and it protects circulating factor VIII from autolysis. Because of its involvement in haemostatic plug formation and its crucial role in coagulation, the bleeding problems associated with vWD are highly heterogeneous. Severe type III vWD is associated with spontaneous bleeding into joints (haemarthrosis), muscles (haematoma) and with severe and prolonged bleeding following trauma. Most cases of vWD, however, are relatively mild and significant bleeding problems may be absent. Where present, bleeding is usually manifest as mucous membrane bleeding including recurrent nosebleeds (epistaxis), heavy or prolonged menstruation (menorrhagia) and easy

Table 19.1 Subtypes of vWD

Subtype	Defining characteristic
Type 1	Partial deficiency of vWF. Autosomal dominant.
Type 2A	Abnormal assembly of high molecular weight multimers. Autosomal dominant.
Type 2B	Increased binding of vWF to platelets, leading to deficiency of high molecular weight multimers and thrombocytopenia. Autosomal dominant.
Type 2M	Decreased binding of vWF to platelets with normal multimer distribution. Autosomal dominant.
Type 2N	Decreased binding of vWF to factor VIII, leading to factor VIII deficiency. Autosomal recessive.
Type 3	Severe deficiency of vWF. Autosomal recessive.
Pseudo vWD	Abnormal platelet GP Ib:IX:V with increased binding of high molecular weight multimers, leading to deficiency of high molecular weight multimers and thrombocytopenia. Autosomal dominant.

bruising. Bleeding from coincident pathology such as duodenal ulcers may be unusually heavy and prolonged. Mild vWD is clinically similar to platelet disorders such as Bernard–Soulier disease.

Diagnosis of vWD. A diagnosis of vWD may be suspected from a clinical examination and family history, but diagnosis requires laboratory testing. Preliminary screening tests show normal prothrombin and thrombin times, but the APTT may be prolonged. The bleeding time or PFA-100 test may be prolonged. Assay of factor VIII reveals a reduced level, but this does not reflect failure of synthesis of factor VIII. Rather, it is due to a deficiency of vWF, with a consequent failure to protect circulating factor VIII from breakdown. Platelet aggregation in response to ADP, adrenaline or thrombin is normal, but is defective in response to ristocetin (see *Box 19.10*). The platelet count is normal except in type 2B where thrombocytopenia is present. Diagnosis of the subtype of vWD requires vWF multimer analysis.

Treatment of vWD. With the exception of the type III variants, vWD is a relatively mild haemorrhagic disorder and treatment is only required for post-traumatic bleeds and to cover surgery. For mild bleeding episodes, the antifibrinolytic agent tranexamic acid may be useful. The most common form of treatment involves the use of the vasopressin analogue DDAVP (1–desamino–8–D–argininylvasopressin) which triggers the release of vWF from the Weibel–Palade bodies of vascular endothelium. This therapy is suitable as a short-term measure only; the endothelial stores of vWF are exhaustible, following which further treatment is ineffective.

DDAVP treatment is most useful in types I and IIA vWD. It is ineffective in type III vWD and triggers acute and severe thrombocytopenia in type IIB vWD. These forms require infusion of cryoprecipitate, which is rich in vWF or high purity vWF concentrates.

Box 19.10 Ristocetin and vWD

Ristocetin is an antibiotic that was used to treat staphylococcal infections, but was withdrawn because it causes platelet aggregation. Following its withdrawal, it was used *in vitro* as an agonist in platelet aggregation studies. Ristocetin-induced platelet aggregation requires the presence of von Willebrand factor. Defective ristocetin-induced platelet aggregation is therefore an indicator of von Willebrand's disease.

Haemophilia

Haemophilia is the second most common inherited haemorrhagic disorder, occurring in all ethnic groups (see also *Box 19.11*). The incidence of this X-linked recessive disorder in the UK is approximately 0.005%. Haemophilia is characterized by a decreased plasma concentration of functionally active factor VIII. The factor VIII activity relates closely to the clinical severity of the condition (see *Table 19.2*).

Box 19.11 Haemophilia is an ancient disease

Haemophilia has probably been recognized as a distinct disease since antiquity. The earliest written evidence of its recognition comes in the Babylonian Talmud which records a decision that the fourth-born son of a particular woman should be exempt from circumcision if her first three sons had all bled to death following this ritual. This is a clear attempt to formally recognize the existence of a severe haemorrhagic disorder that is transmitted vertically to males by symptom-free carrier females.

Table 19.2 Classification of haemophilia

Factor VIII activity (% of normal)	Classification	Incidence (%)	Manifestations
< 0.01	Severe	40	Spontaneous haemarthroses and haematomas
0.01–0.05	Moderate	35	Bleeding after relatively minor trauma
> 0.05	Mild	25	Bleeding after major trauma, e.g. surgery

Genetics of haemophilia. The gene that encodes factor VIII is located on the tip of the q arm of the X chromosome (Xq28). Haemophilia results from mutations of this gene and so is inherited as an X-linked recessive disorder. This mode of inheritance is associated with several clearly defined features:

- hemizygous males express the disease
- heterozygous females are typically symptomless carriers
- homozygous females express the disease
- the sons of a hemizygous male are normal
- the daughters of a hemizygous male are obligate carriers
- the sons and daughters of a carrier female have a 50% chance of inheriting the mutant gene.

The factor VIII gene is large and complex, spanning 186 kb and comprising 26 exons which range in size from 69 to 3106 bp separated by 25 introns. The gene occupies almost 0.1% of the X chromosome. The gene appears to be highly susceptible to mutation: more than 350 different mutations have been identified, many of which are unique to an individual family. About 40% of cases of severe haemophilia result from an inversion involving the tip of the q arm of the X chromosome, involving a breakpoint within intron 22. Another common inversion involving intron 1 is present in about 5% of severe cases. However, most cases of mild–moderate haemophilia are associated with a wide variety of point mutations. Up to 95% of haemophilia patients have identifiable mutations of the factor VIII gene. This means accurate gene tracking and carrier analysis is possible in most families. Precise characterization of genetic defects enables increased accuracy in the detection of female carriers and in antenatal diagnosis of haemophilia.

Factor VIII is synthesized in the liver and the spleen.

Pathophysiology of haemophilia. Primary haemostasis is normal, even in severe haemophiliacs, so bleeding from minor cuts and abrasions is seldom troublesome. More substantial tissue damage results in the formation of weak clots, which are highly susceptible to mechanical or fibrinolytic breakdown. This explains the classical pattern of bleeding into joints and deep tissues that is delayed for some hours after trauma. Most apparently spontaneous bleeds probably result from some ill-remembered minor trauma in the preceding hours.

The most common sites of haemorrhage in haemophilia are the weight-bearing joints such as knees, elbows, ankles, shoulders, wrists and hips. In addition to bearing much of the strain of everyday movement, these joints are particularly susceptible to the knocks and bumps of everyday life. Recurrent bleeding into joint spaces (haemarthrosis) is extremely painful and results in irreversible crippling joint and tissue damage. This is a major cause of illness in haemophiliacs and frequently necessitates joint replacement.

In addition to recurrent haemarthroses, severe haemophiliacs are plagued by frequent, painful bleeding episodes, which most commonly involve the large weight-bearing muscles of the thigh and calf, posterior abdominal wall and the gluteal muscles. Haematomas may take several months to resolve and the affected muscle is frequently damaged permanently, with progressive contraction and loss of power.

Other common bleeding manifestations in haemophiliacs include blood in the urine (haematuria), cerebral bleeds which may be fatal, recurrent nosebleeds and gastrointestinal haemorrhage.

The pattern of bleeding in haemophilia differs according to age. If delivery is not traumatic, bleeds in the first few months of life are uncommon. However, as the child becomes mobile and increasingly adventurous, the falls and bumps that characterize this period of life frequently cause extensive traumatic bruising and haematoma formation and may result in unjust accusations of non-accidental injury. Bleeding in haemophiliacs is not faster than normal but typically continues for longer and may recur several times. For example, dental extractions may bleed intermittently for several weeks. With experience, however, the haemophiliac learns to avoid hazardous situations and to seek medical attention early, thereby limiting the damaging effects of haemorrhage. However, this variation is caused by alteration in behaviour, not by changes in the nature of the disease, which remains constant throughout life.

Because of contamination of factor VIII concentrates used to treat haemophilia in the early 1980s, a significant proportion of haemophiliacs treated in this period were infected with HIV. Similarly, many patients were infected with hepatitis C due to treatment with contaminated concentrate.

Diagnosis of haemophilia. The diagnosis of haemophilia may be suspected from a clinical and family history. Laboratory assessment shows a prolonged APTT and a reduced factor VIII concentration. The prothrombin time, thrombin time, platelet count, platelet function tests and vWF assay are all normal. Definitive diagnosis relies on demonstration of factor VIII deficiency with normal or raised vWF antigen. If the APTT is normalized by the addition of normal plasma, both immediately and following incubation, the presence of a factor VIII inhibitor is excluded.

Carrier detection in haemophilia. One of the most important tasks of the haemostasis laboratory is to offer an assessment of the likelihood that an individual female is a carrier of haemophilia. Typically, such an investigation progresses through the following phases.

- **Formal counselling** of the possible carrier prior to any laboratory investigation. Among the issues that must be explored are the possible implications of the results that might be obtained; the type of tests available for carrier detection and the possibility that the results might be inconclusive. The potential impact of any results on other family members should also be considered.

■ **Family study.** The construction of as complete a family pedigree chart as possible may identify the subject as an obligate carrier such as daughters of confirmed haemophiliacs, mothers of at least two haemophiliac sons born at separate deliveries and mothers of one haemophiliac son where definite evidence of haemophilia in other members of the family exists. Confirmation by DNA-based techniques should still be performed as a precaution. Possible carriers need further investigation. Using the pedigree chart, a probability of carrier status can be derived by examining the relationship of the subject to the closest affected family member and applying a factor of 0.5 for each vertical or horizontal step. For example, in the pedigree chart shown in *Figure 19.1*, the probability that the subject (III2) is a carrier is 0.5×0.5 i.e. 0.25.

■ **Phenotypic assessment** relies on repeated measurements of factor VIII and vWF to demonstrate a reduced level of factor VIII and a normal or increased vWF concentration. Because of random X chromosome inactivation, interpretation of the results is far from straightforward. The presence of a repeatable, reduced factor VIII concentration suggests that the patient is a carrier, but normal levels do not reliably exclude the possibility of being a carrier. Calculation of the factor VIII:vWF ratio facilitates determination of a probability of carrier status. With increasing use and accuracy of genotypic testing, this form of carrier detection has become less important.

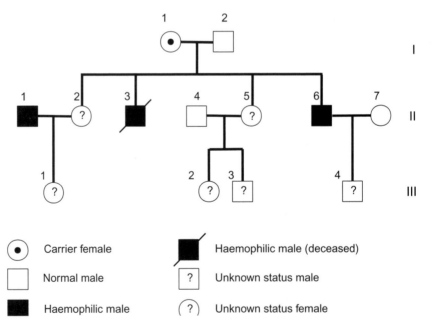

Figure 19.1
Pedigree analysis in haemophilia. Females II2 and II5 have a 50% chance of being a carrier. Female III1 is an obligate carrier because her father is a haemophiliac. If her mother is a carrier, she has a 50% chance of being doubly heterozygous for haemophilia. Female III2 has a 25% chance of being a carrier while her mother's carrier status is unknown. If her mother is a carrier, she has a 50% chance of being a carrier. If her mother is normal, she will be normal. Male III3 has a 25% chance of being a haemophiliac while his mother's carrier status is unknown. If his mother is a proven carrier, he has a 50% chance of being a haemophiliac. If his mother is normal, he will be normal. Male III4 must be normal, since he has inherited his Y chromosome from his father and his X chromosome from his normal mother. All of these probabilities assume the risk of spontaneous mutation is zero.

■ **Genotypic assessment.** The genetics of haemophilia are highly complex. Definitive identification of carrier status used to require identification of the specific gene abnormality in that family, followed by screening in potential carriers. However, a pragmatic approach commonly used today involves screening for the most common mutations first (the intron 22 inversion and other inversions). If these are negative, systematic sequencing of the factor VIII promoter, exons and splice junctions should be performed. This approach can identify mutations in up to 97% of carriers of severe forms of haemophilia.

Antenatal diagnosis in haemophilia. Antenatal diagnosis should only be undertaken in centres with full genetic, haematological and obstetric expertise in such matters. The steps involved in the antenatal diagnosis of haemophilia are similar to those required for carrier detection. Careful pre-investigation counselling of both parents regarding the implications and limitations of possible results is extremely important. Similarly, examination of a family pedigree chart may obviate the need for investigation.

Genotypic assessment for the specific family mutation can be performed in the first trimester of pregnancy using fetal DNA obtained by chorion villus sampling (CVS) or, later, by amniocentesis. Some parents prefer to wait until the second trimester of pregnancy when ultrasound fetal scanning at 16–20 weeks can sex the fetus and so avoid invasive testing of a female fetus (see also *Box 19.12*). At this stage, fetal blood can be sampled and tested for factor VIII activity and also used for genotypic assessment.

Box 19.12 IVF and sex-linked disease

Prospective parents who are at risk of conceiving a haemophiliac son but who are unwilling to undergo antenatal diagnosis may be able to take advantage of recent developments in *in vitro* fertilization. It is now possible to sex pre-implantation conceptuses and to select only females for implantation. Using this approach, half of the children will be entirely unaffected and half will be symptom-free carriers.

Treatment of haemophilia. Treatment of haemophilia involves the infusion of factor VIII concentrate to limit established bleeding or to cover surgery or dental procedures. Prompt and early treatment is essential if secondary tissue damage is to be avoided following a bleed; so most severe haemophiliacs are taught how to administer factor VIII concentrate to themselves at home. Ancillary methods of treatment include the use of fibrinolytic inhibitors and the injection of DDAVP to stimulate the release of vWF from the vascular endothelium. Recombinant human factor VIII concentrate has recently become available and is free of the risk of viral contamination.

One of the most serious problems that bedevils haemophilia treatment is the development of factor VIII inhibitors. An inhibitor is an antibody directed against infused factor VIII and it severely complicates treatment. Massive doses of factor VIII concentrate may achieve a short-term effect in such cases. Alternative treatments include recombinant factor VIIa which is independent of factors VIII or IX and is unaffected by the inhibitor but has a short half-life or activated prothrombin complex (FEIBA – **f**actor **e**ight **i**nhibitor **b**ypassing **a**ctivity) concentrates. Immunosuppressive therapy may be useful in reducing the titre of the inhibitor.

Factor IX deficiency

Factor IX deficiency, also known as Haemophilia B or Christmas disease, results from a deficiency or defect of factor IX, occurs with a frequency of about 15–20 per 1 000 000 and is clinically indistinguishable from haemophilia (see *Box 19.13*). The factor IX gene spans approximately 33.5 kb of the X chromosome at the tip of the long arm, close to the factor VIII gene (Xq27.1–27.2). More than 300 different mutations of the factor IX gene have been characterized, including

---

Box 19.13 Naming Christmas disease

The possibility that haemophilia might consist of more than one defect of coagulation was first raised in 1944 when Argentinian investigators showed that the plasma of two haemophiliacs was mutually corrective. Several similar studies followed until, in 1952, Biggs *et al*. published a report of several patients with the variant form of haemophilia. Since one of the patients was called Christmas and the report appeared in the Christmas issue of the *British Medical Journal*, the name adopted for this condition almost chose itself!

---

point mutations, short deletions or additions and gross deletions. In contrast to haemophilia, the rate of spontaneous mutation of the factor IX gene is low; most patients have a positive family history.

Severe factor IX deficiency (< 1% of normal) most commonly results from gross gene deletions, inversions or nonsense mutations leading to a complete absence of functional factor IX. In general, mild deficiencies with the presence of a dysfunctional protein are caused by point mutations.

The basic approach and underlying principles of carrier detection and treatment in haemophilia B are identical to those for haemophilia.

Fibrinogen disorders

The inherited fibrinogen disorders can be quantitative (afibrinogenaemia and hypo-fibrinogenaemia), qualitative (dysfibrinogenaemia) or both (hypodysfibrinogenaemia).

The normal fibrinogen molecule is a 340 kDa plasma protein that exists as a dimer of three different peptide chains, named Aα, Bβ and γ, linked at their amino termini by disulphide bonds. Fibrinogen is synthesized in hepatocytes by the synchronized expression of three separate genes located at 4q28 (FGA, which expresses the Aα peptide chain, FGB (Bβ) and FGG (γ)). The rate-limiting step in the synthesis of fibrinogen is transcription of the FGB gene. Physiologically, the haemostatic functions of fibrinogen are mediation of platelet adhesion and fibrin clot formation. Conversion of soluble fibrinogen to an insoluble fibrin clot occurs when thrombin cleaves the Aα chain between the arginine and glycine residues at positions 16 and 17, releasing a short peptide chain known as fibrinopeptide A, and also the Bβ chain between the arginine and valine residues at positions 14 and 15 to release fibrinopeptide B. Release of these two fibrinopeptides produces fibrin monomer. Factor XIII then intervenes to crosslink fibrin monomers via the formation of γ-glutamyl-e-lysyl bonds between adjacent molecules, resulting in the formation of a stable, insoluble fibrin mesh.

The inherited quantitative disorders of fibrinogen result from defects in the synthesis, secretion, or intracellular processing of fibrinogen.

Afibrinogenaemia is a rare autosomal recessive disorder, with an estimated frequency of 1 in 10^6 individuals. Most cases are attributable to truncating mutations or splice mutations affecting the FGA gene. The clinical picture in afibrinogenaemia is often unexpectedly mild; in some cases, despite the blood being incoagulable, significant bleeding may be absent. Many cases of afibrinogenaemia are discovered early, following prolonged bleeding of the umbilical stump.

Hypofibrinogenaemia is extremely rare and may represent the heterozygous state for mutations that abolish fibrinogen synthesis or the presence of mutation(s) that reduce the rate of synthesis, secretion or intrahepatocellular processing and storage of fibrinogen. The molecular defects responsible are diverse; mutations of all three genes have been described, including deletions, point mutations, missense mutations and uniparental isodisomy (i.e. both chromosomes inherited from the same parent leading to manifestation of rare recessive disorders). Spontaneous haemorrhage in hypofibrinogenaemia is rare unless the circulating fibrinogen level is < 50 mg/dl: many patients are diagnosed following an episode of post-surgical or post-traumatic bleeding that is unexpectedly severe or prolonged.

Dysfibrinogenaemia results from mutations that cause a functional abnormality of the fibrinogen molecule. Where the abnormal molecule is also deficient, the disorder is known as hypodysfibrinogenaemia. The disorder is rare, but the precise prevalence is difficult to determine because many abnormalities are clinically silent. Because the fibrinogen molecule is central to stable, insoluble clot formation, disorders of its function can be associated with either a haemorrhagic or a thrombotic tendency, but many are clinically silent.

Diagnosis of fibrinogen disorders

Clinically significant fibrinogen disorders usually cause prolongation of the prothrombin, activated partial thromboplastin, and thrombin times. The snake venom reptilase can be used instead of thrombin to perform a reptilase time test. Reptilase cleaves fibrinopeptide A but not B and is a useful test in this setting because it is unaffected by the presence of the anticoagulants heparin, hirudin or direct thrombin inhibitors. However, inherited fibrinogen disorders are rare, while alternative explanations for such results are more common. For example, acquired hypofibrinogenaemia is commonly seen in liver disease, disseminated intravascular coagulation or following L-asparaginase therapy. Similarly, acquired dysfibrinogenaemia may be seen in patients with liver disease, hepatoma renal cell carcinoma or certain autoimmune disorders.

The other inherited coagulation factor deficiencies are summarized in *Table 19.3*.

Table 19.3 Inherited coagulation factor deficiency.

Coagulation disorder	Gene locus	Inheritance pattern	Comment
Prothrombin deficiency	11p11–q12	AD or AR	Extremely rare (< 1 in 10^6). Classified as hypoprothrombinaemia (type I: quantitative defect) or dysprothrombinaemia (type II: qualitative defect). Prothrombin and activated partial thromboplastin times abnormal and thrombin time normal.
Factor V deficiency	1q23	AR	Extremely rare (1 in 10^6). Both quantitative and qualitative defects described. Prothrombin and activated partial thromboplastin times abnormal and thrombin time normal.
Factor VII deficiency	13q34	AR	Rare (1 in 0.5 x 10^6). Bleeding occurs only in severe deficiency. Prothrombin time abnormal but activated partial thromboplastin and thrombin time tests are normal.
Factor X deficiency	13q34	AR	Rare (1 in 0.5 x 10^6). Bleeding clinically severe. Occurs only in severe deficiency. Prothrombin and activated partial thromboplastin times abnormal and thrombin time normal.
Factor XI deficiency	4q35	AD or AR	Sometimes called haemophilia C. Common in Ashkenazi Jewish population (0.3% homozygous). Clinically mild bleeding. Type I caused by splicing mutations; type II by premature stop codon mutations and type III by point mutations resulting in a dysfunctional factor XI molecule. Activated partial thromboplastin time abnormal, prothrombin and thrombin time tests normal.

Coagulation disorder	Gene locus	Inheritance pattern	Comment
Factor XII deficiency	5q33–qter	AR	Usually no bleeding problem. Activated partial thromboplastin time abnormal, prothrombin and thrombin time tests normal.
Factor XIII deficiency Subunit A Subunit B	 6p25–24 1q31–32.1	AR	Extremely rare (< 1 in 10^6). Characterized by normal clot formation, with haemorrhage due to repeated breakdown of unstable clots. Prothrombin, activated partial thromboplastin and thrombin time tests are all normal. Poor wound healing results.
Combined factor V and factor VIII deficiency	18q21.3–q22	AR	Extremely rare (< 200 cases). Affected protein (ERGIC53) acts as a molecular chaperone for the transport from ER to Golgi of factors V and VIII.
Combined deficiency of factors II, VII, IX and X	2p12 16p11.2	AR	Extremely rare. Caused by mutation of genes required for carboxylation of factors II, VII, IX and X, e.g. γ-glutamyl carboxylase or vitamin K epoxide reductase complex, subunit 1 (VKORC1).

AD – autosomal dominant, AR – autosomal recessive

19.2 ACQUIRED DISORDERS OF HAEMOSTASIS

Acquired disorders of haemostasis are far more common than the inherited disorders described above. The acquired disorders of haemostasis are typically multifactorial and are associated with varying assortments of thrombocytopenia, platelet dysfunction, coagulation abnormalities and vascular involvement. Because of this, no attempt will be made to classify these disorders as related to one particular component of haemostasis.

Disseminated intravascular coagulation

Disseminated intravascular coagulation (DIC) is a common complication of a wide range of disorders and is characterized by the widespread activation of all of the haemostatic mechanisms (see *Box 19.14*). Paradoxically, although the early result of DIC is thrombosis, the most obvious feature in most cases is haemorrhage secondary to the consumption of coagulation factors and platelets. Thrombosis is manifest as the formation of occlusive microthrombi throughout the microcirculation, but especially in the kidneys, leading to widespread ischaemic damage. Bleeding manifestations typically involve the gastrointestinal tract and the sites of venepuncture, surgical wounds or indwelling catheters. Subcutaneous and deep tissue haematomas are also common. DIC may present as an acute, life-threatening thrombohaemorrhagic condition or may follow a chronic, less malevolent, course.

Box 19.14 Tissue damage and DIC

Pioneering experiments designed to investigate the role of tissue damage in haemostasis were conducted during the 19th century and revealed apparently paradoxical findings. Rapid injection of tissue extract into animals was immediately fatal, due to widespread thrombosis, while slow infusion of tissue extract prompted death due to uncontrollable haemorrhage. These results are now explicable as two facets of DIC. It was not until the 1950s that the first reports of DIC associated with human clinical conditions appeared.

Pathophysiology of DIC

DIC is seen in association with a wide range of conditions (see *Table 19.4*). The most common triggers of DIC are infection, malignancy and obstetric complications.

DIC occurs in response to varying combinations of three mechanisms.

■ Release of tissue factor or similar procoagulant material into the circulation stimulates activation of the coagulation cascade. This is the predominant triggering mechanism of DIC associated with obstetric complications, surgery, trauma, malignancy, transfusion reaction, liver disease, malaria, tissue rejection and some snake bites.

■ Damage to vascular endothelium results in contact activation of platelets, coagulation, fibrinolysis, complement and the kinin system and can trigger DIC in extensive burns, Gram-negative septicaemia, tissue necrosis and acute or prolonged hypoxia.

■ Direct activation of platelets can occur in some forms of septicaemia or acute viral infections, in the presence of immune complexes and during cardiopulmonary bypass. Secondary platelet activation occurs in response to all forms of DIC.

Whatever the triggering event, the pathophysiology of DIC remains the same. Systemic thrombin generation triggers activation of the coagulation cascade and platelets, resulting in the deposition of microthrombi throughout the body and leading to widespread occlusion of the microcirculation. The resulting ischaemic tissue damage propagates haemostatic activation. Occlusion of the microcirculation of the brain and lungs by microthrombi may be life threatening.

Table 19.4 Acquired conditions associated with DIC

Obstetric complications
Amniotic fluid embolism
Placental abruption
Retained dead fetus
Eclampsia
Septic abortion
Malignancy
Disseminated carcinoma
Acute leukaemia (especially acute promyelocytic)
Infections
Septicaemia (especially meningococci and other Gram negative)
Protozoa (especially *P. falciparum* malaria)
Trauma
Surgical (especially thoracic)
Crush injuries (especially penetrating brain injuries)
Burns
Liver disease
Miscellaneous
Tissue necrosis (necrotizing enterocolitis)
Anaphylactic shock
Acute anoxia
Graft rejection
Cardiopulmonary bypass
Acute intravascular haemolysis (e.g. ABO-incompatible blood transfusion)
Snake bite

Widespread activation of platelets and coagulation leads rapidly and progressively to thrombocytopenia, a drop in the circulating levels of coagulation factors and progressive depletion of circulating antithrombin III, secondary to reticuloendothelial clearance of thrombin–antithrombin complexes. Fibrin deposition and local endothelial injury trigger secondary fibrinolysis, resulting in plasmin generation and digestion of fibrin(ogen), factors V and VIII, and a range of other plasma proteins. Fibrin(ogen) degradation products interfere with fibrin polymerization and platelet function. To cap it all, widespread activation of the complement and kinin systems leads to an increase in vascular permeability, hypotension and shock. These secondary events in the pathogenesis of DIC explain the apparently paradoxical thrombohaemorrhagic state that typifies this condition. Once triggered, DIC can rapidly spiral out of control and result in death. The emphasis, then, must be on speed of recognition, assessment of severity and the prompt initiation of effective therapy. The pathogenesis of DIC is depicted schematically in *Figure 19.2*.

As well as the acute and calamitous events described above, many conditions are associated with a chronic, compensated DIC. This state results from a weak, but sustained, stimulus, where the increased consumption of coagulation factors and platelets is compensated by an increase in their production. The pathophysiology of the chronic condition is identical to that of acute DIC. Conditions associated with chronic DIC include intrauterine death, leukaemia, disseminated carcinoma, graft rejection and vasculitis (see also *Box 19.15*).

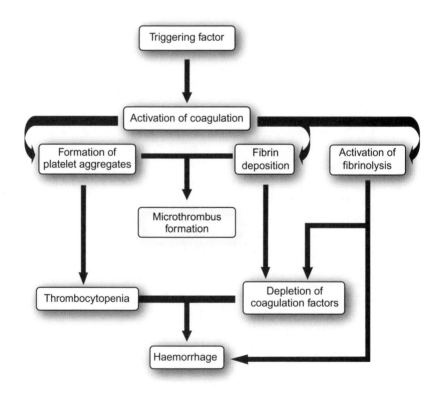

Figure 19.2
Pathogenesis of DIC.

Box 19.15 Snake bite and DIC

The most common cause of DIC worldwide is snake bite. The venoms of a variety of poisonous snakes act by inducing disseminated activation of coagulation. Ironically, many of these venoms have proved to be useful in the investigation of defects of coagulation.

X activation

Russell's viper (*Daboia russelli*) is found in the Indian subcontinent, south-east Asia, southern China and Taiwan.

Prothrombin activation

The common taipan (*Oxyuranus scutellatus*) is found in Australia.

The sawscale viper (*Echis carinatus*) is found in the Middle East, central Asia and the Indian subcontinent.

The mainland tiger snake (*Notechis scutatus*) is found in Australia.

Fibrinogen activation

The common lancehead (*Bothrops atrox*) is found in northern South America.

The Malayan pit viper (*Agkistrodon rhodostoma*) is found in south-east Asia from Thailand to northern Malaysia and on the island of Java.

The eastern diamondback rattlesnake (*Crotalus adamanteus*) is found in the south-eastern USA.

The copperhead or highland moccasin (*Agkistrodon contortrix*) is found in the USA and Mexico.

Fibrinogenolysin

The western diamondback rattlesnake (*Crotalus atrox*) is found in the USA and Mexico.

Platelet activator

The jararaca (*Bothrops jararaca*) is found in southern Brazil, Paraguay and northern Argentina.

Diagnosis of DIC

The laboratory diagnosis of DIC requires the demonstration of the consumption of coagulation factors and platelets, coupled with increased fibrinolysis. However, the results of laboratory testing are highly variable and interpretation can be complex. In the early stages of DIC or in the presence of chronic low-level activation of coagulation and fibrinolysis, the physiological inhibitor systems can balance the activation, leading to compensated DIC. In more advanced cases, consumption of inhibitors allows the activity of the coagulation and fibrinolytic pathways to proceed unhindered, leading to exhaustion of many coagulation factors and platelets, resulting in widespread bleeding. This is known as consumptive coagulopathy or decompensated DIC.

Diagnosis of fully decompensated DIC is fairly straightforward. Laboratory investigation will be prompted by strong clinical suspicion. The coagulation screen will show prolongation of prothrombin time due to coagulation factor deficiency, prolongation of thrombin time due to hypofibrinogenaemia and the presence of fibrin(ogen) degradation products, while the APTT may be normal or prolonged, primarily depending on the level of circulating factor VIII. Thrombocytopenia is common and schistocytes (fragmented red cells caused by fibrin formation in small blood vessels, a phenomenon known as microangiopathic haemolytic anaemia (MAHA)) may be seen on a blood film. The demonstration of reduced fibrinogen concentration, increased D-dimer, fibrin(ogen) split products (FSP) and soluble fibrin monomer (FM) further support the diagnosis. FM suggests the presence of thrombin, FSP the generation of plasmin, and D-dimer, both thrombin and plasmin. Where doubt over the diagnosis exists and time permits, repeat testing will typically show worsening of results.

Diagnosis of compensated DIC is more complex because the results of laboratory testing are variable. Elevation of D-dimer, FSP and FM support such a diagnosis. Compensated DIC can be diagnosed definitively by determination of molecular markers of *in vivo* activation of haemostasis, such as thrombin–antithrombin (TAT) complexes, prothrombin fragment 1+2 (F1+2), or plasmin–antiplasmin (PAP) complexes.

Treatment and management of DIC

Many aspects of the treatment of DIC are highly controversial, partly because the complexity and heterogeneity of the pathophysiology of this disorder make rational treatment selection and objective assessment of effectiveness very difficult. The primary aims of treatment are to eliminate the triggering mechanism for the DIC as quickly and as completely as possible and to maintain life in the meantime by replacement therapy and, in some cases, anticoagulant therapy. Replacement therapy typically involves the administration of large quantities of fresh frozen plasma and cryoprecipitate, which are valuable sources of coagulation factors and natural anticoagulants, platelet concentrates, red cell concentrates and volume expanders such as human albumin solution.

The administration of an anticoagulant such as heparin to a bleeding patient whose blood is apparently incoagulable may seem paradoxical. The rationale for this manoeuvre is that interruption of coagulation should also slow consumption of platelets and secondary fibrinolysis and permit restoration of haemostatic balance. This approach is clearly effective in cases of chronic DIC. Its efficacy is much less certain in acute DIC, however, particularly where septicaemia is involved. In certain cases of severe DIC where standard replacement therapy has proved ineffective, the use of antithrombin III concentrates may be successful.

Haemostatic disorders associated with malignancy

Disturbances of haemostatic function secondary to malignant conditions are both common and diverse but the most common is DIC. Expression of tissue factor by renal, gastric and colonic tumours commonly causes a thrombotic tendency. The monoclonal immunoglobulins that characterize multiple myeloma coat both platelets and coagulation factors, thereby impairing normal function and increasing their rate of clearance. The increased blood viscosity and restricted mobility associated with myeloma also contribute to an increased thrombotic risk. Defective platelet function is common in many haematological malignancies. Prostatic tumours have been shown to promote local fibrinolytic activity, most likely due to release of plasminogen activators. Occasionally, this can result in life-threatening primary hyperfibrinolysis.

Haemostatic disorders associated with liver disease

The liver is the site of synthesis of most of the coagulation factors and natural anticoagulants, although factor VIII appears to be synthesized independently of the others. Acute hepatocellular failure is associated with failure of synthesis of coagulation factors and with an increased incidence of DIC and primary fibrinolysis. In the absence of DIC, the levels of circulating coagulation factor VII correlate well with the severity of the hepatocellular damage. The vitamin K-dependent proteins II, VII, IX, X, protein C and protein S are all reduced in concentration due to a combination of decreased synthesis and impaired γ-carboxylation. Synthesis of dysfunctional coagulation factors may also be present. Thrombocytopenia is a common finding in liver disease and may be associated with DIC or hypersplenism. Defects of platelet function are also relatively common.

Chronic liver disease is associated with thrombocytopenia, platelet dysfunction, failure of synthesis of coagulation factors, dysfibrinogenaemia and increased fibrinolytic activity. In general, the severity of the haemostatic disturbance reflects the severity of the liver disease.

Obstructive jaundice causes impairment of the vitamin K-dependent carboxylation of γ-glutamic acid residues on coagulation factors II, VII, IX, X, protein C and protein S. All other haemostatic proteins are typically normal or elevated. The presence of circulating PIVKAs is one of the earliest and most sensitive markers of hepatic failure.

Haemostatic disorders associated with pregnancy and delivery

Normal, uncomplicated pregnancy is associated with considerable changes in haemostatic function. Most women experience a progressive rise in the concentration of fibrinogen, factor VIII and vWF and a fall in the level of protein S and fibrinolytic activity. The mild hypercoagulable state that results is probably a normal physiological preparation for the rigours of delivery and placental separation.

DIC is a common complication of a number of obstetric disorders such as abruptio placentae, amniotic fluid embolism, retained dead fetus, septic abortion and eclampsia.

■ **Abruptio placentae** is the premature separation of the placenta from the wall of the uterus. The placenta is a rich source of tissue factor. In most cases, evacuation of the uterus results in rapid resolution of the DIC, without the need for massive replacement therapy. The most serious complications of this condition relate to shock, renal failure and thromboembolism.

■ **Amniotic fluid embolism** occurs when a small amount of amniotic fluid is forced into the maternal circulation and presents as an acute and severe DIC with profound respiratory distress secondary to thrombotic occlusion of the pulmonary microcirculation, and uterine haemorrhage. Treatment options include massive replacement therapy and the administration of heparin or the fibrinolytic inhibitor ε-aminocaproic acid (EACA). The mortality rate of this complication is in excess of 80%.

■ **Retained dead fetus** causes a chronic, compensated DIC with a gradual and progressive drop in the platelet count and a rise in the level of circulating FDP. Significant bleeding is typically absent but the danger of rapid acceleration to acute DIC is present.

■ **Septic abortion.** Because of the mild hypercoagulable state which accompanies pregnancy, any severe infective complication such as septic abortion threatens to trigger acute DIC with shock and acute renal failure.

■ **Eclampsia** describes a curious syndrome of pregnancy which is characterized by progressive hypertension, a raised blood urate level secondary to renal impairment, proteinuria, convulsions and chronic, compensated DIC. Occasionally, a hitherto relatively stable case may accelerate abruptly into acute DIC with **H**aemolysis, **E**levated **L**iver enzymes and **L**ow **P**latelets, a condition known as the **HELLP syndrome**. This clinical emergency threatens the life of both mother and baby and requires massive replacement therapy and rapid delivery.

Haemostatic disorders associated with the neonatal period

Most normal neonates show some degree of haemostatic impairment compared to normal adults at delivery, secondary to hepatic immaturity and low levels of vitamin K relative to those of adults. The first weeks of life are the most critical time for haemorrhage due to hereditary and acquired coagulopathies. At full term, the vitamin K-dependent factors II, VII, IX and X are only at around 40% of adult levels and fall further during the first 5 days of life. The circulating fibrinogen level is typically normal but there may be a significant proportion of the fetal variant of fibrinogen, which shows delayed aggregation of fibrin monomers.

Haemorrhagic disease of the newborn

Haemorrhagic disease of the newborn describes an acquired bleeding tendency, sometimes severe, which develops in the first days of life and is secondary to deficiency of the vitamin K-dependent coagulation factors (see also *Box 19.16*). Three forms exist:

■ Early-onset haemorrhagic disease of the newborn is often seen when the mother has ingested anticonvulsants (e.g. phenytoin, barbiturates, carbamazepine), antitubercular

---

Box 19.16 Coagulation factor concentrations

Plasma concentrations of coagulation factors in neonates differ significantly from those in adults. A normal full-term infant attains adult levels by the age of 3 months.

- Factor II 30–40%
- Factor VII 10–45%
- Factor IX 10–15%
- Factor X 10–30%
- Factor XI 20–80%
- ATIII raised
- Fibrinolytic depressed activity

---

drugs (e.g. rifampin, isoniazid) or vitamin K antagonists (e.g. warfarin). Haemorrhage usually occurs within 24 hours of delivery and may be severe.

- Classical haemorrhagic disease of the newborn is characterized by bleeding in the first week of life. Placental transfer of vitamin K is poor, the ability of the fetal liver to store vitamin K is lower than that of a mature liver and breast milk is relatively poor in vitamin K. This all adds up to a relative deficiency of vitamin K in the neonatal period that, in the absence of prophylactic supplementation, can result in haemorrhage in a small number of neonates.
- Late-onset haemorrhagic disease of the newborn is associated with bleeding between 2 and 12 weeks of age, or occasionally later. It is most common in breastfed babies who did not receive vitamin K prophylaxis at birth. Powdered baby milk is supplemented with vitamin K during manufacture and so provides a better dietary source than breast milk.

It is standard practice to administer vitamin K to all neonates within 24 hours of birth. Serious haemorrhagic disease of the newborn is rarely encountered following adequate vitamin K prophylaxis. Treatment consists of the administration of vitamin K_1 and replacement therapy using fresh frozen plasma.

Disseminated intravascular coagulation

Neonatal disseminated intravascular coagulation may be triggered by birth asphyxia, respiratory distress syndrome, trauma, viral or bacterial infection, aspiration of meconium and amniotic fluid or hypothermia. Hepatic immaturity or liver disease may further exacerbate this condition. The pathophysiology of the condition is identical to that seen in adults.

Platelet disorders

The most common acquired abnormality of platelets in neonates is thrombocytopenia, which may be secondary to a variety of conditions including DIC, transplacental passage of maternal anti-platelet antibodies, congenital cyanotic heart disease, giant haemangioma and following exchange transfusion. Neonatal platelet dysfunction may be seen following antibiotic or other drug therapy.

19.3 ACQUIRED PURPURAS

The acquired purpuras are a group of haemostatic disorders manifest as mucous membrane bleeding and a tendency to bruise spontaneously or following minimal trauma. They can be divided into the vascular purpuras and the platelet-associated purpuras, depending on which component is most affected. In most cases, however, the pathogenesis of the purpura is complex and multifactorial.

Vascular purpuras

Henoch–Schönlein purpura (HSP), or allergic purpura, is a self-limited allergic vasculitis, which is seen most commonly in young children and is manifest as a purpuric rash covering the arms, legs and buttocks, with renal impairment and abdominal and joint pain (see *Box 19.17*). Typically, a recent history of upper respiratory tract infection or of penicillin or sulphonamide therapy is present. HSP appears to be caused by IgA immune complex-mediated vascular endothelial damage. Most children with HSP recover with supportive and symptomatic care alone. Renal complications in adults may be more severe and may require steroid therapy or plasmapheresis.

Box 19.17 Naming Henoch–Schönlein purpura

Henoch–Schönlein purpura was originally known as Heberden–Willan disease. The condition was first described in 1802 by William Heberden, although the clinical picture was recognized as early as the 18th century. Robert Willan, a dermatologist, described the cutaneous manifestations of the disease.

The contributions of Henoch and Schönlein came much later: Johann Schönlein described the condition as an entity in 1837 and Eduard Heinrich Henoch reported the first case of a patient with colic, bloody diarrhoea, painful joints and a rash in 1868. Unfortunately for the historical legacy of Drs Heberdan and Willan, their contribution is all but forgotten and the disease is now universally known as Henoch–Schönlein purpura.

The most common vascular purpura, senile purpura, is a benign condition of old age that is caused by a combination of loss of skin elasticity and atrophy of vascular collagen. The condition is manifest as persistent purplish patches on the backs of the hands, forearms and neck that appear spontaneously and leave permanent brown stains when they fade. About 40% of elderly people display this natural phenomenon for which no treatment is required or available.

The apparent excess of easy bruising seen in young women, for which no cause can be found, is known by the spuriously scientific title of purpura simplex. In cases of excessive bruising, for which no cause can be found, the possibility of self-mutilation secondary to psychiatric disturbance, or physical abuse by carers must be considered.

Severe, prolonged vitamin C deficiency, or scurvy, is associated with defects of collagen and a bleeding tendency. Scurvy is associated with chronic malnourishment and, in the developed world, is most commonly seen in alcoholics, the elderly and the poor.

Thrombocytopenic purpuras

Thrombocytopenia is the most common acquired platelet abnormality and can result from three main causes:

- Failure of thrombopoiesis (e.g. hypoplastic anaemia, severe vitamin B_{12} or folate deficiency)
- Accelerated consumption or destruction of platelets (e.g. immune thrombocytopenic purpura, thrombotic thrombocytopenic purpura and haemolytic uraemic syndrome)
- Splenic sequestration of platelets due to hypersplenism or splenomegaly.

Immune thrombocytopenic purpura (ITP) is characterized by antibody-mediated destruction of platelets with thrombocytopenia, extensive petechiae, bruising and mucosal haemorrhagic complications such as epistaxis and menorrhagia. The white cell count, differential count and haemoglobin concentration are all typically normal. Examination of the bone marrow reveals megakaryocytic hyperplasia with an increase in immature, hypolobulated forms. Three forms of immune thrombocytopenic purpura are recognized:

- An acute, self-limited form which is most common in children between the ages of two and six years and is often preceded by an acute viral illness such as rubella, measles or chicken-pox. Treatment is unnecessary in most cases.
- A chronic form with an insidious onset and no history of recent viral illness. This form is most common in young adults and seldom remits spontaneously. Oral corticosteroids are the most common initial treatment, with splenectomy in persistent or recurrent severe ITP.
- A self-limited neonatal form that is associated with the passive transplacental transfer of maternal anti-platelet antibodies.

In all forms of ITP, platelet destruction is mediated by the presence of platelet-bound immunoglobulin with subsequent Fc receptor-mediated phagocytosis by splenic macrophages.

Heparin-induced thrombocytopenia occurs in about 1% of patients treated with unfractionated heparin, and is caused by antibodies directed against heparin:platelet factor 4 complex. The resultant thrombocytopenia, which can occur after several days of uneventful therapy or even after discontinuation of therapy, seldom results in clinically significant bleeding. Instead, the platelet activation that occurs leads to a prothrombotic state with up to a third of patients developing a thrombosis. Prompt heparin discontinuation and substitution of alternative anticoagulation is required.

Thrombotic thrombocytopenic purpura (TTP) is a rare but clinically serious disorder which most commonly affects young adults and is characterized by fever, erratic neurological disturbances such as convulsions, hallucinations and paralysis, renal failure, microangiopathic haemolysis and thrombocytopenia with haemorrhagic manifestations. The haemolysis and thrombocytopenia are secondary to the disseminated deposition of platelet-fibrin microthrombi in arterioles and capillaries. The trigger for the formation of these thrombotic lesions is unknown. It is increased platelet aggregation and consumption, rather than coagulation factor depletion that is the major cause of morbidity and mortality in this condition. TTP has been described secondary to a variety of conditions including pregnancy, bacterial infection, autoimmune disease, neoplasia and drug ingestion.

The treatment for TTP involves intensive supportive care such as haemodialysis, artificial ventilation, plasma exchange and transfusion of fresh frozen plasma.

A closely related condition, haemolytic uraemic syndrome (HUS), most commonly affects infants and young children and is associated with the localized deposition of platelet-fibrin microthrombi in the renal vasculature with thrombocytopenia, microangiopathic haemolysis and renal failure. In many cases, there is a recent history of infection with toxin-producing *Escherichia coli* or *Shigella*. HUS is triggered by immune-mediated damage to vascular endothelium.

Acquired thrombocytopathy

Acquired thrombocytopathies are seen most commonly in association with drug ingestion (e.g. aspirin), uraemia or grossly elevated FDPs. However, ingestion of certain foods has been shown to impair platelet function, and may occasionally be troublesome. Many of the culinary culprits are associated with Asian cooking, e.g. garlic, ginger and black tree fungus.

19.4   ACQUIRED INHIBITORS OF COAGULATION FACTORS

Antibodies directed against coagulation factors may arise following replacement therapy for deficiency states such as haemophilia, or as spontaneous events. The most common inhibitors are directed against factors VIII or IX following treatment. Spontaneous inhibitors also most commonly affect factor VIII but rare instances of inhibitors directed against many other coagulation factors have been reported.

In 5–10% of haemophilia patients an IgG antibody is produced which is directed against factor VIII. Once the inhibitor is formed, further factor VIII infusion acts as an antigenic stimulus, markedly increasing the concentration of the inhibitor. The incidence of inhibitor production is highest in severe haemophiliacs. Factor VIII inhibitors can also occur spontaneously in non-haemophiliacs in association with pregnancy, autoimmune conditions such as rheumatoid arthritis and systemic lupus erythematosus (SLE) and in the elderly, sometimes in the absence of obvious predisposing factors. Males and females have an equal tendency to inhibitor production.

The presence of an acquired inhibitor triggers a progressive and complete destruction of the target coagulation factor, leading to similar clinical consequences to those of severe haemophilia. The long-term treatment of coagulation factor inhibitors is fraught with difficulty but treatment options include the use of immunosuppressive drugs, or attempting to induce immune tolerance using long-term continuous infusion of the affected coagulation factor.

SUGGESTED FURTHER READING

Benjamin, L.W., *et al.* (2009) The laboratory approach to inherited and acquired coagulation factor deficiencies. *Clin. Lab. Med.* **29:** 229–252.

Blomback, M. & Antovic, J. (eds) (2009) *Essential Guide to Blood Coagulation.* Wiley-Blackwell, Oxford.

Cindy, E.N. & Janna, M.J. (2007) Congenital platelet disorders. *Hematol./Oncol. Clin. N. Am.* **21:** 663–684.

Isabelle, I.S., *et al.* (2008) Inherited traits affecting platelet function. *Blood Reviews,* **22:** 155–172.

Jecko, T. & Cheng-Hock, T. (2009) Disseminated intravascular coagulation in obstetric disorders and its acute haematological management. *Blood Reviews,* **23:** 167–176.

Marie, E.P. & Christopher, A.T. (2009) Platelet-related bleeding: an update on diagnostic modalities and therapeutic options. *Clin. Lab. Med.* **29:** 175–191.

Marisa, B.M. (2009) Thrombotic thrombocytopenic purpura and heparin-induced thrombocytopenia: two unique causes of life-threatening thrombocytopenia. *Clin. Lab. Med.* **29:** 321–338.

Paul, H. (2005) Platelet function analysis. *Blood Reviews,* **19:** 111–123.

Peter, L.P. & Annika, M.S. (2009) Molecular diagnostics in hemostatic disorders. *Clin. Lab. Med.* **29:** 367–390.

Richard, T. & Yuri, F. (2009) Laboratory testing for von Willebrand disease: toward a mechanism-based classification. *Clin. Lab. Med.* **29:** 193–228.

Valerie, L.N. (2009) Liver disease, coagulation testing, and hemostasis. *Clin. Lab. Med.* **29:** 265–282.

Valerie, L.N. (2009) Prothrombin time and partial thromboplastin time assay considerations. *Clin. Lab. Med.* **29:** 253–263.

Watson, S.P. & Harrison, P. (2005) The vascular function of platelets. In: *Postgraduate Haematology* (Hoffbrand, A.V., Catovsky, D. & Tuddenham, E.G.D., eds), pp. 808–824. Blackwell Publishing, Oxford.

Yu-Min, P.S. & Eugene, P.F. (2007) Acquired platelet dysfunction. *Hematol./Oncol. Clin. N. Am.* **21:** 647–661.

SELF-ASSESSMENT QUESTIONS

1. Which of the following are inherited haemorrhagic disorders?
    a. Bernard–Soulier disease

       b.   Ehlers–Danlos syndrome
       c.   Thrombotic thrombocytopaenic purpura
       d.   Pseudo von Willebrand's disease
       e.   Protein S deficiency
       f.   Henoch–Schönlein purpura

2.   Complete the table below:

Condition	Gene(s) affected
Congenital amegakaryocytic thrombocytopenia	
	non-muscle myosin heavy chain-9 gene at 22q11.2
Pseudo von Willebrand's disease	
von Willebrand's disease	

3.   Why is the pattern of bleeding seen in von Willebrand's disease different to that in haemophilia?

4.   Define the term 'obligate carrier of haemophilia'.

5.   DIC is seen in association with a wide range of conditions, but what are the three most common triggers?

6.   Which vitamin is deficient in haemorrhagic disease of the newborn?

7.   Name the acquired purpura that is typically a self-limited allergic vasculitis, seen most commonly in young children, and is manifest as a purpuric rash covering the arms, legs and buttocks, with renal impairment and abdominal and joint pain.

Thrombotic disorders

Learning objectives

After studying this chapter you should confidently be able to:

■ **Define the terms thrombus (thrombi), ischaemia and embolus (emboli)**
A thrombus is a blood clot *in vivo*. The term is most often used to describe clinically inappropriate localized blood clots that cause morbidity. Blockage of blood vessels reduces blood flow and oxygen delivery to surrounding areas, which damages tissue – a phenomenon known as ischaemia. Where a thrombus dislodges from its point of origin and is carried in the blood to lodge elsewhere in the body, it is called an embolus.

■ **List selected examples of inherited prothrombotic disorders**
An inherited thrombotic tendency results from any alteration in the haemostatic balance that impairs the capacity of the body to combat clot formation. The two main mechanisms that oppose clot formation are the naturally occurring anticoagulants such as antithrombin III and proteins C and S and the fibrinolytic mechanism. Accordingly, inherited deficiency of any of the natural anticoagulants may result in a thrombotic tendency, as may an inherited defect that impairs the function of the natural anticoagulants or that causes hypofibrinolysis.

■ **List selected examples of acquired prothrombotic risk factors**
Most of the risk factors for arterial and venous thrombosis are acquired, e.g. oral contraceptive use or HRT, pregnancy, malignancy, lupus anticoagulant, obesity, high blood cholesterol and triglyceride levels, increasing age, stress, smoking tobacco, lack of exercise, high-fat diet and medical history. Typically, several risk factors operate together to create an overall thrombotic risk.

■ **Outline the investigation of thrombophilia**
There are no general screening tests for thrombophilia such as the coagulation screen for bleeding disorders. Investigation relies on identifying acquired risk factors such as hypercholesterolaemia, malignancy, hyperhomocysteinaemia, antiphospholipid antibodies, etc. Where inherited thrombophilia is suspected, investigation requires testing for the most common abnormalities by assessment of activated protein C resistance (factor V Leiden), assay of antithrombin, protein C or S using both immunological and functional methods to detect type 1 and type 2 abnormalities and genetic analysis for known gene mutations such as prothrombin G20210A.

■ **Review the prophylaxis and treatment of thrombosis**
Once a venous thrombosis is confirmed, immediate anticoagulation is the treatment of choice, followed by transition to a longer-acting anticoagulant in the medium term. If recurrent thrombosis occurs, anticoagulation may be required for life, although the risk of haemorrhage needs to be balanced against the risk of further thrombosis. Thrombolytic therapy is reserved for patients with acute arterial thrombosis such as myocardial infarction, massive pulmonary embolism and acute thrombotic stroke. Anticoagulants include unfractionated and low molecular weight heparins, warfarin or its analogues, anti-platelet drugs and direct thrombin inhibitors.

A thrombus can be thought of as a blood clot that occurs at the wrong time and in the wrong place. Rather than being formed as a result of blood loss, a thrombus forms because of an imbalance in the haemostatic mechanism. Thrombosis is a major cause of morbidity and mortality because thrombi can block blood vessels, resulting in localized ischaemia, or can shed fragments that form emboli at distant locations, most commonly in the lungs.

Thrombosis can occur in either arteries or veins. The pathogenesis and risk factors of these two types of thrombosis are different. A tendency towards thrombus formation, whether inherited or acquired, is called **thrombophilia**.

20.1   RISK FACTORS FOR ARTERIAL THROMBOSIS

The risk of arterial thrombosis parallels that of a condition called atherosclerosis or 'hardening of the arteries'. Atherosclerosis occurs when fat, cholesterol and other substances build up in the walls of arteries and form plaque. As plaque builds up, the artery loses flexibility, making it harder for blood to flow. In advanced cases, blood flow can be so poor that ischaemia results. This is the cause of angina pectoris, the chest pain or discomfort that occurs when the heart muscle does not get enough blood. Plaques can rupture, forming emboli that travel through the artery and may lodge in the heart, lungs or brain, causing a heart attack, pulmonary embolism or stroke. Platelet deposition and blood clot formation are integral to plaque development and contribute to extension and risk of embolus formation.

Risk factors for atherosclerosis (and arterial thrombosis) include:

- personal or family history of heart disease
- high blood cholesterol and triglyceride levels
- obesity
- high blood pressure
- lifestyle factors (stress, smoking tobacco, lack of exercise, high-fat diet)
- increasing age
- diabetes mellitus
- lupus anticoagulant
- gout
- hyperhomocysteinaemia
- elevated coagulation factor levels (factor VII and fibrinogen).

20.2   RISK FACTORS FOR VENOUS THROMBOSIS

There are three factors that promote venous thrombosis: reduced venous blood flow (stasis), hypercoagulability of the blood and vascular wall damage. Among the known risk factors for venous thrombosis are:

- inherited mutations of haemostatic proteins (e.g. ATIII deficiency, factor V Leiden)
- increased coagulation factor levels
- oral contraceptives or HRT
- pregnancy
- malignancy
- lupus anticoagulant
- increasing age
- obesity
- medical conditions that reduce blood flow or mobility or result in vascular wall damage (e.g. cardiac failure, sepsis, varicose veins).

20.3 INHERITED THROMBOTIC DISORDERS

An inherited thrombotic tendency results from any alteration in the haemostatic balance that impairs the capacity of the body to combat clot formation. The two main mechanisms that oppose clot formation are the naturally occurring anticoagulants such as antithrombin III and proteins C and S, and the fibrinolytic mechanism. Overall, the inherited thrombophilias are estimated to be about three times more common than the inherited bleeding disorders.

Antithrombin deficiency

Antithrombin (AT) deficiency is a relatively common autosomal dominant disorder with an estimated incidence of about 0.05–1.1%. The AT gene is located at 1q23–25. About 4% of patients with recurrent venous thrombosis have AT deficiency. The disorder is manifest as a susceptibility to recurrent deep venous thrombosis (DVT) or pulmonary embolism, which is exacerbated by pregnancy, surgery or oral contraceptive use. In the normal population, thromboembolic problems are most commonly associated with middle and old age whereas in AT-deficient individuals, thrombotic complications typically start in the second or third decade of life. Thromboses in infancy or early childhood are uncommon in AT deficiency.

AT deficiency can be divided into two subtypes (see *Box 20.1*):

- **Type I deficiency** is the more common subtype and results from mutations that interfere with the rate of synthesis of AT, and so is characterized by a relative lack of AT as measured by both functional and immunological assays. Typically, a thrombotic tendency results when the plasma AT concentration falls to less than 50–60% of normal. Up to 80% of cases of inherited AT deficiency are of this type.
- **Type II deficiency** results from point mutations that interfere with the function of AT, and is characterized by a lack of AT as measured by functional assays but a normal concentration as measured by immunological assays.

Box 20.1 AT deficiency

The earliest description of antithrombin deficiency as a cause of a thrombotic tendency was published by Egeberg in 1965. His report described a Norwegian family with an increased incidence of venous thrombosis, which appeared to be associated with trauma, inflammation or pregnancy. Investigation showed that the affected individuals all had an antithrombin level that was 50% of normal as measured by immunological and functional assays.

The three-dimensional structure of AT is critical to its function as an inhibitor of serine proteases. When AT binds to a serine protease, it undergoes a dramatic conformational change that has been likened to a mousetrap springing shut. The ability to undergo this conformational change is central to the inhibitory function of AT. A particular amino acid, the threonine residue at position 85 appears to be critical for the conformational change and mutations at this position have important and predictable consequences. Two identified abnormalities at this position (colourfully named 'wibble' and 'wobble') serve to illustrate:

- in AT wibble, a C to T substitution codes for the replacement of the critical threonine by methionine. The introduction of this bulky but non-charged amino acid causes mild molecular instability, with a tendency for spontaneous conformational change of the AT and resultant functional deficiency. This mutation does not cause a clinically severe thrombotic tendency.
- in AT wobble, substitution of the position 85 threonine by a bulky positively charged lysine residue has a much more serious molecular impact. The severe molecular instability that

results causes a near-total deficiency of AT and is associated with a severe thrombotic tendency.

Acquired deficiency of AT is commonly seen in chronic liver disease (due to reduced synthesis), ascites or nephrotic syndrome (due to increased losses) and in disorders associated with increased coagulation with increased consumption of AT, such as DIC or antiphospholipid syndrome. Circulating AT levels are reduced in pregnancy and during oral contraceptive use.

The relative risk of venous thrombosis in various inherited and acquired thrombophilias is shown in *Table 20.1*.

Once the presence of inherited antithrombin deficiency is established, treatment typically takes one of the following forms:

- Homozygous AT deficiency is associated with a lifelong risk of both arterial and venous thrombosis. Periods of acute risk can be covered using prophylactic infusion of AT concentrate. Long-term anticoagulation with warfarin or low molecular weight heparin may be required.
- Heterozygotes that have not yet experienced thrombosis should be counselled about avoidable factors that are known to predispose to venous thrombosis such as obesity, venous stasis and the use of oral contraceptives, which are known to lower the circulating antithrombin concentration further. Active prophylaxis is not required.
- Acute thrombotic events are managed with a combination of heparin and androgenic steroids, which induces a transient rise in circulating antithrombin concentration. Prophylactic coumarin therapy is usually instigated as quickly as possible and may be required as a long-term measure.

Table 20.1 Relative risk of venous thrombosis in thrombophilia

Thrombophilia	Relative risk*
Antithrombin deficiency	Heterozygous 5
	Homozygous type I lethal *in utero*
	Homozygous type II marked increase in both arterial and venous thrombosis
Protein C deficiency	Heterozygous 7
	Homozygous severe thrombosis at birth
Protein S deficiency	Heterozygous 6
	Homozygous severe thrombosis at birth
Factor V Leiden	Heterozygous 5–7
	Homozygous 80
Prothrombin G20210A	Heterozygous 3
	Homozygous unknown
Hyperhomocysteinaemia	2–4
Oral contraceptive use	4
+ Factor V Leiden	Heterozygous 30–35
	Homozygous > 100
+ Prothrombin G20210A	Heterozygous 16
	Homozygous unknown
* the risk of venous thrombosis in the general population is 1 so heterozygous antithrombin deficiency increases the risk five-fold.	

■ Unavoidable elective surgery in both homozygotes and heterozygotes can be covered by replacement therapy using specific antithrombin concentrates or fresh frozen plasma.

Protein C

The incidence of protein C deficiency is about 0.2% of the general population and accounts for up to 8% of individuals with recurrent venous thrombosis. The protein C gene is located at 2q13–14 (see also *Box 20.2*). Deficiency is typically inherited in an autosomal dominant fashion although a less common autosomal recessive form exists. Protein C deficiency represents an array of genetic defects of the protein C gene that are classified as type I (quantitative) or, less commonly, type II (qualitative) defects. Heterozygous type I protein C deficiency is typically associated with a plasma concentration between 30 and 60% of normal and is accompanied by a variable recurrent venous thrombosis. The risk of thrombosis is not readily predictable from the circulating protein C concentration; other risk factors such as obesity and lifestyle interact to produce an individual risk. Co-inheritance of other thrombophilic gene mutations such as factor V Leiden can explain the severe thrombotic risk in some families. Recent work suggests that isolated heterozygous protein C deficiency produces only a mild thrombotic tendency and may be clinically silent in most cases. It is the impact of other coincident prothrombotic mutations or other factors that interacts with protein C deficiency to produce the excess risk seen in some people.

Box 20.2 Naming of protein C

In 1960, Mammen, Thomas and Seegers reported the presence of an inhibitor of coagulation, which they named autoprothrombin IIa because they thought that it was a degradation product of thrombin. Sixteen years later, Stenflo isolated a novel vitamin K-dependent factor, and named it protein C because it eluted in the third peak of a DEAE chromatographic separation. Protein C was subsequently shown to be identical to autoprothrombin IIa. The first description of an inherited protein C deficiency as the cause of a thrombotic tendency was published by Griffin *et al.* in 1981.

Rare cases of homozygous protein C deficiency have been described and often present as severe DIC in infancy. Treatment with warfarin can result in skin necrosis due to the formation of multiple thrombi in skin blood vessels. This is caused by the fact that protein C and S concentrations fall early in the course of warfarin therapy, creating a transient thrombotic tendency in those with an already reduced plasma concentration.

Treatment of protein C deficiency mirrors that of ATIII deficiency. In the absence of thrombosis, counselling about the disorder and its associated problems may be all that is required. Prophylactic anticoagulant therapy is usually withheld until the first thrombo-embolic event, because some heterozygotes may never have a thrombosis. Surgical cover can be managed using fresh frozen plasma or specific protein C concentrate.

Protein S

Protein S is a vitamin K-dependent protein that circulates in the plasma in two forms (see also *Box 20.3*):

■ About 40% circulates as a free and haemostatically active protein
■ About 60% circulates bound to C4b-binding protein, and has no recognized haemostatic activity.

The overall incidence of protein S deficiency in the general population is unknown but, in a selected thrombotic population, the incidence has been reported as between 1 and 8%. The

---

Box 20.3 Naming of protein S

Protein S was discovered by a PhD student called DiScipio who was working in Seattle at the time. The S in protein S is derived from Seattle, the city of its discovery. The first patients with a thrombotic tendency caused by protein S deficiency were discovered in 1984.

---

protein S gene is located at 3q11.2. Both autosomal dominant and autosomal recessive patterns of inheritance have been described.

Protein S deficiency is clinically indistinguishable from protein C deficiency, including the risk of skin necrosis associated with warfarin therapy. About 70% of cases of protein S deficiency exhibit type I (quantitative) deficiency, where both free and total protein S levels are reduced. In type II (qualitative) deficiency, a dysfunctional protein S is synthesized at a normal rate, so both free and bound protein S levels are normal using immunological assays. An apparently distinct form of deficiency, type III, has been described in which the free protein S concentration is reduced but the C4b-binding protein-bound protein S concentration is normal. This phenomenon has now been explained. The total protein S concentration exceeds that of C4b-binding protein by about 30–40%. The free protein S found in plasma represents the excess that cannot be bound by C4b-binding protein. In cases of mild protein S deficiency, where an excess of protein S over C4b-binding protein still exists, the presentation will be of selective free protein S deficiency. More severe deficiency will cause deficiency of both forms.

Factor V Leiden

Inherited resistance to activated protein C (APCR) is the most common inherited cause of thrombophilia, with an overall incidence of 2–10% (see *Box 20.4*). Up to 60% of Caucasians with confirmed venous thrombosis demonstrate this phenomenon. In more than 90% of cases, APCR can be attributed to a single point mutation in the factor V gene at 1q23, a substitution of the arginine at position 506 by a glutamine. This mutated factor V, known as factor V Leiden after the city of its discovery, is activated normally by thrombin or factor X_a, but is resistant to inactivation by activated protein C, leading to a thrombotic tendency. Factor V Leiden is most common in northern European populations where about 4–7% of the general population is heterozygous and up to 0.25% of the population is homozygous for factor V Leiden. In contrast, factor V Leiden is relatively uncommon in the native populations of Asia, Africa and North America.

Treatment of individuals with factor V Leiden depends upon an assessment of individual thrombotic risk. Prophylactic treatment is not recommended unless there is a proven risk of recurrent venous thrombosis, because of the risk of bleeding associated with anticoagulation.

Box 20.4 Activated protein C resistance

The road to the discovery of factor V Leiden began in the early 1990s when investigations of a patient with recurrent thrombosis in the laboratory of Björn Dahlbäck showed an unexpected result. The addition of activated protein C to patient plasma did not produce the expected prolongation of the clotting time, i.e. the patient appeared to be resistant to activated protein C. This phenomenon was also demonstrated in other family members, suggesting an inherited explanation. The addition of normal plasma normalized the defect. It was soon recognized that the component of normal plasma that produced the normalization was factor V and that all of the patients with this defect had the same mutation of the factor V gene. The original characterization of the mutation was performed in the University of Leiden and so the mutation came to be known as factor V Leiden.

Prothrombin allele G20210A

About 1–2% of Caucasians have a G–A mutation in the prothrombin gene at position 20210. This mutation is in the 3′ untranslated region of the prothrombin gene at 11p11–q12 and results in hyperprothrombinaemia. This mutation is relatively uncommon in the native populations of India, Korea, Africa and North America.

The prothrombin G20210A mutation leads to raised levels of circulating thrombin, and this causes persistent activation of plasminogen activator inhibitor I. The resultant inhibition of fibrinolysis is prothrombotic.

Hyperhomocysteinaemia

Homocysteine is an amino acid produced by metabolism of methionine in the diet, and is required in several biochemical reactions such as synthetic reactions involving methyl group transfer and synthesis of cysteine. Inborn errors of a number of enzymes can lead to increased plasma levels of homocysteine, including methylenetetrahydrofolate reductase (MTHFR; gene locus 1p36.3), cystathionine beta-synthase (CBS; gene locus 21q22.3) and several proteins involved in vitamin B_{12} absorption, metabolism and transport. Hyperhomocysteinaemia is associated with an increased risk of arterial and venous thrombosis.

Administration of folate with or without vitamin B_{12} can reduce plasma homocysteine concentration but it is not known whether this reduces the risk of thrombosis.

Inherited deficiency of fibrinolysis

Hypofibrinolysis may be the result of impaired activation of plasminogen secondary to a variety of causes:

- deficiency of tissue plasminogen activator synthesis or release
- an increased concentration of plasminogen activator inhibitor
- deficiency of plasminogen
- fibrinogen abnormalities (dysfibrinogenaemia, see *Chapter 19*) that are resistant to fibrinolysis
- defects within the factor XII-dependent pathway of fibrinolytic activation.

20.4 ACQUIRED THROMBOPHILIA

Most of the risk factors for arterial and venous thrombosis discussed earlier are acquired. Typically, several risk factors operate together in patients with established thromboembolic disease. The addition of acquired risk factors to the inherited thrombophilias may further increase their relative risk.

The anti-phospholipid syndrome

The anti-phospholipid syndrome (APS) is caused by the spontaneous production of antibodies that are directed against anionic phospholipids. This is manifest *in vitro* as prolongation of phospholipid-dependent coagulation screening tests, which is usually indicative of a bleeding tendency. One example of such anti-phospholipid antibodies is the lupus anticoagulant (see *Box 20.5*). This condition is associated with recurrent venous and arterial thrombosis and recurrent fetal loss. Lupus anticoagulant is found in patients with autoimmune disorders such as systemic lupus erythematosus (SLE), lymphoproliferative diseases and following viral illnesses.

Box 20.5 Anticoagulant or not?

The fact that development of a lupus anticoagulant is associated with thrombosis seems paradoxical. Surely an acquired anticoagulant should cause bleeding? The reason for the inappropriate name lies with the fact that the lupus anticoagulant was first discovered because of its prolongation of phospholipid-based coagulation tests (e.g. prothrombin time, activated partial thromboplastin time and Russell viper venom time) in the laboratory. It seemed in these tests to be acting as an anticoagulant and so was named as such. The clinical effect of a thrombotic tendency was not recognized until after the name had become established.

Screening for APS should be considered in patients with SLE, unexplained recurrent thromboses, a thrombosis before the age of 40 years or women with a recurrent fetal loss in the first and second trimester of pregnancy. The condition also occurs occasionally in otherwise healthy individuals and may be detected as a chance finding as part of routine pre-operative screening. Laboratory testing shows a prolonged APTT that is not corrected by the addition of normal plasma.

Long-term treatment of lupus anticoagulant is with warfarin, but heparin and aspirin can be used to good effect during pregnancy.

20.5 LABORATORY INVESTIGATION OF THROMBOPHILIA

There are no general screening tests for thrombophilia such as the coagulation screen for bleeding disorders. Investigation relies on identifying acquired risk factors such as hypercholesterolaemia, malignancy, hyperhomocysteinaemia, antiphospholipid antibodies, etc. Where inherited thrombophilia is suspected, investigation requires testing for the most common abnormalities by assessment of activated protein C resistance (factor V Leiden), assay of antithrombin, protein C or S using both immunological and functional methods to detect type 1 and type 2 abnormalities and genetic analysis for known gene mutations such as prothrombin G20210A.

20.6 PROPHYLAXIS AND TREATMENT OF THROMBOSIS

Once a venous thrombosis is confirmed, immediate anticoagulation is the treatment of choice, followed by transition to a longer-acting anticoagulant in the medium term. If recurrent thrombosis occurs, anticoagulation may be required for life, although the risk of haemorrhage needs to be balanced against the risk of further thrombosis. Thrombolytic therapy is reserved for patients with acute arterial thrombosis such as myocardial infarction, massive pulmonary embolism and acute thrombotic stroke.

Anticoagulants

Unfractionated heparin

Heparin is a mucopolysaccharide, which is purified for clinical use from bovine lung or porcine intestine (see *Box 20.6*). It cannot be absorbed from the intestine and must therefore be administered intravenously or subcutaneously. Heparin is not a single substance; it consists of a mixture of polysaccharides ranging in molecular weight from 5–30 000 kDa. The anticoagulant effect of heparin is instantaneous, making it the treatment of choice for acute thrombotic episodes. Heparin exerts its anticoagulant effect by binding to antithrombin and potentiating its action against thrombin, X_a and other activated serine proteases.

Box 20.6 Naming of heparin

Heparin was originally isolated from dog liver cells in 1916, hence its name (*hepar* or ἥπαρ is Greek for 'liver'). Heparin's discovery can be attributed to the research activities of two men, Jay McLean, a second-year medical student at Johns Hopkins University and William Henry Howell, his research supervisor.

For the treatment of established thrombosis, high-dose heparin is administered by continuous intravenous infusion. The short *in vivo* half-life of heparin (about one hour or less) facilitates fine adjustment of the anticoagulant effect. The pharmacokinetics of heparin are complex, which means that regular laboratory monitoring of the degree of anticoagulation is required. The most useful laboratory test for monitoring therapy is the degree of prolongation of the APTT. Each laboratory must establish a therapeutic range that equates to an optimal level of anticoagulation. Intravenous heparin therapy is associated with a severe risk of haemorrhage, and a risk of heparin-induced thrombocytopenia. Most patients are transitioned to warfarin therapy as the medium-term anticoagulant. Heparin therapy must be maintained for at least five days after the first dose of warfarin to allow the full oral anticoagulant effect to develop and to overcome the early procoagulant effects of a reduction in the concentrations of the natural anticoagulants protein S and protein C.

Low doses of heparin administered subcutaneously have been shown to offer effective post-operative prophylaxis. The incidence of significant bleeding problems is much lower than for intravenous heparin therapy, although the risk of thrombocytopenia persists.

Heparin is the anticoagulant of choice in pregnancy because it does not cross the placenta and is not teratogenic.

Low molecular weight heparin

Low molecular weight heparins are created by enzymatic or chemical treatment of unfractionated heparin to cleave the higher molecular weight polysaccharide chains. The average molecular weight of polysaccharide chain in a low molecular weight preparation is about 5 000 kDa.

Low molecular weight heparins are administered subcutaneously and have a longer biological half-life than intravenous unfractionated heparin (4–6 hours).

Because of their shorter average chain length, low molecular weight heparins exert a more potent anti-X_a activity than antithrombin activity. The impact of low molecular weight heparins on the APTT is less predictable than for unfractionated heparin, so this test is not useful for monitoring. If monitoring is required, factor X_a assays reflect the anticoagulant effect. Many physicians are happy to administer low molecular weight heparins without laboratory monitoring because their anticoagulant effect is, in general, more predictable. This makes low molecular weight heparins more suitable for outpatient use.

Oral anticoagulants

Oral anticoagulants are suitable for self-administration and so can be used outside of the hospital setting. The most widely prescribed oral anticoagulants, including **warfarin**, are coumarin analogues which act by inhibiting the normal recycling of vitamin K within hepatocytes, thereby preventing the γ-carboxylation of the terminal glutamate residues of the vitamin K-dependent coagulation factors (see also *Box 18.5*). Because the action of warfarin relies on the inhibition of the synthesis of new coagulation factors, its anticoagulant effect is not fully expressed for about 3–4 days after the commencement of therapy. The required degree of anticoagulation is typically maintained by heparin therapy during this period.

Therapeutic anticoagulation requires the induction of a controlled coagulopathy and is therefore fraught with dangers. Successful therapy involves treading the fine line between haemorrhagic and prothrombotic states. It is essential that the required degree of anticoagulation is established early and is subsequently closely controlled. The laboratory monitoring of warfarin therapy utilizes the patient prothrombin time and compares it to a normal (i.e. not anticoagulated) control prothrombin time. Because different laboratory preparations of the thromboplastin reagent used in the measurement of prothrombin time produce different results, they are standardized using a measure called the international sensitivity index (ISI). Each thromboplastin has an ISI value that allows the calculation of the international normalized ratio (INR). The INR is calculated as

$$INR = \left(\frac{Patient\ prothrombintime}{Control\ prothrombintime} \right)^{ISI}$$

The INR is reproducible, regardless of the location of the laboratory undertaking the testing or the thromboplastin reagent used. Because of this, standard recommendations for therapeutic ranges of INR can be established that apply universally. For treatment of established venous thrombosis, an INR of 2.0–3.0 should be maintained.

Warfarin therapy is associated with a significant haemorrhagic risk, even when well-controlled, and bleeding can be life threatening. Warfarin is teratogenic and so is not useful in pregnant women. There is a risk of skin necrosis during warfarin induction in patients with protein C or S deficiency.

Anti-platelet drugs

The deposition of platelets at sites of arterial vascular endothelial damage is an important step in the pathogenesis of arterial thrombosis. The prophylactic administration of anti-platelet drugs such as **aspirin (acetylsalicylic acid)** has been shown to be effective in reducing the rate of re-infarction in myocardial infarction survivors. The major risk associated with any form of antithrombotic therapy is that of inducing haemorrhagic complications. Several large clinical trials have shown that the daily administration of 50–100 mg of aspirin retains the antithrombotic effect while minimizing the risk of haemorrhagic complications. In patients with a history of gastric ulceration, clopidogrel or ticlopidine can be used for prophylaxis. These drugs act by blocking the ADP receptor on the platelet membrane, preventing platelet aggregation and activation of GPIIb/IIIa. In high-risk patients, these drugs can be combined with aspirin to augment the anti-platelet effect.

More recently, direct platelet glycoprotein IIb/IIIa inhibitors such as abciximab, eptifibatide and tirofiban have been used as prophylaxis during cardiac surgery. Rarely, these drugs can cause acute thrombocytopenia, severe enough to require platelet transfusion to avoid bleeding problems.

Danaparoid sodium

Danaparoid sodium is a mixture of three polysulphated glycosaminoglycans: heparan sulphate, dermatan sulphate and chondroitin sulphate. About 90% of the anticoagulant effect is attributable to the anti-X_a activity of heparan sulphate. The biological half-life of danaparoid sodium is about 24 hours. Administration is either intravenous or subcutaneous. Laboratory monitoring is by factor X_a assay. Danaparoid sodium can be used in pregnancy and is useful as a replacement for heparin in cases of heparin-induced thrombocytopenia because it has a low cross-reactivity with the antibodies that cause this condition.

Direct thrombin inhibitors

Hirudin is a natural anticoagulant that is secreted in the salivary glands of the medicinal leech (*Hirudo medicinalis*). The leech uses hirudin to ensure that bites continue to bleed for long enough that it can gorge itself on the issuing blood (see *Box 20.7*). Hirudin is the most potent natural inhibitor of thrombin and acts by binding to thrombin, preventing its interaction with substrates such as fibrinogen and other coagulation factors.

Box 20.7 Discovery and characterization of hirudin

Hirudin was discovered in 1884 by John Berry Haycraft, although it was not isolated until nearly 70 years later. The structure of hirudin was elucidated in 1976. Hirudin is a protein of 65 amino acids and exists in nature as a mixture of several isoforms. Recombinant hirudins such as lepirudin and desirudin are used clinically.

Several chemical derivatives of hirudin are available or being developed, including argatroban and the oral agent dabigatran etexilate. The direct thrombin inhibitors have four advantages over heparin:

- they are not neutralized by platelet factor 4
- they can inactivate thrombin bound to fibrin
- they do not bind to plasma proteins and so are more predictable
- they are not associated with induction of thrombocytopenia, and so are useful for treatment in patients with heparin-induced thrombocytopenia.

Laboratory monitoring of direct thrombin inhibitors is not required.

Thrombolytic drugs

Therapeutic anticoagulants are effective prophylactic antithrombotic agents and can prevent propagation of an established thrombus. However, they do not promote lysis of thrombi. This is the role of the thrombolytic agents such as streptokinase (SK) and tissue plasminogen activator (tPA).

SK is synthesized by β-haemolytic streptococci and activates both free and fibrin-bound plasminogen *in vivo* to release plasmin. The resultant systemic fibrinolysis shows no specificity for the site of the thrombus and so induces a profound hypocoagulable state, which is accompanied by a severe risk of bleeding. SK therapy is associated with a highly significant reduction in morbidity due to ischaemic muscle damage and re-infarction in acute myocardial infarction. The *in vivo* half-life of SK is less than 10 minutes. The repeated use of SK is limited by its immunogenicity and its tendency to induce febrile reactions.

Recombinant human tPA is highly fibrin-specific so exerts its lytic action directly on the formed thrombi and does not induce systemic fibrinolysis. Although tPA is fibrin-specific, it is not thrombus-specific. Digestion of multiple small haemostatic plugs, which form part of the normal defence against wear and tear, may result in serious haemorrhage. Overall, the incidence of haemorrhagic complications during tPA therapy is similar to that for SK therapy. The *in vivo* half-life of tPA is less than 10 minutes.

Box 20.8 ε-aminocaproic acid

Promoters of fibrinolysis such as tPA have found an important role in medicine. However, fibrinolytic inhibitors may be equally useful. For example, ε-aminocaproic acid (EACA) is an analogue of lysine and so acts as an inhibitor of plasmin, which depends on lysine-binding for its function. EACA can be used clinically to delay fibrinolysis and therefore to reduce bleeding following minor surgical procedures, such as dental extraction, in patients with bleeding disorders, e.g. haemophilia. It has also been shown to reduce blood loss in cardiac surgery.

There is no useful laboratory test for monitoring fibrinolytic therapy. The major risk of thrombolytic therapy is intracranial bleeding, which occurs in up to 4% of thrombolysed patients (see also *Box 20.8*).

SUGGESTED FURTHER READING

Bernard, K. & Elizabeth, M.V.C. (2009) Laboratory evaluation of hypercoagulability. *Clin. Lab. Med.* **29:** 339–366.

Charles, E. (2009) Antiphospholipid syndrome review. *Clin. Lab. Med.* **29:** 305–319.

Charles, T.E. (2009) Basic mechanisms and pathogenesis of venous thrombosis. *Blood Reviews,* **23:** 225–229.

Dahlbäck, B. (2008) Advances in understanding pathogenic mechanisms of thrombophilic disorders. *Blood,* **112:** 19–27.

Valerie, L.N. (2009) Anticoagulation monitoring. *Clin. Lab. Med.* **29:** 283–304.

SELF-ASSESSMENT QUESTIONS

1. Which of the following are risk factors for venous thrombosis?
    a. personal or family history of heart disease
    b. lupus anticoagulant
    c. obesity
    d. hyperhomocysteinaemia
    e. pregnancy
2. Complete the following table:

Condition	Gene affected	Inheritance Pattern
AT deficiency		AD
Protein C deficiency		AD or AR
Protein S deficiency	Protein S gene at 3q11.2	
Factor V Leiden	Factor V gene at 1q23	

3. What acquired prothrombotic abnormality is paradoxically associated with prolongation of phospholipid-dependent coagulation screening tests?
4. Which of the following statements about anticoagulants are true?
    a. Heparin has an *in vivo* half-life of about 3 days
    b. The risk of bleeding with subcutaneous low molecular weight heparin is lower than for intravenous unfractionated heparin
    c. warfarin is best administered subcutaneously
    d. the full anticoagulant effect of warfarin is manifest within 2 hours of administration
    e. aspirin has an anti-platelet effect
    f. direct thrombin inhibitors such as argatroban are neutralized *in vivo* by platelet factor 4.

Answers to self-assessment questions

Chapter 1

1. Statements (b) and (c) are true.
2. (b) Each litre of adult male blood contains approximately $4.4–5.9 \times 10^{12}$ red cells.
3. Aged red cells are sequestered primarily by the spleen.
4. Red cell spectrin is a peripheral protein.
5. Platelets are normally the second most numerous blood cell.
6. The outer surface of the platelet membrane is coated in a layer of glycolipids, mucopolysaccharides and adsorbed proteins, called the **glycocalyx**. This layer confers a **negative** charge to the platelet surface, which helps to prevent platelet–platelet and platelet–endothelium adhesion in the resting state. The membrane and glycocalyx make up the **peripheral** zone of the platelet.
7. The DTS is a closed-channel system, while the SCCS is an open-channel system.
8. The three morphologically distinct types of storage granules found in platelets are α-granules, dense granules and lysosomes.
9. Neutrophils are normally the most numerous white cell.
10. Eosinophils are most closely associated with defence against parasitic infestation.
11. Basophils are most closely associated with anaphylaxis.
12. B lymphocytes normally account for 10–30% of the circulating blood lymphocytes and play a central role in **humoral** (i.e. **antibody**-mediated) immunity. B lymphocytes also play a role in processing and presenting antigen to **T** cells. T lymphocytes account for 40–80% of the circulating blood lymphocytes and are responsible for **cell**-mediated immunity. The **thymus** gland is responsible for T cell education. NK cells play an important role in fighting **cancer** and **viral** infections.

Chapter 2

1. The earliest recognizable blood cell precursors are formed in the yolk sac of 2 week old embryos.

2. The three embryonic haemoglobins are haemoglobin Gower I $(\zeta_2\varepsilon_2)$, haemoglobin Portland $(\zeta_2\gamma_2)$ and haemoglobin Gower II $(\alpha_2\varepsilon_2)$.
3. Red marrow is actively haemopoietic whereas yellow marrow is fatty and does not produce blood cells. However, during periods of prolonged haemopoietic stress, yellow marrow can revert to haemopoietic red marrow. Red marrow is found mainly in the flat bones such as the pelvis, sternum, skull, ribs, vertebrae and scapulae, and in the epiphyseal ends of the long bones such as the femur and humerus. Yellow marrow is found in the hollow interior of the middle portion of long bones.
4. In order of increasing maturity: CFU-GEMM, myeloblast, promyelocyte, myelocyte.
5. Chronic renal failure is associated with anaemia because of inappropriately reduced synthesis of erythropoietin, the glycoprotein hormone responsible for regulating erythropoiesis.
6. Post-natal antigen-independent differentiation in B cells occurs in the **bone marrow**, while for T cells it occurs primarily in the **thymus gland**.

Chapter 3

1. There are significant changes in plasma volume and red cell mass in pregnancy. Typically, the red cell mass of a pregnant woman increases, but the increase in plasma volume is usually greater, leading to a dilution effect that causes an apparent reduction in [Hb], RBC and Hct, but does not reflect a true anaemia.
2. Five per cent of a population will have an [Hb] outside of the reference range for that population.
3. The following are common features of acute, severe anaemia: fatigue, tachycardia and vertigo.
4. Erythropoietin is the hormone responsible for stimulation of red cell production.
5. Variation in red cell size on a blood film is called anisocytosis.
6. Variation in red cell shape on a blood film is called poikilocytosis.

7. The variation in red cell colour seen in reticulocytosis is called polychromasia.
8. Thalassaemia is a microcytic anaemia due to impaired globin synthesis.
9. An adequate supply of vitamin B_{12} and folate co-enzymes is essential for optimal DNA and RNA synthesis. Folate deficiency causes retardation of DNA and, to a lesser extent, RNA synthesis. The result is a macrocytic anaemia.

Chapter 4

1. Iron is absorbed optimally from the duodenum and upper jejunum.
2. Absorption of inorganic iron is enhanced by any factor that increases its solubility. For example, Fe^{2+} compounds are generally more soluble than their Fe^{3+} counterparts, so the presence of reducing agents such as ascorbic acid (vitamin C) improves absorption.
3. About one quarter of the total body iron is in storage, mainly in the liver, tissue macrophages and bone marrow.
4. Severe iron deficiency is associated with anaemia which can lead to breathlessness on exertion.
5. Inorganic iron in food is released by proteolytic enzymes and hydrochloric acid in the stomach and reduced from Fe^{3+} ions to Fe^{2+} ions, which are absorbed more readily. Gastrectomy predisposes to the development of iron deficiency because of the absence of stomach acid and decreased gastrojejunal food transit times.
6. Negative iron balance describes the state where the rate of absorption of iron is insufficient to meet daily requirements, and iron is mobilized from body stores to meet the shortfall. Latent iron deficiency is the state where the body is deficient in iron but erythropoiesis is still normal and no adverse physiological effects are obvious. Iron-deficient erythropoiesis occurs when iron stores are exhausted and is marked by the development of the signs of iron deficiency. Iron deficiency anaemia describes the state where erythropoiesis is so impaired due to iron deficiency that anaemia develops.
7. The three main causes of an increased iron requirement are chronic loss of blood, growth and pregnancy, and increased loss of iron due to chronic intravascular haemolysis.
8. The hallmarks of iron-deficient red cells are microcytosis and hypochromasia.
9. Retarded haemoglobin synthesis allows more divisions to occur before developing red cells are released into the circulation, resulting in microcytosis.

10. Most cases of acquired clonal sideroblastic anaemia are classified as refractory anaemia with ring sideroblasts (RARS), a myelodysplastic syndrome.
11. Hereditary haemochromatosis results from an irregularity of intestinal iron absorption in which feedback control over the rate of absorption of dietary iron is impaired. Haemosiderosis results from chronic blood transfusion.

Chapter 5

1. Vitamin B_{12} is absorbed optimally in the terminal ileum and folates are absorbed optimally from the upper jejunum.
2. Vitamin B_{12} and folate are stored primarily in the liver.
3. Severe folate deficiency is associated with megaloblastic anaemia, which can result in breathlessness on exertion.
4. Total gastrectomy is associated with depletion of the vitamin B_{12} body stores due to lack of intrinsic factor.
5. N-5-methyltetrahydrofolate cannot be conjugated with glutamate until it has donated its methyl group to homocysteine, a reaction that requires methylcobalamin as co-enzyme. In the absence of methylcobalamin, absorbed folate cannot be converted to a metabolically active form, a phenomenon known as the methyltetrahydrofolate trap.
6. Vitamin B_{12} deficiency in pregnancy is uncommon in the developed world because body stores are typically sufficient to last for around 3 years, far longer than the duration of pregnancy.
7. Deficiency of folic acid is especially common in pregnancy (in the absence of supplementation) because dietary intake often fails to meet the increased demand for folate imposed by the growth of maternal blood volume and the developing fetus.
8. Serum folate assay provides an estimate of folate concentration as a snapshot in time. Serum folate levels can vary widely over a relatively short time period. On the other hand, because red cells survive for around 120 days, analysis of red cell folate provides a picture of the average folate level over a 120-day period and so provides a more informative picture.
9. The following statements are true: (b), (c) and (d).
10. Homocysteine is converted to methionine in the presence of methyl cobalamin as a co-enzyme and N-5-methyltetrahydrofolate as the methyl donor. In vitamin B_{12} and folate deficiency, this reaction is retarded and so plasma homocysteine levels rise.
11. Chromosomal breaks are more common in megaloblastic tissue because of attempts to repair misincorporation of uracil into DNA instead of

thymine by the enzyme uracil-DNA-glycosylase. Normally, a series of other enzymes mediate the repair of the mutilated DNA by incorporating thymine in place of the excised uracil. However, when thymine is in short supply, suboptimal repair of DNA leads to fragmentation of the helical structure, impaired mitosis and premature cell death.

Chapter 6

1. The rate-limiting step of haem synthesis is the combination of glycine and succinyl Co-A to produce δ-aminolaevulinic acid (δ-ALA).
2. The synthesis of δ-aminolaevulinic acid, the conversion of coproporphyrinogen III to protoporphyrinogen IX, the conversion of PPG IX to protoporphyrin IX and the insertion of the central ferrous ion to complete the synthesis of haem are all conducted within mitochondria. The remaining reaction steps occur in the cytoplasm.
3. Haemoglobin Gower I ($\zeta_2\epsilon_2$), haemoglobin Portland ($\zeta_2\gamma_2$) and haemoglobin Gower II ($\alpha_2\epsilon_2$).
4. The ferrous ion of the haem group is protected from the oxidative effects of water within the hydrophobic haem pocket. Contact with water would convert the Fe^{2+} to Fe^{3+}, destroying the oxygen-binding capability of the haemoglobin molecule.
5. The normal mean alveolar pO_2 is around 100 mmHg.
6. When severe anaemia is present, increased oxygen demand due to exertion is difficult to meet because the oxygen-carrying capacity of the blood is so reduced. This leads to an exaggerated cardiovascular response with shortness of breath and palpitations.
7. Pallor of the mucous membranes can be caused by a reduction in the level of oxyhaemoglobin in the underlying blood due to anaemia.
8. No, because δ-globin is a minor component of overall globin synthesis so its absence would likely be physiologically insignificant.
9. The frequencies of the different deletions that give rise to α thalassaemia vary widely in different races. Deletion of both α-globin genes on one chromosome 16 is uncommon in African-Americans; the most common deletion in this population is of only one α-globin gene. Haemoglobin H disease is rare in this population and haemoglobin Barts hydrops fetalis exceedingly so.
10. The ineffective erythropoiesis in thalassaemia results from an imbalance of α- and β-globin synthesis. In a moderately severe β thalassaemia, there will be an excess of α-globin. Coincident inheritance of heterozygous α^0 thalassaemia is likely to lessen the

degree of globin imbalance and so ameliorate the condition.
11. The presence of haemoglobin M increases methaemoglobin formation and so reduces oxygen-carrying capacity. Peripheral cyanosis is a sign of tissue hypoxia.
12. Hypoxia is a known trigger of sickling and oxygen levels are lower at altitude. A short flight may cause no problems, particularly if plenty of water is drunk throughout.

Chapter 7

1. Haemolytic disorder is the umbrella term for all disorders (other than haemorrhage) characterized by a reduction in red cell lifespan. Haemolytic anaemia describes a haemolytic disorder in which the reduction in red cell lifespan is so severe that it cannot be compensated for by an increase in the rate of erythropoiesis, leading to anaemia.
2. The four most abundant red cell membrane phospholipids are phosphatidyl choline (lecithin), phosphatidyl ethanolamine, sphingomyelin and phosphatidyl serine.
3. The following are integral proteins: (a) AE1, (c) glycophorin C and (e) glucose transport protein.
4. Band 5 is more commonly known as actin.
5. Normally, α spectrin is synthesized at around 3–4 times the rate of β spectrin.
6. The spleen is the major site of haemolysis in HS.
7. The five major forms of hereditary elliptocytosis include common HE, haemolytic HE, hereditary pyropoikilocytosis, HE with spherocytosis and HE with stomatocytosis.
8. Progressive red cell water depletion in hereditary xerocytosis is explained by markedly increased Na^+ transport into the cell, resulting in the ingress of water and loss of the normal biconcave shape.
9. PCH is caused by the Donath–Landsteiner antibody, which has anti-P blood group specificity. Haemolysis in PCH is biphasic; the Donath–Landsteiner antibody binds to red cells at temperatures below 15 °C, so exposure to cold triggers antibody binding but no haemolysis because complement is inactive at these temperatures. However, following warming, rapid complement-mediated intravascular haemolysis ensues.
10. Prophylactic injection of IgG anti-D has been shown to effectively prevent maternal production of anti-D in response to fetal immunization and so precludes the most serious form of HDN.
11. The four forms of DI-IHA include penicillin-type

immune haemolysis, in which the drug binds non-specifically to the red cell surface, stimulating production of IgG anti-drug antibodies; immune complex formation with compound neoantigen formation; the α-methyldopa-type immune response, where the drug stimulates production of a warm-reactive autoantibody and rifampicin-type immune haemolysis, in which the drug forms a stable complex with plasma protein and induces synthesis of anti-drug antibody immune complexes, triggering complement-mediated intravascular haemolysis.

Chapter 8

1. Mature red cells have no nucleus, mitochondria or ribosomes, which means they cannot synthesize protein and their means of energy is inefficient. This means that a deficiency or defect of an enzyme in the glycolytic pathway can be catastrophic.
2. Mature red cells have no mitochondria, the site of oxidative phosphorylation.
3. Conversion of ATP to ADP is the major source of energy production in mature red cells.
4. There are three main requirements for energy within normal red cells: maintenance of intracellular cation balance, maintenance of cell shape and the phosphorylation of glucose and fructose-6-phosphate.
5. 2,3-DPG is physiologically vital because it modulates the oxygen affinity of haemoglobin A.
6. Reducing power is required by the red cell to combat oxidation of membrane lipid and methaemoglobin formation and to detoxify oxidants.
7. The most common enzyme defect of the Embden–Meyerhof pathway is pyruvate kinase deficiency, which accounts for more than 90% of cases of glycolytic enzyme deficiency that are associated with haemolysis. The most common enzyme defect of the hexose monophosphate pathway is G-6-PD deficiency.
8. Hexokinase deficiency leads to a reduction in 2,3-DPG, which increases the oxygen affinity of haemoglobin A, resulting in a clinically more severe anaemia than expected from the haemoglobin concentration. Conversely, pyruvate kinase deficiency leads to an increase in 2,3-DPG concentration, which ameliorates the anaemia.
9. The normal form of G-6-PD is designated G-6-PD^B or Gd^B and the normal gene is denoted *Gd^B*. This form of G-6-PD is present in 99% of Caucasians and in about 70% of people of African descent. A functionally normal variant G-6-PD isoenzyme, Gd^A is found in about 20% of people of African descent.
10. Ingestion of oxidant drugs, ingestion of broad beans

and infection are the three most common triggers of acute haemolysis in G-6-PD deficiency.
11. The term favism relates to forms of G-6-PD deficiency that are sensitive to broad bean ingestion, most commonly G-6-PD^{MED} and G-6-PD^{CANTON}. However, the term is also often used (incorrectly) to mean any form of G-6-PD deficiency.

Chapter 9

1. Autoimmune neutropenia is caused by the acquisition of antibodies directed against neutrophil antigens, resulting in splenic sequestration and destruction. Most cases occur in infants 6–12 months of age and the condition frequently remits spontaneously. In adults, autoimmune neutropenia usually occurs in patients with other autoimmune conditions such as rheumatoid arthritis, systemic lupus erythematosus or Sjögren's syndrome. Neonatal alloimmune neutropenia is caused by IgG maternal antibodies directed against fetal neutrophil antigens in a similar manner to haemolytic disease of the newborn. The condition remits in the first months of life and seldom requires clinical intervention.
2. LAD-1 is caused by mutations of the CD18 gene at 21q22.3, with a consequent deficiency of all three integrins on the neutrophil surface. LAD-2 is an autosomal recessive disorder caused by mutation of the SLC35C1 gene at 11p11.2, which encodes a GDP-fucose transporter. The result is impaired fucosylation of P-selectin glycoprotein ligand 1 (PSGL-1) on the neutrophil surface. LAD-3 is caused by mutations in the FERMT3 gene at 11q13, which encodes kindlin 3, an intracellular regulator of integrin activation.
3. (a) Classical CGD is caused by a mutation of the *CYBB* gene at Xp21.1, resulting in deficiency of both gp91-*phox* and p22-*phox*.
4. The following statements about Pelger–Huët anomaly are true: (c) and (d).
5. (c) Undritz anomaly is associated with neutrophil hypersegmentation.
6. The affected genes are:
   a. Jordan's anomaly: the ABHD5 gene at 3p21 or the PNPLA2 gene at 11p15.5.
   b. Chédiak–Higashi syndrome: the LYST gene at 1q42.1–42.2.
   c. Pelger–Huët anomaly: the laminin B-receptor gene at 1q42.1.
   d. May–Hegglin anomaly: MYH9 gene at 22q11.2.
7. Development of severe basophilia in a patient with CML is a poor prognostic indicator.

Chapter 10

1. (b) Alkylating agents and (c) topoisomerase inhibitors are strongly implicated in the development of secondary malignancy.
2. Epstein–Barr virus.
3. The specific translocation t(15;17)(q22;q21) involves the *PML* gene on chromosome 15q22 and the retinoic acid receptor gene *(RARα)* on chromosome 17q21, and results in the formation of two novel fusion genes, both of which are transcribed.
4. *ABL* and *RAS* function as proto-oncogenes while *RB, P53* and *VHL* function as tumour suppressor genes.
5. a. The restriction checkpoint is located at the end of G_1 phase and functions as a decision point on whether to permit entry into S phase.
    b. The G_2 checkpoint acts as the decision point at the interface between G_2 and M phase. The role of this checkpoint is to prevent damaged DNA from being passed on to the next generation.
    c. The purpose of the mitotic spindle checkpoint (also known as the anaphase checkpoint) is to ensure that, when cells divide, each daughter cell is correctly allocated one copy of each chromosome.
6. Cyclophosphamide and melphalan are alkylating agents, decitabine is an epigenetic modifier or hypomethylating agent, 5-fluorouracil and cytosine arabinoside are antimetabolites, bortezomib is a proteasome inhibitor and thalidomide is an immunomodulating agent.

Chapter 11

1. (a) M3; acute promyelocytic leukaemia (b) M5a; acute monoblastic leukaemia (c) L3; Burkitt leukaemia / lymphoma.
2. The following cytogenetic abnormalities are commonly associated with AML: (a) t(8;21)(q22;q22); *(AML1/ ETO)* and (c) t(15;17)(q22;q12); (PML/*RARα*).
3. The following are poor prognostic indicators in AML: (a) age > 60 years, (b) antecedent haematological disorder and (d) absent Auer rods.
4. M3; acute promyelocytic leukaemia is commonly associated with disseminated intravascular coagulation.
5. ALL is more common in children than AML.
6. T ALL often presents with a mediastinal mass.
7. L3; Burkitt leukaemia / lymphoma is characterized by the presence of surface immunoglobulin on the leukaemic blasts.
8. The following numerical chromosomal changes are associated with an unfavourable prognosis in childhood ALL: (b) extreme hyperdiploidy (65–84 chromosomes) and (c) near haploidy (23–29 chromosomes).
9. (c) The t(12;21)(p13;q22); *(TEL/AML1)* translocation is associated with a good prognosis in children with ALL.
10. L-asparaginase is most associated with a temporary increase in thrombotic risk during remission induction in childhood ALL.
11. The Philadelphia chromosome is far more common in adults than in children with ALL.

Chapter 12

1. The most commonly seen cytogenetic abnormality in CLL is (c) del13q14.
2. (b) del11q22–23 is associated with several high-risk features in CLL and is an indicator of unfavourable prognosis.
3. *miR-15* and *miR-16-1*.
4. Diffuse marrow infiltration is indicative of more advanced disease.
5. Rai stage I.
6. Binet stage B.
7. CD11c (a monocyte and neutrophil marker), CD25 (an activated T cell marker) and CD103 (an intraepithelial T cell marker).
8. (b) 2′-deoxycoformycin and (e) 2-chlorodeoxy-adenosine are both purine analogues.

Chapter 13

1. The FAB classification system recognizes refractory anaemia (RA), refractory anaemia with ring sideroblasts (RARS), refractory anaemia with excess of blasts (RAEB), refractory anaemia with excess of blasts in transformation (RAEB-t) and chronic myelomonocytic leukaemia (CMML).
2. The FAB subtypes of MDS suggested by the results are:
    a. > 5% blasts in the peripheral blood: **RAEB-t**
    b. a blood monocyte count of > 1.0×10^9/l: **CMML**
    c. 10% blasts in the marrow, < 5% blasts in the peripheral blood: **RAEB**.
3. The following are associated with a poor prognosis in MDS: (a) abnormalities of chromosome 7 and (c) complex or multiple cytogenetic abnormalities.
4. RAEB-t is the most likely and RA the least likely FAB subtype of MDS to transform into AML.
5. RA affects the red cell line, whereas in RCMD dysplasia affects at least two cell lines.
6. The WHO subtype of MDS being described is RAEB-1.

7. An IPSS score of 2.0 belongs to the intermediate-2 risk group.
8. A WHO score of 3 belongs in the high risk group.

Chapter 14

1. (c) Polycythaemia vera is a malignant disease.
2. Serum erythropoietin levels are usually normal in relative polycythaemia, because this is due to reduced plasma volume.
3. Primary familial polycythaemia is inherited as an autosomal recessive disorder, and is caused by mutations in the von Hippel–Lindau gene.
4. Substitution of a phenylalanine for a valine at position 617 of the JAK2 molecule is identifiable in almost all cases of PV and around half of cases of essential thrombocythaemia and primary myelofibrosis.
5. 'Tear-drop' poikilocytosis is a red cell abnormality most commonly seen in chronic idiopathic myelofibrosis.
6. The splenomegaly in chronic myeloid leukaemia is most likely the result of extramedullary haemopoiesis.
7. The Philadelphia chromosome is manifest as a minute chromosome 22 and results from reciprocal translocation of chromosome 9 and 22 t(9;22) (q34;q11).
8. The chromosome 9 breakpoint is located at 9q34 and involves the *abl* gene, adhesion and stress response. The chromosome 22 breakpoint is located at 22q11 and involves the *bcr* gene.
9. (a) Blast phase chronic myeloid leukaemia is typically Philadelphia positive. All of the others (chronic neutrophilic leukaemia, atypical chronic myeloid leukaemia, juvenile myelomonocytic leukaemia and chronic eosinophilic leukaemia) are, by definition, Philadelphia negative.

Chapter 15

1. True.
2. Reed–Sternberg (R–S) cells and lymphocyte-predominant (LP) cells, respectively.
3. HD is more common in the Mediterranean region than in Japan.
4. Stage II.
5. X.
6. Serum albumin < 4 g/dl; haemoglobin < 10.5 g/dl; male gender; stage IV disease; age ≥ 45 years; total white cell count > 15.0 × 10^9/l; absolute lymphocyte count < 0.6 × 10^9/l or < 8% of the total white cell count.
7. Indolent forms of NHL are generally considered to be incurable using current standard therapies.

8. Ann Arbor stage ≥ III; patient age > 60 years; LDH raised; ECOG performance status ≥ 2; at least two extranodal sites involved.
9. (b) DLBCL is an aggressive form of NHL.

Chapter 16

1. Multiple myeloma is a B cell disorder.
2. ROTI is defined as any of the following: increased serum calcium levels; renal insufficiency; anaemia; bone lesions; other organ or tissue impairment relatable to myeloma.
3. The three criteria required for a diagnosis of symptomatic multiple myeloma are: identification of an M protein in serum and/or urine; a clonal proliferation of plasma cells in the bone marrow and/or a biopsy-proven plasmacytoma; evidence of any ROTI.
4. This patient has ISS Stage 2 disease.
5. IgA, IgD, IgE, IgG and IgM.
6. The most common subtype of multiple myeloma is IgG.
7. The following are adhesion molecules: (a) ICAM-1; (c) CD44.
8. Osteo**clasts** resorb bone while osteo**blasts** replace bone.
9. Bence Jones protein.
10. Smouldering myeloma is the same as indolent myeloma apart from having 10–30% plasma cells in the bone marrow and an absence of bone disease.
11. MGUS is not a malignant disease.

Chapter 17

1. About two thirds of cases of Fanconi anaemia are attributable to mutations in the *FANCA* gene.
2. Diamond–Blackfan syndrome is an inherited pure red cell aplasia.
3. Type II CDA or HEMPAS is associated with a positive Ham's test.
4. Most cases of cyclic neutropenia are attributable to a mutated *ELA2* gene, which encodes neutrophil elastase.
5. Congenital amegakaryocytic thrombocytopenia is attributable to mutations of the c-*MPL* gene, which encodes the thrombopoietin receptor.
6. Parvovirus B19 is the cause of fifth disease and can be associated with a transient arrest of erythropoiesis.
7. Severe aplastic anaemia is defined as a hypocellular bone marrow (< 25% cellularity) with any two peripheral blood cytopenias (absolute neutrophil count < 0.5 × 10^9/l, platelet count < 20 × 10^9/l, reticulocyte

count $< 0.06 \times 10^{12}/l$), that is not explained by marrow infiltration or any other cause.

8. PNH is caused by an acquired somatic mutation of the *PIGA* gene in one or more haemopoietic stem cells. Since it does not affect germ cells, it is not heritable.

9. PNH is caused by an acquired mutation of the *PIGA* gene, which encodes phosphatidylinositol glycan class A, a protein involved in the synthesis of the GPI anchor.

10. Aerolysin is a bacterial toxin that binds specifically to the GPI anchor on blood cells. An inactive, fluorescent-conjugated form of aerolysin can be used in flow cytometric determination of deficiency of the GPI anchor and so can diagnose PNH with great sensitivity.

Chapter 18

1. The five main systems involved in haemostasis are the vascular system, blood platelets, the coagulation cascade, the physiological inhibitors of coagulation and the fibrinolytic system.

2. The three concentric layers in the structure of blood vessels are called the tunica adventitia, the tunica media and the tunica intima.

3. (e) All of the following substances are synthesized by vascular endothelial cells: vWF, PGI₂, thrombomodulin and TFPI.

4. The following substances are stored in platelet α granules: (b) thrombospondin, (c) fibrinogen, (e) PF4, (f) vWF, (g) β-TG and (h) coagulation factor V.

5. The principal platelet membrane glycoprotein receptor for sub-endothelial-bound vWF is GPIb-IX-V.

6. Aspirin acetylates platelet cyclo-oxygenase.

7. The following coagulation factors are vitamin K-dependent: (b) VII and (d) II.

8. Factor XIII is a transglutaminase.

9. The main physiological inhibitor of activated coagulation serine proteases is antithrombin III (ATIII) or heparin cofactor I.

10. Three components of the protein C inhibitory pathway include proteins C and S and thrombomodulin.

11. Both plasminogen and plasmin have a very strong affinity for fibrinogen and fibrin. This means that a fibrin clot will also contain plasminogen activator and plasminogen bound up within it.

Chapter 19

1. The following are inherited haemorrhagic disorders: (a) Bernard–Soulier disease and (b) Ehlers–Danlos syndrome.

2.

Condition	Gene(s) affected
Congenital amegakaryocytic thrombocytopenia	c-*MPL* gene at 1p34
May–Hegglin anomaly	non-muscle myosin heavy chain-9 gene at 22q11.2
Pseudo von Willebrand's disease	**GPIb gene at 17pter–p12**
von Willebrand's disease	**vWF gene at 12p13.3**

3. Von Willebrand's disease is associated with mucous membrane bleeding because vWF is required for platelet adhesion, a component of primary haemostasis. The coincident deficiency of VIII is not an important cause of bleeding unless it is severe. For example, in type III vWD, the pattern of bleeding is similar to that of haemophilia (i.e. bleeding into muscles and joints). Haemophilia is associated with haematoma and haemarthrosis because it is a severe defect of coagulation. Typically, primary haemostasis is normal in haemophiliacs.

4. An obligate carrier of haemophilia is a female whose carrier status can be deduced without doubt from a family study. For example, the daughter of a haemophiliac is an obligate carrier because she must have inherited his affected X chromosome.

5. The most common triggers of DIC are infection, malignancy and obstetric complications.

6. Vitamin K is deficient in haemorrhagic disease of the newborn.

7. Henoch–Schönlein purpura (HSP), or allergic purpura, is a self-limited allergic vasculitis, which is seen most commonly in young children and is manifest as a purpuric rash covering the arms, legs and buttocks, with renal impairment and abdominal and joint pain.

Chapter 20

1. The following are risk factors for venous thrombosis: (b) lupus anticoagulant, (c) obesity and (e) pregnancy.

2.

Condition	Gene affected	Inheritance pattern
AT deficiency	**AT gene at 1q23–25**	AD
Protein C deficiency	**Protein C gene at 2q13–14**	AD or AR
Protein S deficiency	Protein S gene at 3q11.2	**AD or AR**
Factor V Leiden	Factor V gene at 1q23	**AD**

3. Antiphospholipid antibodies such as the lupus anticoagulant are prothrombotic despite prolongation of laboratory tests that employ phospholipid.

4. The following statements about anticoagulants are true:

(b) The risk of bleeding with subcutaneous low molecular weight heparin is lower than for intravenous unfractionated heparin;

(e) aspirin has an anti-platelet effect;

(f) direct thrombin inhibitors such as argatroban are neutralized *in vivo* by platelet factor 4.

Index

Use of bold denotes main entries